Laboratory Profiles of Small Animal Diseases

A Guide to Laboratory Diagnosis

Laboratory Profiles of Small Animal

of Small Animal

Third Edition Diseases

A Guide to Laboratory Diagnosis

Charles H. Sodikoff, DVM, MS

with 192 illustrations

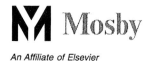 Mosby

An Affiliate of Elsevier

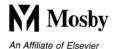

Mosby

An Affiliate of Elsevier

Publisher: John A. Schrefer
Executive Editor: Linda L. Duncan
Senior Developmental Editor: Teri Merchant
Project Manager: Linda McKinley
Senior Production Editor: Julie Eddy
Book Design Manager: Kathi Gosche
Educational Design Concept: K. Rebecca Robins
Cover photos: IDEXX

THIRD EDITION

NOTICE

Pharmacology is an ever-changing field. Standard safety precautions must be followed, but as new research and clinical experience broaden our knowledge, changes in treatment and drug therapy may become necessary or appropriate. Readers are advised to check the most current product information provided by the manufacturer of each drug to be administered to verify the recommended dose, the method and duration of administration, and contraindications. It is the responsibility of the licensed prescriber, relying on experience and knowledge of the patient, to determine dosages and the best treatment for each individual patient. Neither the publisher nor the editor assumes any liability for any injury and/or damage to persons or property arising from this publication.

Permissions may be sought directly from Elsevier's Health Sciences Rights Department in Philadelphia, USA: phone: (+1)215-238-7869, fax: (+1)215-238-2239, email: healthpermissions@elsevier.com. You may also complete your request on-line via the Elsevier Science homepage (http://www.elsevier.com), by selecting 'Customer Support' and then 'Obtaining Permissions'.

Mosby, Inc.
An Affiliate of Elsevier
11830 Westline Industrial Drive
St. Louis, Missouri 63146

Printed in the United States of America

International Standard Book Number 0-323-00956-5

05 CC/KPT 9 8 7 6 5 4

To my wife Karen Rebecca Sodikoff,
who made me see that complex ideas become useful
only when they are
understandable and presented in a clear manner.

Preface

In this era of high-cost specific testing such as ultrasound examination and CT scans, clinical pathology still remains the best tool for screening an animal for disease. It discloses underlying pathology that is often hidden from visual-based tools (that is, endoscopy, radiology, ultrasound, and physical examination).

I wrote this book to help small animal practitioners rapidly interpret the results of blood chemistry assays, hematologic studies, urinalyses, and special tests. It is a standard practice for panels of 12 to 30 tests to be run on a single blood sample and another 5 to 12 tests on a urine sample. In a busy practice, harried circumstances encourage veterinarians to simply rule out diseases by a single positive or negative test rather than making use of the entire test panel. Because of this, much information is wasted unless interrelated tests are sequentially evaluated.

Format

Laboratory Profiles of Small Animal Diseases allows busy practitioners to integrate clinical signs with laboratory findings in arriving at a diagnosis. It also provides a systematic approach for integrating laboratory abnormalities to disclose a probable diagnosis.

Sections 1 through 8 explain the various laboratory tests and the significance of their results. Sections 9 through 11 present flow charts that approach a diagnosis in three different ways. In Section 9, a laboratory abnormality is combined with other laboratory tests to suggest a diagnosis. In Section 10, the laboratory tests are used to help rule out causes for a common clinical sign. In Section 11, the laboratory tests are presented in flow sheet format to define certain pathologic conditions. This section also shows how dynamic testing can disclose the development of disease before the animal is clinically ill. Section 12 presents laboratory profiles of many common diseases of dogs and cats. These profiles include clinical signs, significant results of blood chemistry assays, hematologic examination, urinalysis, and other assays. This section also lists special tests to aid diagnosis of each disease.

Changing Methods of Interpretation

When the first edition of this book was written in 1982, panel testing was still new, but today it is an accepted approach to clinical pathologic diagnosis. The second edition in 1995 introduced several new tests. In this edition more than 80 new tests are included and Section 11, Dynamic Testing, is new.

I would like to differentiate between static and dynamic testing. *Static laboratory testing* is the standard approach of diagnosing disease. The patient's laboratory values are compared with a set of normal values from a generally healthy population. This is the approach most textbooks use to discuss testing for organ dysfunction. It has its limits because it does not consider age, breed, or environmental factors.

Dynamic laboratory testing is a method of evaluation based on changes over time in an individual animal's own laboratory values. It provides a good method for detecting disease early, monitoring response to therapy, and disclosing age-based changes.

In this approach, laboratory tests are repeated so that trends may be detected (for example, dropping RBCs or a rising BUN) before the test values deviate from the normal values for the general population. If an animal establishes its own normal values, small changes become important. For example, if the kidney function test "creatinine" rises from 1 to 2, it suggests early renal disease that necessitates further workup with a urinalysis. If an RBC count within the normal range drops 10% from the previous test, further tests are performed to find the cause for this pending anemia.

Charles H. Sodikoff, DVM, MS

How to Use This Book

Step 1

If you are inexperienced with clinical pathology, first become familiar with the meaning of results for the common tests that are available from your laboratory. Although hundreds of possible tests exist, you will use only about 30 of them routinely. Compare the test results on the laboratory panel with the marginal notes in this book for the basic meaning of an abnormal test. You should do this for the clinical chemistries, hematology, and urine tests. For more detailed information, refer to the main text.

Step 2

When you find multiple test abnormalities, see whether these tests can be correlated by following the flow sheets in Section 9. Combinations of certain tests often direct you to a pathway that suggests a specific diagnosis. Because the chemistry tests focus on the liver, kidneys, and metabolic diseases and the blood counts center on response, you may discover several unrelated areas of pathology.

Step 3

If a disease pattern is suggested by multiple abnormal tests, you should go to Section 12 and note any special tests that you may need to confirm a diagnosis. These special tests are described in Sections 1 to 8.

Step 4

If the laboratory panel is normal and cannot answer your questions why an animal shows specific clinical signs of disease, you should go to Sections 10 and 11 to see whether special tests exist that may help. Those sections will also help you find out whether your normal findings do indeed rule out the specific diseases you are considering.

Step 5

If the laboratory panel is normal and no special tests seem appropriate, you can retest a few days later and note any changing patterns. Trends may become apparent that suggest a pending problem (for example, anemia, kidney failure, liver dysfunction, or hyperthyroidism).

The Laboratory

Choosing a Commercial Laboratory

Metropolitan areas usually offer a variety of veterinary laboratories that are capable of performing laboratory tests on animal blood. Most of the hematology and clinical chemistry tests are done on large automated machines that are calibrated for animal samples. If possible, you should choose a laboratory that is operated by veterinary pathologists or internists that direct technicians trained in interpreting animal blood samples. These veterinary-directed laboratories offer assistance with diagnosis on routine panels and special animal-specific tests often for a lower price than you would pay for performing the tests in your own inhospital laboratory.

The major advantage of commercial laboratories is their ability to run large panels at a very low cost. Their machines often provide tests such as electrolytes that are unavailable on smaller veterinary hospital units. Their major disadvantage is that the results are delayed for a few hours or are unavailable during certain periods such as weekends, evenings, or holidays.

Choosing an In-Hospital Laboratory System

A good in-hospital laboratory system offers the clinician the advantages of immediate results and availability at all hours. With a little training, technicians can perform hematology and chemistry tests that are more accurate than commercial laboratories and provide a profit center that separates a medical practice from a vaccination or spay clinic. On a cost basis, however, the expense of buying or leasing a chemistry analyzer or hematology machine plus the cost of reagents is more expensive than a commercial laboratory. It takes 2 to 3 tests per day (>40 tests per month) to break even on the cost of the equipment. If your hospital exceeds this volume, however, or has a special need such as after-hours emergency work, oncology cases, or a large number of surgical patients, an in-hospital unit is feasible.

The complexity of an in-hospital laboratory depends on the size of the practice. In most cases a system that provides a 12-panel test and a 3-part CBC is sufficient. A hospital staff with no special training can run most of these units.

Comparing Laboratory Results

Please note that normal values may vary with your particular laboratory. In addition, values run in the hospital on whole blood within a few minutes of drawing the sample may vary by 10% from the sample sent to an external laboratory. Alterations listed in the disease profiles of this book may not be observed in every case of a specific disease. The general pattern rather than the exact laboratory profile should be used as an aid in diagnosis.

Contents

Section 1
Serum Chemistry Tests

Routine Chemistry Tests

Alanine Transferase

↑ ALT indicates hepatic cell damage or necrosis

Alanine transferase (ALT), formerly known as SGPT, is present in large quantities in the cytoplasm of canine and feline hepatocytes. This enzyme enters the blood when liver cells are damaged or destroyed and circulates for a few days.

This enzyme is a sensitive indicator of active liver damage but does not indicate the cause or reversibility of the damage. Increased serum ALT activity indicates recent or ongoing liver cell damage. An increase of at least three times normal indicates significant liver damage within the previous 2 to 5 days.

	Dogs	Cats
Normal	<100 IU/L	<80 IU/L
My lab	_____	_____

Albumin

↑ albumin suggests dehydration

malnutrition malabsorption, enteritis, and glomerulonephritis cause ↓ albumin

Albumin is a serum protein that affects osmotic pressure, binds calcium, and transports fatty acids and many drugs.

Starvation, parasitism, chronic malabsorptive disease, chronic liver disease, exudative enteritis, and glomerulonephritis decrease serum albumin levels.

Hypoalbuminemia with normal serum globulin levels suggests decreased albumin production, increased loss, or sequestration. If both albumin and globulin levels are low, hemorrhage, exudation, and dilution are likely causes.

Severe dehydration often increases serum albumin levels.

	Dogs	Cats
Normal (SU)	2.5-3.5 g/dl	2.1-3.4 g/dl
Normal (IU)	25-35 g/L	21-34 g/L

Alkaline Phosphatase

cholestatic liver disease and excessive exogenous corticosteroids are major causes ↑ AP activity in dogs

Alkaline phosphatase (AP) is found in both liver and bone. Elevated AP activity in the serum indicates increased production by the liver parenchyma, bile ducts, and growing bone or decreased excretion in bile and urine. The enzyme is induced by bile stasis and in the dog by corticosteroid or anticonvulsant drugs. Elevated AP activity does not suggest liver or bone necrosis.

The major causes of increased serum AP activity in dogs are cholestatic liver disease or excessive exogenous corticosteroids. Serum AP activity increases after an episode of acute pancreatitis because of secondary cholangitis. It also increases if liver disease causes a disruption of hepatobiliary architecture with local impairment of bile flow.

Cats have less AP than dogs and the kidneys rapidly excrete slight excesses. Any increased AP activity in cats is significant and suggests cholestasis.

Normal values in puppies and kittens are higher than in adults because of active bone growth. Diseases causing bone remodeling in adults cause slight elevations of less than two times normal.

Persistence of AP activity unrelated to continued disease might be due to decreased clearance secondary to diseases such as renal failure, cirrhosis, or the formation of macroenzymes.

	Dogs	Cats
Normal (SU)	<200 IU/L	<200 IU/L
My lab	_____	_____

Alkaline Phosphatase, Cortical-Induced (CIALP)

normal levels of AP make a diagnosis of glucocorticoid excess unlikely in the dog

Corticosteroid-induced alkaline phosphatase is an isoenzyme that increases total serum ALP in the dog. It offers negative predictive value in diagnosing hyperadrenocorticism. Its absence makes a diagnosis of glucocorticoid excess unlikely. High levels may be present with extraadrenal disease, so it is not a good screening test for adrenal disease.

Normal	None

Alpha-2 Acid Glycoprotein (AGP)

↑ AGP is a very early indicator of disease

Alpha-2 acid glycoprotein (AGP) is an acute phase protein manufactured in the liver and found in the blood. Detection of elevated levels of AGP indicates illness or other stressors even though an animal appears clinically normal. AGP indicates disease before antibodies are created by the immune system and before clinical symptoms are apparent. AGP is elevated by inflammation, infectious diseases, surgery, malignant tumors, autoimmune diseases, liver cirrhoses, and with all types of stress in general.

The AGP test is species specific and is available in kit form. It can be used as a prognostic indicator to detect subclinical disease and changes in homeostasis and to monitor immune system function, chemotherapy, and vaccine efficacy. In monitoring cancer therapy, continued high levels of AGP where the level was initially high suggests that treatment is not working or not appropriate. Levels above 1000 mg/ml of serum indicate a poor prognosis, especially if subsequent measurements show increasing levels.

	Dogs	Cats
Normal adult	260-450 mg/ml	270-470 mg/ml
Normal immature	<250 mg/ml	<250 mg/ml

Alpha Glutathione S-Transferase (GST)

↑ GST indicates early hepatocyte injury

Alpha glutathione S-transferase (GST) is a superior marker of hepatocyte injury from toxicity, ischemia, and other liver injury. It is unique to hepatocytes, found in high concentrations, and is readily released in response to injury. It comprises 5% of the soluble protein of hepatocytes. Its rapid release into and removal from the circulation provides immediate information regarding liver status. It is a valuable tool in research evaluation of liver damage.

Amino Acid Ratio

branched-chain AA ↓ with gluconeogenesis

Protein catabolism, gluconeogenesis, and increased insulin activity reduce serum levels of branched-chain amino acids. Hepatic insufficiency from portosystemic shunts or liver fibrosis (cirrhosis) increases serum levels of aromatic amino acids. The ratio of branched-chain to aromatic amino acids is termed the amino acid (AA) ratio.

aromatic AA ↑ with hepatic insufficiency

The AA ratio is decreased with hepatic encephalopathy. CNS signs occur because increased levels of aromatic amino acids increase production of inhibitory neurotransmitters, while decreased levels of branched-chain amino acids decrease production of stimulatory neurotransmitters.

Normal branched-chain:aromatic AA ratio >3

Ammonia

↑ ammonia indicates hepatic insufficiency

Increased baseline blood ammonia levels or persistently high blood ammonia levels after oral administration of ammonium chloride (available as a urine acidifier) indicate hepatic insufficiency. This test is helpful in evaluating animals with chronic weight loss, abnormal CNS signs, and a small liver. Abnormalities correlate with serum bile acid assays.

Congenital and acquired hepatic shunts, bile duct obstruction, cholangiohepatitis, and cirrhosis increase blood ammonia levels.

Protocol for Ammonia Loading Test
1. Give ammonium chloride PO at 100 mg/kg.
2. Collect a blood sample 30 to 45 minutes after administration of ammonium chloride.

Interpretation
At 30 to 45 minutes after administration, blood ammonia levels should not exceed the following normal values.

	Dogs	Cats
Normal (SU)	<120 μg/dl	<100 μg/dl
Normal (IU)	<70 μmol/L	<59 μmol/L

Amylase

↑ amylase is an indicator of acute pancreatitis

Pancreatic inflammation, necrosis, or pancreatic duct occlusion releases amylase into the blood and peritoneal cavity. This elevates serum amylase levels to two to three times normal. Increased absorption from upper intestinal inflammation and decreased renal excretion mildly elevate serum amylase activity.

When associated with abdominal pain, increased serum amylase activity suggests acute pancreatitis. Macroamylasemia causes increased levels but is not associated with disease.

Since many cats with acute pancreatitis have amylase within the normal range, trypsin-like immunoreactivity (TLI) is a better test.

	Dogs	Cats
Normal (SU)	<3000 IU/L	<2000 IU/L
My lab	_____	_____

Anion Gap

↑ anion gap usually means metabolic acidosis

The anion gap can be used to screen for metabolic acidosis when blood pH cannot be measured. It is calculated with the equation:

$$\text{Anion gap} = (Na + K) - (Cl + HCO_3)$$

Anion gap increases when unmeasured anions (lactic acid, keto acids) or exogenous substances (salicylates, ethylene glycol) are present.

The most common cause of increased anion gap in dogs and cats is metabolic acidosis from lactic acidosis, renal failure, diabetes mellitus, ketosis, or hypovolemic shock.

If an increased anion gap cannot be explained by these conditions, consider intoxications (ethylene glycol, salicylate, metaldehyde), dehydration, drug therapy (penicillin), alkalosis, and laboratory error.

Normal	15-20
Acidosis	>20

Aspartate Transferase (AST)

↑ AST activity suggests muscle necrosis or liver necrosis

Aspartate transferase (AST), formerly known as SGOT, is a mitochondria-bound enzyme. It is found in several body tissues but is especially high in liver and striated muscle.

Serum AST activity is elevated with skeletal muscle necrosis and hepatocellular necrosis. Elevated serum AST activity with no ALT elevation indicates muscle necrosis. In liver damage, AST activity rises more slowly than ALT and indicates more complete cellular disruption because it leaks from the cell only with necrosis, not membrane instability. Increased serum AST activity suggests muscle necrosis or liver necrosis. In liver disease the serum AST returns to normal more rapidly than ALT.

Rising levels indicate continued severe insult to the hepatocytes. The normal plasma half-life is approximately 12 hours in dogs or 2 hours in cats. Persistence of high but stable serum levels past two to three normal half-lives may be due to continued cellular injury, increased synthesis by normal hepatic tissue, or the formation of macroenzymes. Hemolysis and lipemia can falsely elevate serum AST activity.

	Dogs	Cats
Normal	<90 IU/L	<80 IU/L
My lab	_____	_____

Bicarbonate (HCO₃, CO₂)

↓ bicarbonate
usually means
acidosis

Bicarbonate is measured as CO_2 or HCO_3 on routine blood panels. Values can increase in respiratory acidosis or metabolic alkalosis, and decrease in metabolic acidosis or respiratory alkalosis.

	Dogs	Cats
Normal	18-24 mEq/L	18-24 mEq/L
Acidosis	<18 mEq/L	<18 mEq/L
My lab	_____	_____

Bile Acid

↑ bile acids
screen for con-
genital macro-
scopic and
microscopic vas-
cular shunts

↑ bile acids with
↑ alkaline phos-
phatase occur
with cholangio-
hepatitis not
steroid induction

Serum bile acid assays are used to evaluate the excretory system of the liver. They are helpful in determining the cause of chronic weight loss, abnormal CNS signs, and a small liver.

Test paired serum samples (fasting and 2 hours after eating). Congenital and acquired hepatic shunts, bile duct obstruction, cholangiohepatitis, and cirrhosis increase serum bile acid levels. Occasionally, the fasting bile acid values are higher than the postprandial values. This is due to stimulation of the gallbladder by stomach juices that pass into the intestine. If either value exceeds the upper postprandial values, shunting is indicated.

In young animals with seizures but no obvious liver disease, bile acids are used to check for congenital macroscopic and microscopic vascular shunts.

In animals with persistently increased ALT or other indications of hepatobiliary disease, abnormally high bile acids indicate shunting because of the increased resistance of hepatic portal blood flow from intrahepatic disease. This is a good indication of active liver disease. Low levels of bile acids with high alkaline phosphatase levels would suggest steroid hepatopathy rather than cholangitis.

	Dogs	Cats
Preprandial (SU)	<10 μmol/L	<5 μmol/L
Postprandial (IU)	<25 μmol/L	<15 μmol/L
Severe liver dysfunction	>35 μmol/L	>35 μmol/L

Total Unconjugated Bile Acids (TUBA)

↑ TUBA indicate small intestinal bacterial overgrowth

TUBA is a test for small intestine bacterial overgrowth. Normally, bile acids are conjugated with taurine (cat and dog), secreted into the duodenum, and reabsorbed through the portal circulation. If excess bacteria are present in the small intestine, the bile acids are deconjugated and reabsorbed. Separation and quantification of conjugated and unconjugated bile acids is analyzed by special equipment. High levels of TUBA indicate small intestinal bacterial overgrowth.

Biliprotein

↑ biliprotein causes persistent conjugated bilirubin levels with no urinary bilirubin

Biliprotein (delta-bilirubin) is a fraction of conjugated bilirubin irreversibly bound to albumin. Variable amounts form in icteric dogs and cats. Its rate of degradation parallels the 14-day half-life of albumin. In some animals this accounts for persistently high conjugated bilirubin levels despite resolution of the liver disease and low levels of urinary bilirubin.

Bilirubin

↑ total bilirubin indicates liver disease or hemolytic disease

Bilirubin is derived from catabolism of hemoglobin and circulates in conjugated and unconjugated forms.

Increased levels of conjugated bilirubin indicate liver disease. The direct van den Bergh reaction indicates water-soluble conjugated (direct) bilirubin in serum. Any bilirubin in the urine is conjugated bilirubin.

Unconjugated bilirubin is not water soluble and does not pass into the urine. Increased levels of unconjugated bilirubin in conjunction with anemia suggest hemolysis.

Total Bilirubin (Conjugated Plus Unconjugated)		
	Dogs	Cats
Normal (SU)	<0.6 mg/dl	0.2 mg/dl
Normal (IU)	<8 μmol/L	<8 μmol/L

	Direct (Conjugated) Bilirubin	
	Dogs	Cats
Normal (SU)	<0.14 mg/dl	<0.15 mg/dl
Normal (IU)	<2 μmol/L	<2 μmol/L
My lab	_____	_____

Bromsulfophthalein (BSP) Retention

↑ BSP retention indicates decreased liver circulation, liver fibrosis, or hepatic insufficiency

Bromsulfophthalein (BSP) retention is a liver function test that has been largely replaced by the serum bile acid assay.

Hepatic insufficiency, icterus, and poor hepatic perfusion increase BSP retention. The dye is retained with heart failure, portosystemic shunts, portal vein obstruction, and loss of functional liver parenchyma.

Protocol
1. Inject 5% BSP solution (50 mg/ml) IV at 5 mg/kg
2. Obtain a blood sample 30 minutes after injection.

Interpretation

	Dogs and Cats
Normal	<5% Retention at 30 minutes
Abnormal	>5% Retention at 30 minutes

Blood Urea Nitrogen (BUN, SUN)

↑ BUN means azotemia or uremia

An increased blood level of nitrogenous waste products is called *azotemia*. When the increase is of renal origin or when accumulation of nitrogenous waste causes clinical signs, the condition is called *uremia*.

Increased blood urea nitrogen (BUN) levels can have prerenal, renal, or postrenal causes. Heart disease, hypoadrenocorticism, dehydration, and shock are common prerenal causes. Urethral obstruction, bladder rupture, and urethral laceration are common postrenal causes.

Glomerular, tubular, or interstitial renal disease that raises the BUN indicates that over 70% of nephrons are nonfunctional.

Urinalysis, with determination of specific gravity and evaluation of sediment can be used to differentiate prerenal azotemia from azotemia of renal origin.

BUN levels are decreased with starvation or chronic liver disease.

	Dogs	Cats
Normal (SU)	10-25 mg/dl	10-30 mg/dl
Normal (IU)	6 U/L	<5 U/L
My lab	_____	_____

BUN:Creatinine Ratio

↑ BUN:creatinine ratio suggests prerenal azotemia

A fall in the GFR normally causes the blood urea nitrogen (BUN) and creatinine to rise in equal proportions. The enhanced salt and water avidity associated with prerenal states causes a disproportionate rise in the plasma ratio of BUN to creatinine. A ratio higher than 20:1 suggests prerenal azotemia.

In normal animals the BUN:creatinine ratio is usually greater than 5. When the liver fails to convert ammonia to urea, this ratio can fall. A low ratio is a rough suggestion of chronic liver failure, especially when other signs of liver disease are present. To confirm poor ammonia conversion, follow up with an ammonia tolerance test.

Normal	>5-20

Calcium

lymphosarcoma is a common cause of hypercalcemia

Parathyroid hormone (PTH), calcitriol, and calcitonin control calcium levels in extracellular fluid and bone.

Hypercalcemia can be a sign of a wide variety of diseases. Osteolytic bone lesions (septic osteomyelitis, bone tumors), pseudohyperparathyroidism, hyperparathyroidism, hypervitaminosis D, lymphosarcoma, perianal-gland tumors, hemoconcentration, hypoadrenocorticism, renal failure, and hyperproteinemia can increase serum calcium levels. The most common cause of hypercalcemia is lymphosarcoma.

↓ albumin is the most common cause of hypocalcemia

The clinical features of *hypocalcemia* depend on the underlying cause, the rate of development and the presence of acidemia. Necrotizing pancreatitis, hypoalbuminemia, thyroid surgery, ethylene glycol poisoning, hypoparathyroidism, renal failure, and puerperal tetany can decrease serum calcium levels. The most common cause of hypocalcemia is hypoalbuminemia.

Calcium values can be falsely low in EDTA or oxylated samples.

	Dogs	Cats
Normal (SU)	8-12 mg/dl	8-12 mg/dl
Normal (IU)	2-3 mmol/L	2-3 mmol/L
My lab	_____	_____

Calcium, Ionized

acidosis and alkalosis affect levels of ionized calcium

Ionized calcium is the physiologically active form of serum calcium. In normal animals and during hypercalcemia, ionized calcium is usually 50% to 60% of total calcium. In renal failure the ionized values can be reduced by reactions with phosphorus or raised because of acidosis.

Where hypocalcemia occurs without hypoalbuminemia, the ionized calcium is usually low. Accurate assays require ion specific electrodes and careful collection of serum in nonserum separator tubes. Samples must be submitted within 72 hours to the laboratory in airtight containers. Any loss of CO_2 may cause a pH shift and decrease the ionized calcium by shifting the free to the bound form.

Hypercalcemia
Renal failure usually causes a normal to low ionized calcium with a concurrent high parathormone. However some dogs with severe renal secondary hyperparathyroidism have high ionized calcium. Primary hyperparathyroidism causes high ionized calcium with high parathormone levels.

Hypocalcemia
Clinical signs of hypocalcemia develop if the total serum calcium is below 6.5 mg/dl and the ionized calcium is decreased. Cases with hypoalbuminemia and low total serum calcium usually have a normal ionized calcium but ionized calcium is low in some patients with hypoalbuminemia.

	Dogs	Cats
Normal	55%	60%

Calcium-Albumin Adjustment

calcium values must be corrected for albumin levels

In animals with hypoalbuminemia and hyperalbuminemia, the serum calcium value should be corrected to provide a measure of true hypocalcemia and hypercalcemia.

The following equation is used to adjust calcium values in dogs with abnormal albumin levels but it is not accurate with cats. In cats only a rough estimate can be made; low calcium is expected with low albumin and high calcium with high albumin.

$$\text{Adjusted Ca} = (\text{Ca} - \text{albumin}) + 4$$

	Dogs	Cats
Normal (SU)	8-12 mg/dl	8-12 mg/dl
Normal (IU)	2-3 mmol/L	2-3 mmol/L

Calcium × Phosphorus Product

↑ Ca × P indicates ↑ danger of calcification

Concurrent elevations in serum calcium and phosphorus are likely to cause soft tissue mineralization, such as calcification of the kidney. The risk is increased when the product of calcium × phosphorus is greater than 60.

Normal Ca × P	<60

Chloride

chloride is not a diagnostic test when used alone, but it supplements other tests

Common causes of *hypochloremia* are vomiting and hypoadrenocorticism.

Common causes of *hyperchloremia* include administration of chloride-containing compounds, dehydration, and hyperchloremic metabolic acidosis.

The ratio of serum chloride to phosphorus (Cl:P ratio) is used to differentiate some causes of hypophosphatemia. Chloride values are used to calculate the anion gap.

	Dogs	Cats
Normal (SU)	105-115 mEq/L	117-123 mEq/L
Normal (IU)	105-115 mmol/L	117-123 mmol/L
My lab	_____	_____

Chloride:Phosphorus Ratio

↑ Cl:P ratio sug-
gests primary
hyperparathy-
roidism

The ratio of serum chloride to phosphorus (Cl:P ratio) is used to distinguish the hypophosphatemia of hyperparathyroidism from that of pseudohyperparathyroidism (hypercalcemia of malignancy).

↓ Cl:P ratio sug-
gests malignancy

A Cl:P ratio >33:1 suggests primary hyperparathyroidism because of concurrent hyperchloremic acidosis.

A ratio <33:1 suggests hypercalcemia from malignancy.

Cholesterol

cholesterol is not
a diagnostic test
when used
alone, but it
supplements
other tests

Cholesterol is primarily produced in the liver and excreted in bile. Hypercholesterolemia occurs in obstructive biliary disease, hypothyroidism, hyperadrenocorticism, acute nephritis, nephrotic syndrome, and primary dyslipoproteinemias.

Hepatocellular disease, diabetes mellitus, and anorexia decrease cholesterol production and reduce serum cholesterol levels.

	Dogs	Cats
Normal (SU)	120-255 mg/dl	90-200 mg/dl
Normal (IU)	2.9-7.8 mmol/L	1.8-3.9 mmol/L
My lab	_____	_____

Chylomicron Test

clearing indi-
cates postpran-
dial lipemia

Lipemia can be caused by triglycerides in the form of chylomicrons or very-low-density lipids. These cause the blood to become lactescent (resembling cream of tomato soup).

This test determines if lipemia is from chylomicrons related to a recent meal or from very-low-density lipids produced by metabolism.

Protocol
Collect a blood sample and refrigerate it for 6 hours.

Interpretation
Chylomicrons rise to the top, forming a creamy layer. Very-low-density lipids remain suspended in the blood, forming an opaque layer.

Creatine Phosphokinase, Creatine Kinase (CPK, CK)

↑ CK indicates muscle necrosis or rarely a CNS lesion

Creatine kinase (CK), also called creatine phosphokinase (CPK), is found in high levels in the CNS and striated muscle. Muscle trauma, IM injection, myositis, and occasionally CNS damage cause elevated serum CK activity. Increased CK activity parallels rises in AST activity with muscle necrosis.

	Dogs	Cats
Normal (SU)	<120 IU/L	<120 IU/L
My lab	_____	_____

Creatinine

creatinine >2 indicates uremia from >50% loss of kidney function

Creatinine is a nonprotein nitrogenous product of muscle metabolism. Serum creatinine levels are much less affected by diet and protein catabolism than are BUN levels.

As with BUN, serum creatinine levels are elevated by conditions that reduce glomerular filtration. Isosthenuria (specific gravity 1.010 ± 0.002) suggests a renal cause, but a higher urine specific gravity suggests prerenal or postrenal causes.

Because the rate of creatinine excretion in the urine is constant, the urine creatinine level can be used to quantify other excreted hormones or proteins.

	Dogs	Cats
Normal (SU)	1-2 mg/dl	0.8-2 mg/dl
Normal (IU)	<115 μmol/L	<115 μmol/L
My lab	_____	_____

Fibrinogen and Acute-Phase Proteins

↑ acute-phase proteins may indicate pregnancy in dogs

Inflammation, suppuration, and early pregnancy (28 to 37 days in dogs) increase serum levels of fibrinogen and acute-phase proteins.

Liver disease, neoplasia, major surgery, and disseminated intravascular coagulation decrease their levels.

A pregnancy test for dogs is based on elevated levels of these proteins.

	Dogs	Cats
Normal (SU)	100-400 mg/dl	110-400 mg/dl

Fructosamine for Monitoring Diabetics

↑ fructosamine indicates persistent hyperglycemia

Fructosamine concentration is proportional to blood glucose concentration over the life span of the glycosylated protein being measured (e.g., 1 to 2 weeks for feline and canine albumin). Therefore, serum fructosamine concentration provides an assessment of an individual's average blood glucose concentration over the proceeding few weeks.

Serum fructosamine levels can be used to monitor glycemic control in dogs and cats with diabetes mellitus. Fructosamine concentration reflects metabolic control of diabetics more objectively than sporadic blood glucose measurements.

In screening for diabetes mellitus, normal levels of fructosamine in a hyperglycemic animal rule out a diagnosis of diabetes.

	Dogs	Cats
Normal	258-343 μmol/L	175-400 μmol/L
Well regulated	<450	<450
Poorly regulated	>600	>600

Fructosamine for Monitoring Hypoproteinemia

hypoalbumin-
emia with normal
fructose amine
indicates acute
protein loss

Fructosamine is primarily albumin linked to glucose by the process of glycosylation. The level of fructosamine depends on the average blood glucose concentration and the age of the albumin molecule (life span 1 to 2 weeks). Because albumin normally becomes glycosylated during its serum life span, fructosamine may be used to determine the age of the circulating albumin.

Concurrent hypoalbuminemia and normal serum fructosamine indicate hypoalbuminemia of less than 1 week. Concurrent hypoalbuminemia and hypofructosaminemia indicate persistent hypoalbuminemia of more than 1 week, and concurrent normal albumin and hypofructosaminemia indicate recovery from either hypoalbuminemia or hypoglycemia.

	Dogs	Cats
Normal	258-343 μmol/L	175-400 μmol/L

Gamma Glutamyl Transpeptidase (GGT)

↑ GGT indicates
cholestatic liver
disease or corti-
sol excess (in
dogs)

Gamma glutamyl transpeptidase (GGT) is an induced liver enzyme that indicates disease of the portal biliary system. Increases in GGT activity parallel those of AP, but GGT is not found in bone.

Glucocorticoids and bile stasis induce GGT production. In cats, GGT activity tends to increase more than AP activity with cholestasis.

Increased GGT activity suggests cholestatic liver disease or cortisol excess (in dogs).

	Dogs	Cats
Normal (SU)	<10 IU/L	<10 IU/L
My lab	_____	_____

Globulin

↑ globulin suggests chronic inflammation or gammopathy

Serum globulin levels are usually estimated from the total serum protein and albumin levels. If globulin levels are increased, serum protein electrophoresis can determine if the increase is attributable to inflammation or neoplasia.

Inflammation and certain diseases (feline infectious peritonitis in cats, ehrlichiosis in dogs) cause *polyclonal gammopathies.*

Lymphocyte and plasma-cell disorders (lymphosarcoma and multiple myeloma) cause *monoclonal gammopathies* with a narrow peak.

Marked hyperglobulinemia can cause problems because of increased serum viscosity.

	Dogs	Cats
Normal (SU)	2-4 g/dl	2-5 g/dl
Normal (IU)	20-40 g/L	20-50 g/L
My lab	_____	_____

Glucagon Tolerance Test

insulinoma causes ↑ insulin: glucose ratio

↑ glycogen storage or pre-diabetes causes persistently ↑ glucose

↓ glycogen storage causes no rise in glucose

Glucagon causes release of glucose from glycogen and can be used to test for glycogen-storage problems or abnormal glucose metabolism from insulin excess or deficiency. The glucagon tolerance test detects excessive or insufficient glycogen storage and glucose use caused by excessive or insufficient insulin.

Animals with an insulinoma respond to glucagon injection with hyperglycemia, followed by a rapid drop in blood glucose to below the pretest level *(rebound hypoglycemia).*

The glucagon tolerance test can be used as an indirect test in animals with signs of hyperadrenocorticism or an enlarged liver. Glucagon injection causes marked hyperglycemia in animals with excessive glycogen stores (as in hyperadrenocorticism). The hyperglycemic response to glucagon is diminished in animals with severe hepatic insufficiency, portacaval shunts or starvation.

Protocol
1. Fast the animal for 12 hours.
2. Obtain a preinjection blood sample, then give glucagon IV at 0.03 mg/kg.
3. Obtain blood samples at 15, 30, 60, and 90 minutes after injection.

Interpretation
Normal response:

- Blood glucose rises to 200 mg/dl, then falls to <100 mg/dl by 60 minutes.

Insulinoma:

- Blood insulin >50 µU/ml at 15 minutes after glucagon injection.
- Blood glucose <135 mg/dl at 15 minutes after glucagon injection.
- Insulin:glucose ratio >75 at 15 minutes after glucagon injection.
- Blood glucose <50 mg/dl at 90 minutes after glucagon injection.

Excessive glycogen storage or prediabetic state:

- Normal pretest blood glucose level, with glucose >200 mg/dl at 15 and 30 minutes after glucagon injection.
- Blood glucose levels remains elevated beyond 90 minutes.

Reduced glycogen storage:

- Blood glucose levels remain at pretest levels at 15 and 30 minutes and do not rise.

Glucose

↑ glucose is seen in stress and diabetes mellitus

↓ glucose is usually a laboratory error

In dogs, persistent marked hyperglycemia is usually caused by diabetes mellitus. Endogenous epinephrine release and sample collection after a recent meal may cause transient hyperglycemia.

In cats, diabetes mellitus, epinephrine release, and systemic disease can cause marked and usually persistent hyperglycemia. Exogenous corticosteroids and progestins cause slight hyperglycemia (see Type II Diabetes Mellitus) and delay glucose use. Muscle activity (convulsions or shivering) also results in transient hyperglycemia.

Insulin-secreting pancreatic neoplasms, starvation, hypoadrenocorticism, hypopituitarism, shock, nonpancreatic tumors, and severe exertion can cause hypoglycemia.

The most common cause of low glucose values is inappropriate handling of the blood specimen. To avoid this artifact, blood should be collected in a sodium fluoride tube, or, if collected in a clot tube, the serum should be immediately separated from the clot so that glycolysis is inhibited.

	Dogs	Cats
Normal (SU)	60-120 mg/dl	75-160 mg/dl
Normal (IU)	3-3.5 μmol/dl	3-5.6 μmol/dl
My lab	_____	_____

Glucose Tolerance Test

persistently ↑ glucose indicates prediabetes, cortisol excess

rapid glucose ↓ indicates insulin excess

The glucose tolerance test is indicated for patients with mild hyperglycemia (glucose 125 to150 mg/dl). It is used to detect prediabetic states and insulinoma.

Protocol
1. After a 24-hour fast, administer 50% glucose solution IV at 0.5 ml/kg (1 ml/lb).
2. Collect a pretest blood sample and samples every 30 minutes for 3 hours after glucose injection.

Interpretation
Normal
Blood glucose levels return to normal 60 to 90 minutes after injection.

Abnormal Hyperglycemia
A high blood glucose level at 90 minutes after injection can indicate hyperadrenocorticism, diabetes mellitus, or severe liver disease.

Abnormal Hypoglycemia
A rapid drop in blood glucose levels after injection suggests an insulinoma. Determine the blood insulin:glucose ratio of the hypoglycemic sample to detect an insulinoma.

Normal	<100 mg/dl 90 minutes after injection

Heparin Stimulation Test For Lipoprotein Lipase

clearing indicates postprandial lipemia from a recent meal

no clearing indicates lipoprotein lipase deficiency

The heparin stimulation test differentiates postprandial lipemia from pathologic lipemia. Heparin activates lipoprotein lipase, causing clearance of postprandial hypertriglyceridemia.

Lipoprotein lipase can be deficient in diabetes mellitus, acute pancreatitis, hypothyroidism, corticosteroid excess, and idiopathic hyperlipoproteinemia in Schnauzers.

Protocol
If blood is lipemic:

1. Administer heparin IV at 100 IU/kg (50 IU/lb).
2. Collect blood after 15 minutes.
3. Observe for clearing of turbidity (fat) in the blood sample.

Interpretation
Clearing indicates adequate lipoprotein lipase and postprandial hyperlipidemia. No clearing indicates pathogenic lipemia from deficiency of lipoprotein lipase.

Lipase

↑ lipase suggests acute pancreatitis

Lipase is a pancreatic enzyme normally secreted into the duodenum during digestion. It can be pathologically activated within the pancreas by lipemia or pancreatic trauma.

Pancreatic necrosis sometimes elevates serum lipase activity from two to seven times normal within 48 hours. Lipase activity also rises with increased absorption from upper intestinal inflammation and from decreased excretion with renal failure. Serum lipase activity remains elevated longer after pancreatic insult than does serum amylase activity.

Kidney failure and macrolipasemia raise lipase levels but are not associated with pancreatitis.

	Dogs	Cats
Normal (SU)	<800 IU/L	<250 IU/L
My lab	_____	_____

Lipoprotein Electrophoresis

electrophoresis is rarely used to classify lipoproteins

Unexplained persistent fasting hyperlipidemia can be studied by electrophoretic separation of lipid-carrying proteins. Electrophoresis can be used to classify lipoproteins but provides no information on the underlying cause of hyperlipidemia.

Classification
Chylomicrons contain triglycerides derived from dietary fat and synthesized in the intestinal mucosa.

Very-low-density lipoproteins (VLDLs) are high in triglycerides and are synthesized in the liver.

Low-density lipoproteins (LDLs) are high in cholesterol. They are formed from VLDLs through removal of triglycerides by lipoprotein lipase.

High-density lipoproteins (HDLs) are the primary carriers of cholesterol in dogs. They are synthesized in the liver.

Macroenzymes

↑ serum enzymes with no disease may be due to macroenzymes

Macroenzymes are complexes of serum enzymes with proteins that have a higher molecular weight and longer plasma half-life than the normal enzyme. The presence of macroenzymes is suggested by finding increased serum enzyme activity not associated with symptoms. They may account for persistence of enzymemia after the liver or pancreatic disease has been controlled.

Macroenzymes can cause diagnostic errors and the performance of unnecessary tests or invasive procedures.

Magnesium (Mg)

↓ Mg is a common electrolyte disorder in critically ill dogs and cats

Most of the magnesium in the body is intracellular with 50% in the bones. Potassium, magnesium, and calcium are closely linked. When one of these positively charged elements is low, another positively charged element is driven into the intracellular space causing a decrease in extracellular blood levels. Severe hypomagnesemia impairs PTH secretion producing hypocalcemia.

Magnesium deficiency occurs from decreased digestive intake or increased renal loss. It is a common electrolyte disorder in critically ill dogs and cats and predisposes them to a variety of cardiovascular, neuromuscular, and metabolic problems.

Hypokalemia is often associated with and is a good indicator of possible hypomagnesemia. Low blood magnesium supports a diagnosis of total body magnesium deficiency, but a normal level does not rule out deficiency.

Hypermagnesemia is rare unless the animal has received drugs containing magnesium.

	Dogs	Cats
Normal	1-2.2 mg/dl	1.8-2.5 mg/dl
	0.8-1.8 mEq/L	1.5-2.1 mEq/L
My lab	_____	_____

Osmolality

hyponatremia causes ↓ serum osmolality; ↓ ADH causes ↓ urine osmolality

Hyponatremia is the usual cause of serum hypoosmolality; it becomes dangerous at <240 mOsmol/kg.

Hypernatremia, hyperglycemia, azotemia, and ethylene glycol cause hyperosmolality. Hyperosmolality is dangerous at >350 mOsmol/kg.

Urine osmolality less than serum osmolality indicates insufficient antidiuretic hormone (vasopressin).

hypernatremia, hyperglycemia, azotemia, ethylene glycol cause ↑ serum osmolality

Osmolality can be measured by freezing point or with vapor pressure osmometers, or it can be calculated using the equation:

$$\text{Osmolality} = 2\,(Na + K) + (glucose \div 18) + (BUN \div 2.8)$$

If osmolality is both measured and calculated, a difference between the two values could indicate exposure to a toxic substance, such as ethylene glycol (antifreeze).

	Dogs	Cats
Serum (SU)	250-310 mOsmol/kg	280-310 mOsmol/kg
Urine (IU)	>500	>500
My lab	_____	_____

Phosphorus

↑ P is common in hemolysis, renal disease, hypoparathyroidism, and growing animals

Diet, hormones, and renal function affect serum phosphorus (P) levels. Because RBCs contain significant amounts of P, hemolysis of blood samples or delayed removal of the serum from the clotted blood sample can falsely elevate the phosphorus value.

Serum phosphorus levels are elevated with renal failure, hypoparathyroidism, nutritional secondary hyperparathyroidism, hypervitaminosis D, and hyperthyroidism in cats. Uremia is the most common cause of hyperphosphatemia.

↓ P is common in early hyperparathyroidism, alkalosis, and neoplasia

Serum phosphorus levels are decreased with alkalosis, hyperparathyroidism, and pseudohyperparathyroidism (hypercalcemia of malignancy).

	Dogs	Cats
Normal (SU)	2.2-5.6 mg/dl	2-6.5 mg/dl
Normal (IU)	0.94-1.6 mmol/L	0.8-1.6 mmol/L
Age <1 yr (SU)	5-9 mg/dl	6-9 mg/dl
My lab	_____	_____

Plasma Protein

↑ total protein is a rough screen for dehydration

Total plasma protein alterations are generally nonspecific.

Glomerular disease, liver disease, starvation, and malabsorption can decrease total plasma protein levels.

Severe dehydration, lymphosarcoma, myeloma, and infection increase the total plasma protein level.

	Dogs	Cats
Normal (SU)	5.5-7.8 g/dl	5.5-7.9 g/dl
Normal (IU)	55-78 g/L	55-79 g/L
My lab	_____	_____

Potassium

↓ K is caused by translocation in alkalosis and by excessive loss

Potassium (K) is found primarily in the intracellular fluid and is excreted by the kidneys under the influence of aldosterone.

Translocation or excessive loss of K can cause hypokalemia. Potassium can be translocated from plasma to body cells with acute alkalosis, insulin-mediated cellular uptake of glucose, and hypothermia. Vomiting, diarrhea, or polyuria also causes potassium loss.

↑ K has many causes, for example, adrenal failure, dehydration, and acidosis

Renal failure, urethral obstruction, dehydration, and hypoadrenocorticism can cause hyperkalemia severe enough to result in cardiac arrest. Serum potassium levels can be high and intracellular levels low in acidosis because of translocation.

	Dogs	Cats
Normal (SU)	3.6-5.8 mEq/L	3.7-4.6 mEq/L
Normal (IU)	3.6-5.8 mmol/L	3.7-4.6 mmol/L
My lab	_____	_____

Renal Disease Index (1/Cr)

plotting 1/Cr indicates rate of kidney deterioration

Plotting the reciprocal of the serum creatinine concentration is a simple method for estimating the rate of progression of chronic renal failure. The linear decline of the reciprocal of the serum creatinine concentration occurs with increasing age and is correlated with decreasing nephrons in cases of chronic renal failure.

Changes in the slope of this line may provide a means of evaluating response to treatment.

Normal	$> \frac{1}{2}$

Renal Failure Index (RFI)

↑ RFI indicates renal azotemia

The RFI is used to differentiate between prerenal, renal, and postrenal causes of azotemia. In acute renal failure the urine excretion of sodium is increased. This is not documented by fractional sodium excretions and may not be clearly differentiated when urine sodium is measured without taking creatinine values into consideration.

RFI = Na urine/(Cr urine/Cr plasma)

	Prerenal	Renal
RFI	<1	>2

Sodium

↓ Na with no apparent loss may indicate aldosterone deficiency

Sodium (Na) levels are high in extracellular fluid and bone. Serum sodium levels are controlled by aldosterone, which promotes sodium retention by the kidneys.

Diarrhea, vomiting, renal disease, diabetes mellitus, hypoadrenocorticism, and uroabdomen can cause low serum sodium levels (hyponatremia).

↑ Na usually indicates dehydration

Water loss from the respiratory, urinary, or intestinal tract occasionally results in dehydration severe enough to increase serum sodium levels (*hypernatremia*).

Mineralocorticoids, osmotic diuretics, or sodium-containing drugs may cause iatrogenic sodium retention.

	Dogs	Cats
Normal (SU)	140-152 mEq/L	146-155 mEq/L
Normal (IU)	140-152 mmol/L	146-155 mmol/L
My lab	_____	_____

Sodium:Potassium Ratio

↓ Na:K ratio
suggests hypo-
adrenocorticism

The ratio of serum sodium (Na) to potassium (K) is the Na:K ratio.

If the Na:K ratio is <23, check for substances that dilute the serum (hyperlipidemia, hyperglycemia) or for conditions that cause Na loss (vomiting, diarrhea). Also check for cause of potassium retention or translocation (renal failure, acidosis, shock, uroabdomen).

If none of these is present, hypoadrenocorticism (Addison's disease) is the likely cause and should be confirmed with an ACTH stimulation test for plasma cortisol levels.

Normal Na:K ratio	>30
Possible hypoadrenocorticism	24-27
Hypoadrenocorticism	<23

Triglycerides

↑ triglycerides
cause lipemic
serum

Hypertriglyceridemia produces lipemic or lactescent ("milky") serum. This may occur normally for up to 12 hours after a meal (*postprandial hyperlipidemia*) and typically clears after IV injection of heparin (see Heparin Stimulation Test for Lipoprotein Lipase).

Fasting hyperlipidemia is usually caused by diabetes mellitus, hypothyroidism, cortisol excess, cholestasis, and idiopathic conditions in some miniature Schnauzers.

Hyperlipidemia is both a cause and a result of acute pancreatitis.

	Dogs	Cats
Normal (SU)	<150 mg/dl	<60 mg/dl
Normal (IU)	<1.14 mmol/L	<0.6 mmol/L
My lab	_____	_____

Viscosity Test for Hyperproteinemia

↑ viscosity indicates hyper-globulinemia or gammopathy

Serum viscosity can be measured with a manual red or white blood cell pipette. Increased serum viscosity indicates *hyperglobulinemia* and a possible *gammopathy.*

Protocol
1. Fill the pipette with serum and measure the time required for the fluid to flow from the top mark on the pipette to a second mark.
2. Repeat the procedure with water.
3. Divide the flow time of serum by the flow time of water to determine the relative serum viscosity.

Relative Serum Viscosity	
Normal	<2.5
Equivocal	2.5-3
Abnormal	>3

Adrenal Function Tests

ACTH Assay

ACTH is ↑ with pituitary tumor

ACTH assays can determine the cause of hyperadrenocorticism. Normal to high serum ACTH levels with high serum cortisol levels indicate a pituitary tumor or a defect in the negative-feedback mechanism.

Low serum ACTH levels with high serum cortisol levels indicates a primary adrenal problem. This test is useful, but it is difficult to find a laboratory to perform it.

Interpretation

Normal values	20-40 ng/L
My lab	_____

In dogs with high serum cortisol levels:

- An ACTH value >40 ng/L suggests pituitary neoplasia.
- An ACTH level <20 ng/L is highly suggestive of adrenal neoplasia.
- An ACTH level of 20-40 ng/L is inconclusive.

ACTH Stimulation

↑ post ACTH cortisol is consistent with hyperadrenocorticism

↓ post ACTH cortisol is diagnostic of adrenocortical insufficiency

Most animals with pituitary-dependent hyperadrenocorticism are hyperresponsive to ACTH stimulation. Animals with hyperadrenocorticism caused by adrenocortical tumors do not respond as well to ACTH stimulation although their blood levels of cortisol are markedly increased.

Animals with adrenal insufficiency resulting from primary hypoadrenocorticism or secondary (iatrogenic) hypoadrenocorticism are hyporesponsive to ACTH stimulation.

The protocol differs for dogs and cats and with the type of ACTH used. A markedly elevated post-ACTH cortisol level is consistent with but not diagnostic of hyperadrenocorticism. It can be caused by adrenal hyperplasia. A subnormal post-ACTH cortisol level is diagnostic of adrenocortical insufficiency.

Cats
Synthetic ACTH:

- Inject 0.125 mg of synthetic ACTH (Cortrosyn 0.25 mg/ml) IM.
- Collect three blood samples: preinjection, 30 and 60 minutes.

ACTH gel:

- Gives inconsistent results in cats.

Dogs
Synthetic ACTH:

- Inject 0.25 mg of synthetic ACTH per dog IM.
- Collect two blood samples: preinjection, 1 hour.

ACTH gel:

- Inject 2.2U/K(1U/lb) ACTH gel IM.
- Collect three blood samples: preinjection and 2 hours.

Interpretation
Cats
Post ACTH

<5 μg/dl	Hypoadrenocorticism
6-12 μg/dl	Normal
13-16 μg/dl	Suggestive hyperadrenocorticism
>16 μg/dl	Usually pituitary tumor

Dogs
Post ACTH

<5 μg/dl	Hypoadrenocorticism
6-18 μg/dl	Normal
18-24 μg/dl	Suggestive hyperadrenocorticism
>24 μg/dl	Usually pituitary tumor

Combined ACTH-Stimulation/ Dexamethasone Suppression

The ACTH-stimulation test and the dexamethasone suppression test may be run on the same day. Start with the high-dose dexamethasone suppression test by giving 0.1 mg dexamethasone/kg. Obtain a blood sample in 2 hours. Immediately after the sample, administer ACTH IM (2.2U/k gel, 0.25 mg synthetic, or per dog). Obtain samples 1 and 2 hours for ACTH gel or 30 minutes and 1 hour for synthetic.

Normal	
Dexamethasone suppression 2 hours	<1.5 μg/dl
ACTH Stimulation	<18 μg/dl
Values over these suggest hyperadrenocorticism	

Dexamethasone Suppression Tests

dexamethasone suppresses pituitary secretion of ACTH

Pituitary ACTH regulates cortisol secretion through hypothalamic pituitary feedback. A high level of endogenous cortisol or administration of dexamethasone inhibits secretion of ACTH.

In animals with high serum cortisol levels caused by stress or pituitary tumors, dexamethasone administration reduces cortisol levels.

With adrenal tumors, dexamethasone administration does not suppress cortisol secretion and serum cortisol levels remain high.

Dexamethasone Suppression, Low-Dose

low-dose dexamethasone suppression differentiates stress from hyperadrenocorticism

The low-dose dexamethasone suppression test helps differentiate cortisol levels elevated by stress or chronic disease from elevations caused by spontaneous hyperadrenocorticism. This test is more sensitive than the ACTH stimulation test because it suppresses levels that result from chronic stress. Cortisol levels in animals with pituitary or adrenal tumors are usually resistant to low-dose dexamethasone suppression.

Protocol
1. Collect a pretreatment blood sample.
2. Inject dexamethasone phosphate IV at 0.005 mg/lb (0.01 mg/kg).
3. Collect blood samples: preinjection, 4 and 8 hours in dogs and at 4, 6, and 8 hours in cats.

Interpretation

	Dogs	Cats
Normal response cortisol	<1 μgdl	<1 μgdl
Hyperadrenocorticism cortisol	>2 μg/dl	>2 μgdl
My lab	_____	_____

In some dogs with pituitary-dependent hyperadrenocorticism, the decrease in cortisol levels is transitory and occurs at 2 to 4 hours postinjection. Levels return to resting preinjection values at 6 to 8 hours postinjection. In animals that only partially suppress cortisol levels, retest with a high-dose dexamethasone suppression test.

Dexamethasone Suppression, High-Dose

↓ posttreatment cortisol indicates a pituitary tumor

The high-dose dexamethasone suppression test is used to distinguish between a pituitary tumor and an adrenal tumor. In animals with an adrenal tumor, dexamethasone does not suppress cortisol levels. In most animals with a pituitary tumor, plasma cortisol levels are reduced by at least 50%.

Protocol
1. Collect a pretreatment blood sample.
2. Inject dexamethasone phosphate IV at 0.05 mg/lb (0.1 mg/kg).
3. Collect blood samples: preinjection, 4 and 8 hours in dogs and at 4, 6, and 8 hours in cats.

Interpretation
- With pituitary tumors, cortisol is <50% of pretreatment levels.
- With adrenal tumors, cortisol is >50% of pretreatment levels.

Dexamethasone Suppression, Very-High-Dose

↓ plasma cortisol indicates pituitary hyperadrenocorticism

Very-high-dose dexamethasone suppression clearly distinguishes a pituitary tumor from an adrenal tumor. The very high dosage, however, can cause thromboembolism, pancreatitis, heart failure, or hypertension. In animals with pituitary-dependent conditions, plasma cortisol levels fall to less than 1.5 µg/dl.

Protocol
1. Collect a pretreatment blood sample.
2. Inject dexamethasone phosphate IV at 0.5 mg/lb (1 mg/kg).
3. Collect a blood sample 6 to 8 hours after injection.

Interpretation
- With pituitary tumor, cortisol is 1.5 µg/dl or <50% of the pretreatment value.
- With adrenal tumor, cortisol is >1.5 µg/dl or >50% of the pretreatment value.

In some dogs with pituitary tumors, even very large doses of dexamethasone do not suppress cortisol levels.

Aldosterone

↓ aldosterone indicates hypoadrenocorticism

Angiotensin and ACTH stimulate secretion of aldosterone, the principal mineralocorticoid of the adrenal cortex. In most cases, aldosterone deficiency is suggested by a low serum sodium (Na) level, a high serum potassium (K) level, and a Na:K ratio <23. Aldosterone levels can be determined after ACTH stimulation. Aldosterone levels after ACTH injection should be at least twice the resting value unless the resting value was in the high-normal range.

Check with your diagnostic laboratory to determine the protocol for this test.

Protocol Using ACTH Gel
1. Fast the animal overnight and collect a preinjection blood sample.
2. Inject ACTH gel (Acthar, 40 U/ml) IM at 1 U/lb.
3. Collect blood samples 1 and 2 hours postinjection. Assay samples for aldosterone.

Interpretation

Normal pre-ACTH aldosterone	5-345 pg/ml
1 hour post-ACTH	91-634 pg/ml
2 hours post-ACTH	71-758 pg/ml

Normal response is doubling of the pre-ACTH value, unless this pretreatment value is high-normal.

Cortisol, Indirect Assay

↓ eosinophils after ACTH injection indicates normal adrenal function

Neutropenia, lymphocytosis, and eosinophilia suggest cortisol insufficiency. To confirm this, the adrenal response to ACTH can be indirectly evaluated by performing absolute neutrophil, lymphocyte, and eosinophil counts before and 1 to 4 hours after IV or IM injection of 0.025 mg of ACTH (Cosyntropin).

If ACTH administration increases neutrophil numbers and decreases lymphocyte and eosinophil numbers, adrenal function is usually normal.

Persistent lymphocytosis and eosinophilia suggest adrenocortical insufficiency and should be verified by assaying plasma cortisol levels (see ACTH stimulation).

Normal response is >30% increase in ratio of neutrophils to lymphocytes, and a 50% decrease in eosinophil numbers.

Cortisol, Serum

↑ cortisol suggests stress or adrenal hyperfunction

↓ cortisol after ACTH indicates adrenal hypofunction

Serum cortisol levels can be measured to check for hyperadrenocorticism or hypoadrenocorticism. Stimulation or suppression tests are usually necessary because there is considerable overlap between normal dogs and those with adrenal disease.

Because hospitalization and other stress can artificially raise baseline cortisol levels, an ACTH stimulation test or a dexamethasone suppression test gives the most accurate assessment of serum cortisol levels.

	Dogs	Cats
Normal (SU)	0.5-4 μg/dl	1-4 μg/dl
Normal (IU)	28-110 nmol/L	48-110 nmol/L
My lab	_____	_____

Old Thyroid Function Tests

Over the years many tests have been developed to diagnose thyroid deficiency. In most areas the following tests have been replaced either because materials are unavailable or newer tests give better information. If newer tests are unavailable these tests may still be useful.

Free T_4
Free T_4(fT_4) is the portion that produces negative feedback on the pituitary gland. It most accurately reflects thyroid function but offers no diagnostic advantage over the T_4 assay.

	Dogs	Cats
Normal (SU) fT_4	1-2 ng/dl	1-2.5 ng/dl
Normal (IU) fT_4	79-158 pmol/L	79-198 pmol/L
My lab	_____	_____

Reverse T_3

Reverse triiodothyronine (rT_3) is the inactive form of T_3. The main use of rT_3 is to diagnose hypothyroidism from nonthyroidal causes. In a variety of illnesses, T_3 levels decrease because of conversion to rT_3. When serum T_4, T_3, and rT_3 levels are low, the animal is hypothyroid.

When serum T_4 and T_3 levels are low but the rT_3 level is high, nonthyroidal illness is probably the cause. This test is rarely performed.

	Dogs	Cats
Normal rT_3	19-45 ng/dl	?

Triiodothyronine (T_3)

Assay of triiodothyronine (T_3) is rarely helpful in diagnosing thyroid dysfunction. Dogs with a high T_3 level (>250 ng/dl) are likely to have antithyroid antibodies and could be clinically hypothyroid.

For therapeutic monitoring, obtain a blood sample 3 hours after giving T_3 (Cytobin) or 4 to 8 hours after giving T_4

(Synthroid, Soloxine). The dose can then be increased or decreased to achieve a euthyroid state.

	Dogs	Cats
Normal (SU) T_3	100-200 ng/dl	75-150 ng/dl
Normal (IU) T_3	1.5-3 nmol/L	1.2-3.3 nmol/L

Thyroid K Value

The K value is calculated using serum cholesterol and free T_4 values. With the K value, a single blood sample can be used to diagnose some cases of hypothyroidism. This test has been replaced by the T_4d test.

Interpretation
- A thyroid K value above +1 is normal.
- A thyroid K value of −4 to +1 is nondiagnostic and could be due to primary hypothyroidism, or hypothyroidism of disease.
- A thyroid K value of less than −4 indicates primary hypothyroidism.

Thyroid-Stimulating Hormone Response Test

The thyroid-stimulating hormone (TSH) response test is the most reliable method of diagnosing hypothyroidism in a private veterinary clinic, but the test reagent is difficult to obtain. To minimize the cost of this test, bovine thyrotropin can be reconstituted and stored frozen for at least 3 months.

Protocol
1. Collect a preinjection blood sample for T_4 assay.
2. Administer TSH IV at 0.1 IU/kg, up to 1 U for an individual dog or cat.
3. Collect another blood sample 6 hours after TSH injection. Assay samples for T_4.

	Dogs	Cats
Normal T_4 post-TSH (SU)	1.5-4.5 μg/dl	1-3 μg/dl
Normal T_4 post-TSH (IU)	19-51 nmol/L	13-39 nmol/L

In normal animals, the T_4 level doubles and is at least in the low end of the normal range.

A post-TSH T_4 level <1.5 μg/dl is diagnostic for hypothyroidism.

Current Thyroid Function Tests

Free T$_4$ Dialysis (fT$_4$d)

↓ fT$_4$d confirms hypothyroidism

Free T$_4$ by dialysis is more accurate than total T$_4$, TSH, free T$_4$ by ELISA, or T$_3$ for diagnosing thyroid disease in the dog. A low fT$_4$d is over 90% sensitive, accurate, and specific for the diagnosis of hypothyroidism. Because this test is more expensive and time consuming than other tests, it is best used as a confirmatory test on animals that have a low total T$_4$. In autoimmune thyroiditis the fT$_4$d is low even though the total T$_4$ is high. In the euthyroid-sick syndrome, fT$_4$d is normal even though the total T$_4$ is low.

My lab _____

TSH Assay

primary hypothy-roidism, ↓ fT$_4$d and ↑ TSH

secondary hypo-thyroidism ↓ fT$_4$d and ↓ TSH

Although not as diagnostic in dogs as in man, TSH assays give a good indication of primary thyroid disease versus secondary (pituitary) thyroid disease. This test is useful in patients with suspected hypothyroidism or a low total T$_4$. Accuracy is increased if run in conjunction with free T$_4$ by dialysis. In primary hypothyroidism, fT$_4$d is low and TSH is high. In secondary hypothyroidism fT$_4$d is low and TSH is also low.

Normal   0.1-0.45 ng/ml

Post Pill TSH Monitoring

normal T$_4$ and ↓ TSH indicate adequate re-placement

Animals that are adequately treated with l-thyroxine should suppress pituitary TSH. Normal levels of TSH indicate adequate therapy. As the test is improved we may be able to measure low TSH levels to indicate excessive thyroid replacement.

Thyrotropin-Releasing Hormone (TRH) Stimulation Test

TRH increases T_4 in normal cats but not in hyperthyroid cats

Thyrotropin-releasing hormone (TRH) administration increases serum T_4 in normal cats but not in hyperthyroid cats. The thyrotropin-releasing hormone stimulation test is easier to perform than the T_3 suppression test in detecting mild hyperthyroidism in cats. If the TRH response test results are equivocal, scintigraphy of the thyroid or a T_3 suppression test should be performed.

Protocol
Sample T_4 before and 4 hours after administering 0.1 mg of TRH/kg BW, intravenously. Dosages greater than 0.1 mg/kg cause adverse reactions (salivation, urination, vomiting, defecation, miosis, tachycardia, and tachypnea).

Calculate

$$\frac{(\text{Post-TRH } T_4 - \text{basal } T_4)}{\text{Basal } T_4} \times 100$$

Normal	>50%
Hyperthyroid	<50%

Antithyroid Hormone Antibody

antithyroglobulin antibodies indicate immune-mediated thyroid disease

Antithyroid antibodies may be formed to thyroglobulin, T_3, or T_4. Antithyroglobulin antibodies are seen in 50% of hypothyroid dogs and indicate immune-mediated thyroid disease. Antibodies to T_3 or T_4 are less frequently detected.

T_4/T_3 Autoantibody Test

T_4 autoantibodies cause total T_4 and free T_4 (RIA) assays to be elevated and mask hypothyroidism

T_4 and T_3 antibodies detect hypothyroidism in cases that show a high T_4. All dogs with autoantibodies against T_3 and/or T_4 also have autoantibodies against thyroglobulin, but not all dogs with autoantibodies against thyroglobulin have autoantibodies against T_3 and/or T_4. The prevalence of anti-T_3 autoantibodies is much higher than the prevalence of anti-T_4 autoantibodies. T_4 autoantibodies can cause total T_4 and free

T_4 (RIA) assays to be elevated and mask hypothyroidism. They serve as markers for autoimmune thyroiditis.

Normal	
Anti-T_3 antibodies	<10 units
Anti-T_4 antibodies	<20 units

Thyroglobulin Autoantibody Test

↑ antithyroglobulin antibodies are an early marker of thyroid disease

Autoantibodies against thyroglobulin occur in 30% to 60% of dogs with hypothyroidism and are an indicator of autoimmune thyroiditis. Not all dogs with autoantibodies against thyroglobulin have autoantibodies against T_3 and/or T_4. Although 13% of euthyroid dogs have antithyroglobulin autoantibodies, these antibodies may serve as a marker for early autoimmune thyroid disease before enough thyroid gland has been destroyed to cause clinical hypothyroidism. This early marker may help veterinarians and breeders reduce the incidence of hypothyroidism through genetic counseling.

Tetraiodothyronine (T_4)

↑ T_4 indicates hyperthyroidism

↓ resting T_4 does not confirm hypothyroidism

High resting serum tetraiodothyronine (T_4) values indicate *hyperthyroidism.* Hyperthyroidism is common in cats and is usually diagnosed by T_4 levels two to ten times normal.

Resting T_4 levels are of little help in diagnosing *hypothyroidism.* Primary thyroid diseases (congenital underdevelopment, thyroiditis, atrophy, and neoplasia) decrease T_4 levels. Secondary disease from deficiency of pituitary thyrotropin (TSH) and nonthyroidal illness also decrease T_4 levels. A low resting T_4 level could suggest hypothyroidism, but a TSH test or T_4d test is needed to differentiate hypothyroidism from nonthyroidal disease.

	Dogs	Cats
Normal (SU) T_4	1.5-4.5 pmol/L	1-3 pmol/L
Normal (IU) T_4	19-51 nmol/L	13-39 nmol/L

T$_3$ Suppression Test

↓ T$_3$ suppression diagnosis early hyperthyroidism

The T$_3$ suppression test is used to diagnose mild or early hyperthyroidism in cats with high normal or slightly elevated resting serum T$_3$ values. After administration of T$_3$, serum T$_4$ levels fall in normal cats but remain high in cats with hyperthyroidism.

T$_3$ Suppression Test
1. Measure the serum T$_4$ level before T$_3$ administration.
2. Give 25 µg of T$_3$ PO (½ of a 50-µg Cytomel tablet) TID for 2 days (6 doses total).
3. On day 3, give a final (seventh) 25-µg dose of T$_3$ and measure the T$_4$ level in a blood sample collected 24 hours after the last dose.

Normal	50% decrease from pretreatment T$_4$ values or <1.5 µ/dl
Hyperthyroidism	No decrease in T$_4$ values

Special Tests

Caffeine Liver Clearance Test

caffeine is used to evaluate the drug metaboliz-ing capacity of the liver

A commercially available automated enzyme-multiplied immunoassay technique (EMIT) can be used to determine serum caffeine concentration after oral or IV administration. This allows capacity limited substances such as caffeine to be used to evaluate the drug metabolizing capacity of the liver. A decreased excretion is a measure of the loss of liver parenchyma.

Protocol
- Administer caffeine PO or IV at 5 mg/kg.
- Sample at 4 and 8 hours.

Normal values   Consult with lab

Hypertonic Saline Test (Hickey-Hare Test)

↑ urine specific gravity indicates medullary washout

The hypertonic saline test distinguishes between renal medullary washout from psychogenic polydipsia and diabetes insipidus. IV infusion of a concentrated salt solution reestablishes the osmotic gradient in the kidney. If polyuria is due to medullary washout, infusion of hypertonic saline allows the kidney to concentrate urine.

Protocol
1. Give water PO at 10 ml/lb to induce diuresis.
2. After 30 minutes, empty the bladder and measure the urine volume and specific gravity.
3. Through an indwelling IV catheter, infuse 2.5% saline solution at 10-12 ml/lb/minute for 45 minutes.
4. Record the urine volume and specific gravity every 15 minutes during IV infusion and again 45 minutes after infusion ends.

Interpretation

Pituitary diabetes insipidus	No change in urine volume or specific gravity
Renal diabetes insipidus	No change in urine volume or specific gravity
Renal medullary washout	Decreased urine volume and high specific gravity (>1.020)

Vasopressin Response

↑ urine specific gravity after vasopressin indicates pituitary diabetes insipidus

The vasopressin (antidiuretic hormone) response test is a rapid, safe way to differentiate causes of polydipsia with hypotonic urine. In animals with pituitary-dependent diabetes insipidus, vasopressin injection increases the urine specific gravity. In animals with medullary washout, renal diabetes insipidus or renal failure, vasopressin does not increase the urine specific gravity.

Repository Vasopressin Test
1. Do not withhold food and water during the test period.
2. Measure the specific gravity of a urine sample before treatment.
3. Inject vasopressin in oil IM:
      2.5 units for animals <15 lb
      5 units for animals ≥15 lb
4. Empty the bladder 3 to 6 hours after vasopressin injection. Discard the urine.
5. Measure the specific gravity of urine obtained 9, 12, and 24 hours after vasopressin injection.

Interpretation
- In animals with diabetes insipidus, urine specific gravity exceeds 1.020 after 9 to 24 hours.
- Animals with renal insufficiency have a urine specific gravity below 1.020 after vasopressin injection.
- If renal medullary washout is suspected, inject 5 units of vasopressin once daily for 2 to 4 days and note if the urine specific gravity rises above 1.025.

Normal urine specific gravity is >1.020 after 9 hours

Aqueous Vasopressin Test
1. Empty the bladder and discard the urine.
2. Give aqueous vasopressin solution IM at 0.5 unit/kg (maximum of 5 units).
3. Measure the urine specific gravity at 30, 60, and 90 minutes after vasopressin injection.

Interpretation
- Animals with pituitary-dependent diabetes insipidus have a urine specific gravity >1.015 after 90 minutes.
- Animals with renal insufficiency or medullary washout have a urine specific gravity <1.015.

Normal urine specific gravity is >1.020 after 90 minutes.

Water Deprivation Test

↑ urine specific gravity after water deprivation rules out diabetes insipidus

The water deprivation test is an economical way to differentiate diabetes insipidus from psychogenic polydipsia and renal failure. This test endangers the animal if polyuria continues over several hours without access to water. Failure to concentrate urine suggests central diabetes insipidus, renal diabetes insipidus, or renal medullary washout.

Protocol
1. Withhold water. Empty the urinary bladder and check the urine specific gravity hourly.
2. End the test and provide water if:

- Urine specific gravity rises above 1.025
- BUN level is increased
- The animal loses more than 5% of its body weight
- The animal becomes dehydrated (increased PCV, increased total plasma protein level)
- Skin elasticity is decreased

Interpretation
An increased urine specific gravity (>1.025) rules out diabetes insipidus.

Normal urine specific gravity	>1.025
Diabetes insipidus, renal diabetes insipidus, or medullary washout	<1.012

Water Deprivation Test, Modified

↑ urine specific gravity after water deprivation rules out diabetes insipidus

To eliminate the problem of urinary washout when testing for diabetes insipidus, restrict the patient's water intake several days before being tested.

First day give 120 ml/kg.
Second day give 90 ml/kg.
Third day give 60 to 80 ml/kg.
Fourth day give no water.

Empty the bladder and take urine samples hourly as in regular water deprivation test. If urine does not concentrate or animal becomes dangerously dehydrated, allow patient free access to water and administer 2 to 5 units of ADH IM. Collect additional urine samples every 30 minutes for up to 2 hours.

Interpretation
1. Normal urine concentration with water deprivation indicates kidney washout.
2. Normal urine concentration after ADH indicates central diabetes insipidus.
3. Inability to concentrate urine suggests nephrogenic diabetes insipidus.

Insulin

↑ glucose,
↓ insulin
indicates insulin-dependent diabetes mellitus

↑ glucose,
↑ insulin
indicates non-insulin-dependent diabetes mellitus

↓ glucose,
↑ insulin indicates insulinoma

Insulin levels usually parallel blood glucose levels. When the blood glucose level is high, the insulin level should also be high. When the blood glucose level is low, the insulin level should also be low. These patterns are important in diagnosing causes of hypoglycemia and hyperglycemia.

Interpretation
- A low blood glucose level with a high insulin level (>26 μU/ml) suggests an insulinoma.
- A high blood glucose level with a low insulin level (<26 μU/ml) suggests insulin-dependent diabetes mellitus.
- A high blood glucose level with a normal to high insulin level suggests non-insulin-dependent diabetes mellitus.

Normal Insulin Patterns

<26 μU/ml fasting blood sample

<20 μU/ml during hypoglycemia

26-150 μU/ml after glucose loading

My lab _____

Insulin:Glucose Ratio

↑ insulin with ↓ glucose suggests insulinoma or insulin overdose

The ratio of blood insulin to blood glucose (insulin:glucose ratio) indicates if the insulin response to blood glucose levels is appropriate. An increased insulin:glucose ratio suggests excessive insulin with low blood glucose. This occurs with an insulinoma or with an overdose of exogenous insulin.

The insulin:glucose ratio can be calculated in 2 ways:

$$\text{Insulin:glucose ratio} = \text{insulin } (\mu\text{U/ml})/\text{glucose (mg/dl)}$$

Normal	0.3
Insulin excess	>0.3
Insulin deficiency	<0.2

or

$$\text{Amended insulin:glucose ratio} = \frac{\text{Insulin}}{(\text{Glucose} - 30)} \times 100$$

Normal	<30
Abnormal	>30

Insulin-Like Growth Factor-1 (IGF-1, Somatomedin C)

in diabetic cats, IGF-1 is not a reliable test for excess GH

IGF-1, also known as *somatomedin C*, is polypeptide hormone and an indirect test for excess growth hormone in the dog. It is produced predominantly in the liver in response to growth hormone (GH) release from the pituitary gland. Many of the growth-promoting effects of GH are because of its ability to release IGF-1 from the liver, which in turn acts on several different tissues to enhance growth.

IGF concentrations increase in feline diabetes mellitus without a rise in growth hormone. Thus, total IGF concentrations are not a reliable indicator of acromegaly in diabetic cats.

Estrogen

estrogen assays
are rarely used in
dogs and cats

Serum estrogen assay can help detect estrogen-secreting tumors.

In the bitch, serum estradiol levels are usually <10 pg/ml in anestrus, 10 to 20 pg/ml in proestrus, and 50 to 100 pg/ml in late proestrus. It does not appear to be a useful assay in canine or feline reproduction.

Progesterone

progesterone
<2 ng/ml indi-
cates ovulation
has not yet
occurred

Serum progesterone levels remain below 2 ng/ml until the LH surge triggers ovulation. Because ovulation occurs 2 days after the LH surge, a rise in progesterone levels can be used to predict the optimal time for mating.

To anticipate estrus, begin testing every other day after proestrus is indicated by vaginal cytology or a serosanguineous vulvar discharge.

Interpretation
- Progesterone 2 to 5 ng/ml indicates impending ovulation.
- Levels >2 to 5 ng/ml indicate the luteal surge is occurring and ovulation should occur within 2 days.
- Levels of 6 to 10 ng/ml indicate ovulation has already occurred and the fertile period is nearly ended.
- Levels >15 ng/ml occur after the fertile period.
- Progesterone levels cannot be used to confirm pregnancy in dogs or cats.
- Progesterone >10 ng/ml occur in pregnancy, pyometra, pseudopregnancy.
- Levels are >10 ng/ml during pregnancy and drop below 10 ng/ml just before parturition. To predict whelping, begin daily testing the week before expected parturition. Parturition should occur within 24 hours after the serum progesterone level falls below 2 ng/ml.

Relaxin Canine Pregnancy Test

pregnancy may be diagnosed with the serum relaxin test as early as 21 days after breeding

Relaxin is a specific marker of pregnancy in the bitch. It can be detected in the blood 21 days after implantation and 25 days postovulation. It is never present in the blood of pseudopregnant animals. A commercial kit (ReproCHECK) is an ELISA test that shows blue with a positive specimen. The test is run on plasma or anticoagulated blood but not on serum or EDTA anticoagulated samples.

Gastrin

↑ gastrin may indicate gastrinoma

Gastrin is a hormone secreted by G-cells in the stomach and duodenum or by neoplastic cells in the pancreas. Serum gastrin levels normally decrease when gastric acidity increases. Serum gastrin levels are elevated when gastric contents are alkaline.

High dietary calcium, gastric outlet obstruction, gastric dilatation, liver disease, renal failure, and occasionally gastrinomas of the pancreas cause high serum gastrin levels. High (>500 pg/ml) or moderately elevated gastrin levels with an acidic gastric pH suggest a gastrinoma.

	Dogs	Cats
Normal range	45-125 pg/ml	28-135 pg/ml
My lab	_____	_____

Gastrin Stimulation Test

The gastrin stimulation test is used to confirm a diagnosis of a gastric secreting tumor in an animal where the fasting gastrin level is below 500 pg/ml

Fast the animal for 24 hours then feed 200 g Prescription diet p/d (Hill's) mixed with 200 g of beef broth and determine serum gastrin levels at 30 and 90 minutes after feeding. Gastrin response to secretin or calcium gluconate may also be used.

Normal Serum Gastrin Levels
30 minutes = 200 pg/ml or less
90 minutes = 100 pg/ml or less

Growth Hormone Stimulation

↓ growth hormone causes growth abnormality and dermatitis

Immature dogs or cats with abnormal growth could have a deficiency of growth hormone. Growth hormone-responsive dermatitis occurs in adult Chows, Pomeranians, miniature Poodles, and Keeshonds.

Protocol
1. Give xylazine IV at 0.01 mg/kg (0.005 mg/lb) or clonidine IV at 0.003 mg/kg (0.0015 mg/lb).
2. Collect blood samples every 15 minutes for 90 minutes. Assay for growth hormone levels.

Interpretation
Blood levels of growth hormone peak at 15 to 30 minutes and return to normal at 90 minutes. A reduced response indicates growth hormone deficiency.

Normal resting GH value	0-10 ng/ml
Peak GH value after stimulation	25-40 ng/ml at 15-30 minutes
Abnormal	<25 ng/ml at 15-30 minutes
My lab	_____

Parathyroid Hormone (PTH)

↑ PTH indicates hyperparathyroidism

PTH acts on bone and kidney, the classic target organs of calcium homeostasis and on muscles, heart, immune system, and pancreatic islets. It maintains normal serum calcium levels by enhancing calcium uptake from the bones, kidneys, and intestines, and increasing phosphorus excretion by the kidneys. In cases of uremia PTH causes muscle dysfunction, cardiomyopathy, leukocyte and T-cell dysfunction, and insulin secretion. Suppression of PTH is important in controlling progressive renal failure in uremic patients. Excess PTH causes hypercalcemia with a Cl:P ratio >33. Animals with pseudohyperparathyroidism secondary to malignancy have normal to decreased PTH levels. Increased PTH occurs with parathyroid adenomas and renal failure.

Parathyroid trauma during thyroid surgery is the most common cause of decreased PTH with concurrent hypocalcemia.

	Dogs	Cats
Normal	2-13 pmol/L	2-13 pmol/L
My lab	_____	_____

Parathyroid Hormone-Related Protein (PTHrP)

↑ PTHrP and hypercalcemia indicate malignancy

PTHrP is secreted by a variety of malignant tumors but lymphosarcoma and anal sac adenocarcinoma are the most common types. High levels in association with hypercalcemia indirectly indicate malignancy. Low or undetectable PTHrP during episodes of hypercalcemia indicate the hypercalcemia is not due to malignancy. Persistently high levels following cancer treatment indicate inadequate control of the tumor. Excess PTHrP causes hypercalcemia with a Cl:P ratio <33.

Sodium Sulfanilate Clearance

↓ sodium sulfanilate clearance with ↓ renal blood flow, renal disease or urinary obstruction

Renal clearance of sodium sulfanilate reflects the glomerular filtration rate and can be used to detect early renal dysfunction. Sodium sulfanilate clearance is often reduced before azotemia or urine concentration changes become evident.

Protocol
1. Fast the animal for 12 hours.
2. Give a 10% solution of sodium sulfanilate IV at 0.2 ml/kg.
3. Collect heparinized blood samples 30, 60, and 90 minutes after injection. Have samples analyzed for sulfanilate levels.
4. Plot blood sulfanilate levels at 30, 60, and 90 minutes on semi-log paper.
5. Calculate the half-life (time required for sodium sulfanilate level to fall by one-half).

Interpretation
A prolonged half-life indicates decreased glomerular filtration rate.

	Dogs	Cats
Normal	50-80 minutes	38-52 minutes

References

Chew DJ et al: *Kirk's current veterinary therapy XII*, Philadelphia, 1995, WB Saunders.

Concannon PW, Gimpel T, Newton L, Castracane VD: Postimplantation increase in plasma fibrinogen concentration with increase in relaxin concentration in pregnant dogs, *Am J Vet Res* 57(9):1382-1385, 1996.

Crenshaw KL et al: Serum fructosamine concentration as an index of glycemia in cats with diabetes mellitus and stress hyperglycemia, *J Vet Intern Med* 10(6):360-364, 1996.

Flanders JA et al: Adjustment of total serum calcium concentration for binding to albumin and protein in cats, *J Am Vet Med Assoc* 194(11):1609-1611, 1989.

Galasso PJ, Litin SC, O'Brien JF: The macroenzymes: a clinical review, *Mayo Clin Proc* 68(4):349-354, 1993.

Golden DL et al: Application of an enzyme-multiplied immunoassay technique for determination of caffeine elimination kinetics as a test of liver function in clinically normal dogs, *Am J Vet Res* 55(6):790-794, 1994 (experimental study).

Gordon ER, Seligson D, Flye MW: Serum bilirubin pigments covalently linked to albumin, *Arch Pathol Lab Med* 120(7):648-653, 1996.

Grauer GF: Acute renal failure. In Morgan RV, ed: *Handbook of small animal practice*, ed 3, Philadelphia, 1997, WB Saunders.

Jensen AL: Glycated blood proteins in canine diabetes mellitus, *Vet Rec* 14:137(16):401-405, 1995.

Jensen AL: Serum fructosamine as a screening test for diabetes mellitus in non healthy middle aged to older dogs, *J Am Vet Med Assoc* 41:480-484, 1994.

Jover R et al: Salivary caffeine clearance predicts survival in patients with liver cirrhosis, *Am J Gastroenterol* 92(10):1905-1908, 1997.

Khanna C et al: Hypomagnesemia in 188 dogs: a hospital population-based prevalence study *J Vet Intern Med* 12(49):304-309, 1998 (retrospective study).

Kintzer PP: TSH and TRH stimulation testing, *Canine Pract* 22(1):47-48, 1997.

Lewitt MS et al: Regulation of insulin-like growth factor-binding protein-3 ternary complex in feline diabetes mellitus, *J Endocrinology* 166(1):21-27, 2000.

Mooney CT, Little CJ, Macrae AW: Effect of illness not associated with the thyroid gland on serum total and free thyroxine concentrations in cats, *J Am Vet Med Assoc* 208(12):2004-2008, 1996.

Nagode LA, Chew DJ, Podell M: Benefits of calcitriol therapy and serum phosphorus control in dogs and cats with chronic renal failure, *Vet Clin North Am Small Anim Pract* 26(6):1293-1330, 1996.

Ogilvie GK et al: Concentrations of alpha-2-acid glycoprotein in dogs with malignant neoplasia, *J Am Vet Med Assoc* 203(8):1144-1146, 1993.

Paradis M et al: Serum-free thyroxine concentrations, measured by chemiluminescence assay before and after thyrotropin administration in healthy dogs, hypothyroid dogs, and euthyroid dogs with dermatopathies, *Can Vet J* 37(5):289-294, 1996.

Peterson ME, Broussard ID, Gamble DA: Use of the thyrotropin-releasing hormone stimulation test to diagnose mild hyperthyroidism in cats, *J Vet Intern Med* 8:279-286, 1994.

Peterson ME, Melian C, Nichols R: Measurement of serum total thyroxine, triiodothyronine, free thyroxine, and thyrotropin concentrations for diagnosis of hypothyroidism in dogs, *J Am Vet Med Assoc* 211(11):1396-1402, 1997.

Remaley AT, Wilding P: Macroenzymes: biochemical characterization, clinical significance, and laboratory detection, *Clin Chem* 35(12):2261-2270, 1989.

Ritz E, Stefanski A, Rambausek M: The role of the parathyroid glands in the uremic syndrome, *Am J Kidney Dis* 26(5):808-813, 1995.

Rothuizen J, van den Ingh T: Covalently protein-bound bilirubin conjugates in cholestatic disease of dogs, *Am J Vet Res* 49(5):702-704, 1988.

Scott-Moncrieff J et al: Comparison of serum concentrations of thyroid stimulating hormone in healthy dogs, hypothyroid dogs, and euthyroid dogs with concurrent disease, *J Am Vet Med Assoc* 212(3):387-391, 1998.

Sevelius E: Diagnosis and prognosis of chronic hepatitis and cirrhosis in dogs, *J Small Anim Pract* 36(12):521-528, 1995.

Solter PF et al: Hepatic total 3 alpha-hydroxy bile acids concentration and enzyme activities in prednisone-treated dogs, *Am J Vet Res* 55(8):1086-1092, 1994.

Steinetz BG, Goldsmith LT, Harvey HJ, Lust G: Serum relaxin and progesterone concentrations in pregnant, pseudopregnant, and ovariectomized, progestin-treated pregnant bitches: detection of relaxin as a marker of pregnancy, *Am J Vet Res* 50(1):68-71, 1989

Steinetz BG, Goldsmith LT, Harvey HJ, Lust G: Use of Serum relaxin for preganancy diagnosis in the bitch. In Bonagura JD: *Kirk's current veterinary therapy*, ed 13, Philadelphia, 2000, WB Saunders.

Thoresen SI, Bredal WP: An evaluation of serum fructosamine as a marker of the duration of hypoproteinemic conditions in dogs, *Vet Res Commun* 22(3):167-177, 1998.

Turgut K et al: Pre- and postprandial total serum bile acid concentration following acute liver damage in dogs, *Zentralbl Veterinarmed A* 44(1):25-29, 1997.

Young DW: Antibodies to thyroid hormone and thyroglobulin in canine autoimmune lymphocytic thyroiditis, *Canine Pract* 22(1):14-15, 1997.

Section 2
Digestion Tests

Obsolete Fecal Tests

As new diagnostic tests are developed, they replace older tests that are less accurate. These older tests may be useful when the more advanced tests are unavailable.

Fecal Trypsin

Fecal trypsin analysis is a qualitative test for proteolytic activity by gelatin digestion. This can be done by incubating a strip of unexposed radiographic film in a test tube containing an alkaline solution of fresh feces (1 part feces + 9 parts 5% sodium bicarbonate) for 2 hours. To increase the accuracy of results, negative findings should be confirmed on at least three random fecal samples. This is a convenient method to test for trypsin secretion by the pancreas, but the test produces false results 25% of the time.

Normal   Clearing of gelatin on film

Fecal Proteolytic Activity (FPA)

FPA may be measured by radial enzyme diffusion. This is a qualitative test for digestive enzymes of cats and dogs. Normal animals have detectable fecal protease activity, while those with exocrine pancreatic insufficiency do not.

Although the test may be done on a single sample, to increase the sensitivity of the test, feces should be collected over a 3-day period and stored in the refrigerator. This test may be set up in a clinic or can be sent to reference labs.

Normal   Clearing of zone on plate

Xylose Absorption Test

Xylose is a sugar that is absorbed intact from the duodenum. Xylose absorption is used to distinguish between maldigestion and malabsorption.

Protocol
1. Fast the patient for 12 hours.
2. Collect a pretest sample.
3. Administer 5% xylose solution PO at 10 ml/kg.
4. Collect anticoagulated blood samples every 30 minutes for 90 minutes.

Interpretation
The serum xylose level in normal dogs peaks at 60 minutes and decrease at 90 minutes. Dogs with serum xylose levels above 50 mg/dl at 60 minutes or above 45 mg/dl at 90 minutes are normal. Dogs with malabsorption have a flat absorption curve that peaks below 50 mg/dl. Dogs with maldigestion have a normal curve.

Normal xylose	>45 mg/dl at 30-90 minutes
Malabsorption	<44 mg/dl at 30-90 minutes

Bentiromide (Bt-PABA) Test

This is a useful test in the dog for maldigestion. In the normal dog, pancreatic chymotrypsin acts on bentiromide to yield free para-aminobenzoic acid (PABA), which is absorbed passively through the intestine and is measured in the blood. The diagnostic laboratory can supply bentiromide for testing.

Protocol
1. Withhold pancreatic enzyme supplementation for 3 days before the test.
2. After a 12-hour fast, collect a heparinized blood sample.
3. Give 1% bentiromide solution PO by stomach tube at 4 ml/kg followed by 100 ml water.
4. Collect heparinized blood samples 60 and 90 minutes after administration.

Interpretation

Normal dogs have a plasma PABA level of at least 400 μ/dl. Lower levels indicate a pancreatic enzyme deficiency or malabsorption.

Normal PABA at 60-90 minutes	>400 μg/dl
Maldigestion	<125 μg/dl
Malabsorption	125-400 μg/dl

Currently Available Digestive Tests

Fat Absorption Tests

Fat absorption requires normal bile and pancreatic enzyme secretion for digestion as well as normal lymphatic absorption. Vegetable oil is fed to test a patient's ability to digest and absorb lipids.

Protocol
1. Fast the patient for 12 hours and check a pretest sample of lipemia.
2. Give vegetable oil (2 to 5 ml/kg) by stomach tube or mixed with a meal.
3. Check an anticoagulated blood sample for lipemia at hourly intervals for 3 hours.
4. If no lipemia is observed, do a second test after incubating the oil with a pancreatic enzyme supplement 1 tsp. (Viokase/ 10 ml oil) for 30-60 minutes.

Normal	Lipemia following oil
Maldigestion	Lipemia following oil + enzymes
Malabsorption	No lipemia following oil + enzymes

Vitamin A Absorption Test

vitamin A absorption indicates malabsorption or maldigestion

Vitamin A absorption requires normal bile and pancreatic enzyme secretion for digestion as well as normal fat absorption. This test cannot differentiate maldigestion from malabsorption.

Protocol
1. Feed 200,000 units vitamin A and immediately take a blood sample.
2. Collect a second sample after 6 to 8 hours.
3. Assay for vitamin A in both samples.

The concentration in normal dogs increases three to five times.

Normal	>3 times baseline sample
Maldigestion	<3 times baseline sample
Malabsorption	<3 times baseline sample

Fecal Cytology

check the cyto-logic smear for neutrophils, tumor cells, or RBCs

When the feces is abnormal, in addition to routine fecal examinations for intestinal parasites, it should be examined microscopically to assess intestinal mucosal damage.

Cytology can indicate active inflammation, hemorrhage, or neoplasia.

Protocol
1. Stain a dry fecal smear with Wright's stain or mix Schalm's new methylene blue stain with a small fleck of feces on a slide that is covered with a cover slip.
2. Examine the specimen for the presence of neutrophils, eosinophils, blood or tumor cells.

Interpretation
Many neutrophils indicate colitis or proctitis. Few or no neutrophils are present in feces of normal animals or from those with intestinal inflammation from viral infections, bacterial overgrowth, or nonspecific irritants. RBCs can indicate ulceration. Tumor cells indicate intestinal neoplasia.

Normal feces	No neutrophils
Bowel inflammation	Many neutrophils

Serum Trypsin-Like Immunoreactivity (TLI)

↓ TLI indicates pancreatic insufficiency

↑ TLI indicates acute pancreatitis

The TLI test measures the amount of trypsinogen that leaks out of the pancreas. Normally there are trace amounts of this inactive enzyme in the blood, even though it is excreted in the urine. Since this enzyme is not found in other organs, it acts as a pancreas-specific marker. This enzyme enters the blood directly from the pancreas and is not lowered in small intestinal disease. In cases of pancreatic insufficiency, the serum TLI concentration is reduced. In cases of acute pancreatitis the serum TLI is increased.

A species-specific assay must be used. Since the kidney excretes this enzyme, falsely elevated values occur with uremia. In cats, testing TLI for an increase is the test of choice for acute pancreatitis. In the dog, increases occur earlier and decreases sooner than amylase and lipase, so all three enzymes should be tested. In cats, TLI values below 8 µg/L and in dogs values below 2 µg/L confirm a diagnosis of pancreatic insufficiency.

	Dogs	Cats
Normal	5-35 µg/L	17-49 µg/L
My lab	_____	_____

Serum Cobalamin (Vitamin B$_{12}$)

↓ serum cobalamin levels are usually due to chronic malabsorption

Absorption of cobalamin occurs only in the ileum. Since cobalamin is usually abundant in canine and feline diets, subnormal serum levels are usually due to chronic malabsorption. Malabsorption may be caused by generalized intestinal disease that affects the ileum, bacterial overgrowth proximal to the ileum, and exocrine pancreatic insufficiency.

To confirm that low serum levels are due to intestinal disease, run concurrent assays for folate and TLI. Cobalamin values below 225 are suggestive of malabsorption. Normal values vary with the type of assay.

Normal values for a common veterinary radioassay are:

	Dogs	Cats
	225-860 ng/L	200-1680 ng/L
My lab	_____	_____

Serum Folate

↓ folate levels indicate chronic proximal small intestinal disease

↑ folate levels occur with bacterial overgrowth in the proximal small intestine

Absorption of folate occurs in the proximal small intestine. Subnormal folate levels may be caused by chronic proximal small intestinal disease. Increased serum folate concentrations occur with bacterial overgrowth in the proximal small intestine. This is commonly seen with exocrine pancreatic insufficiency but may also occur with intestinal disease. Normal values vary with the assay method. Since folate is high in RBCs, hemolysis may cause falsely increased values.

	Dogs	Cats
	7-17 ng/L	13-38 ng/L
My lab	_____	_____

Alpha 1-Protease Inhibitor (Alpha 1-PI)

↑ fecal alpha 1-PI indicates protein losing enteropathy

Fecal alpha 1-protease inhibitor provides a reliable marker for the diagnosis of protein losing enteropathy (PLE). Protein loss occurs when there is excessive loss of plasma and intercellular fluid into the lumen of the gut as a result of mucosal ulceration, lymphatic obstruction, or mucosal inflammation. These protein rich fluid exudates contain albumin and other proteins including alpha 1-protein inhibitors. Most proteins are digested; however, alpha 1-protease inhibitor is resistant to digestion and passes down the GI tract. It can then be detected in fecal extracts using species specific immunologic assay.

This test reveals the excessive loss of protein into the GI tract before the concentration of albumin in serum becomes abnormal.

Normal   Not detected

Tests of the Future

Differential Sugar Absorption

↑ complex sugar absorption indicates ↑ intestinal permeability

Sugar absorption of lactulose and xylose increases with small intestinal disease. A diseased intestine becomes abnormally leaky, since its barrier function is impaired.

New methods of analysis may increase the accuracy of these tests, but currently the tests await wide availability.

Breath Hydrogen Test

↑ breath hydrogen suggests carbohydrate malabsorption

The pulmonary excretion of hydrogen after a carbohydrate meal can diagnose carbohydrate malabsorption in the small intestine. The test provides semiquantitative information on the degree of malassimilation, which, in turn, assists interpretation of the clinical significance of intestinal biopsies. Normal values will depend on the laboratory and the sugar used.

Sucrose Absorption/Excretion Test

↑ sucrose absorption indicates gastric erosions or ulcerations

Sucrose is not normally absorbed from the stomach, and it is digested in the small intestine. When there is diffuse gastric mucosal damage or gastric ulcers, it is absorbed and passed into the urine. Increased sucrose permeability is useful in predicting presence of endoscopically relevant gastric damage and NSAID-induced ulcers. Healing of these lesions can be monitored by sequential measurements of sucrose permeability.

Administer 1 tablespoon table sugar (sucrose).
Collect urine over the next hour.
Check urine sample for sucrose.

Normal   Negative

References

Hall EJ, Batt RM: Differential sugar absorption for the assessment of canine intestinal permeability: the cellobiose/mannitol test in gluten-sensitive enteropathy of Irish Setters, *Res Vet Sci* 51(1):83-87, 1991.

Meddings JB, Kirk D, Olson ME: Noninvasive detection of nonsteroidal antiinflammatory drug-induced gastropathy in dogs, *Am J Vet Res* 56(8):977-981, 1995.

Melgarejo T, Williams DA, Asem EK: Enzyme-linked immunosorbent assay for canine alpha 1-protease inhibitor, *Am J Vet Res* 59(2):127-130, 1998.

Muir P et al: Evaluation of carbohydrate malassimilation and intestinal transit time in cats by measurement of breath hydrogen excretion, *Am J Vet Res* 52(7):1104-1109, 1991.

Sorensen SH et al: Blood test for intestinal permeability and function: a new tool for the diagnosis of chronic intestinal disease in dogs, *Clin Chim Acta* 264(1):103-1156, 1997.

Washabau RJ et al: Evaluation of intestinal carbohydrate malabsorption in the dog by pulmonary hydrogen gas excretion, *Am J Vet Res* 47(6):1402-1406, 1986.

Section 3
Urine Tests

Acid Loading Test

alkaline urine after inducing acidosis indicates a renal tubular defect

The acid loading test is used to diagnose renal tubular acidosis. In patients with distal renal tubular acidosis, the kidneys are unable to acidify the urine. In slightly acidemic patients with alkaline urine, ammonium chloride can be given to confirm that the kidneys cannot acidify the urine.

Protocol
1. Collect a urine sample.
2. Administer ammonium chloride PO at 100 mg/kg every 15 minutes for 4 doses.
3. Collect urine samples every hour for 6 hours after administration of ammonium chloride.

Interpretation
Alkaline urine after acid loading confirms distal renal tubular acidosis. Urine pH is normally <5.5 at 3 to 4 hours. Urine pH >5.6 at 3 to 4 hours indicates distal tubular acidosis.

Normal urine pH after 4 hours	<5.5
Distal tubular acidosis	<5.6

Bilirubin

↑ urine bilirubin indicates liver disease; this is a very sensitive test for liver disease in cats

A small amount of bilirubin can be found in the urine of normal dogs, but none is normally present in feline urine. Amounts greater than 2+ in dogs or 1+ in cats in urine with a specific gravity greater than 1.020 are an early indicator of liver disease. Only conjugated bilirubin is passed in the urine, so bilirubinuria usually indicates liver disease, such as bile duct obstruction, hepatic necrosis, hepatitis, hepatic tumors, or cholangiohepatitis. In hemolytic anemias, some indirect bilirubin may be conjugated by the kidney of dogs to produce bilirubinuria.

	Dogs	Cats
Normal	Trace	None

Bladder Tumor Antigen Test (VBTA Test)

the VBTA test detects early stages of transition cell carcinoma

The BTA test is a qualitative, rapid, latex agglutination, dipstick test that is run on voided urine. It measures a glycoprotein (basement membrane) antigen complex associated with bladder cancer. Pyuria (>30 WBC/HPF), hematuria (>30 RBC/HPF), 4+ protein, or 4+ glucosuria may interfere with the test results by creating false-positive reactions. Urine parameters that had no effect on efficacy included collection method (cystocentesis or freecatch), pH, specific gravity, crystalluria, bilirubinuria, bacteriuria, and casts.

Casts

casts indicate active renal disease

Casts are cylindric protein accumulations that precipitate in the distal and collecting tubules of the kidney. They are flushed from these areas and pass into the urine.

Several kinds of casts can form. All casts signify renal disease, such as nephritis, pyelonephritis, amyloidosis, or nephrosis.

Normal	No casts in urine
Acute nephritis	Many casts
Acute nephrosis	Many casts

Catheterization

Urine samples collected by catheterization are helpful in localizing urinary tract problems. With sequential placement of a catheter, samples may be taken from the urethra, prostate area, and bladder. This is especially valuable for detecting sites of hemorrhage or locations of abnormal cells that indicate a tumor or infection.

Cold Urine Crystal Analysis

↑ crystals in cold
urine indicate the
potential for
urolith formation

Analysis of crystals in a cold urine specimen provides an estimate of the crystal production potential of a particular diet and the risk of crystalluria if the urine pH should rise.

Protocol
1. Feed a test diet for 2 weeks.
2. Fast overnight.
3. Obtain a urine sample by cystocentesis and check the pH.
4. Freeze and thaw the urine to precipitate the crystals.
5. On microscopic examination, note the amount and type of crystals.

Interpretation
See discussion in *Crystals* section.

Color

red-brown urine
indicates hemor-
rhage, hemoglo-
bin, or myoglobin

Urine is usually clear to pale yellow. A yellow-orange color suggests bilirubinuria. A red to brown color suggests hematuria, hemoglobinuria, or myoglobinuria. If no RBCs are present, the cause of red-brown urine can be determined in the following way:

Protocol
1. Centrifuge the urine sample.

Interpretation
With hematuria, the supernatant is clear and the sediment is red.

2. If the supernatant remains red or brown, add 2.5 g of ammonium sulfate to 5 ml of the supernatant.
3. Mix and centrifuge.

Interpretation
With hemoglobinuria, the supernatant is clear.

With myoglobinuria, the supernatant remains red or brown.

Cortisol:Creatinine Ratio

↑ C:Cr ratio suggests hyperadrenocorticism

Adrenocortical function can be evaluated by determining the ratio of cortisol to creatinine in the urine. High levels of cortisol in the urine (ratios >20) indicate hyperadrenocorticism. When the urine cortisol level is high, ACTH stimulation or a dexamethasone suppression test is needed to confirm hyperadrenocorticism because stress can also raise the urine cortisol level. A ratio <20 rules out hyperadrenocorticism.

Normal cortisol:creatinine ratio   <20

Exogenous Creatinine Clearance (CrC)

infrequently used test

The renal clearance of creatinine allows the calculation of glomerular filtration rate (GFR). Because 24-hour urine specimens are hard to obtain, exogenous creatinine clearance is easier than endogenous clearance, but it is still laborious to obtain.

Protocol
- Give no food for 12 hours, but give free access to water.
- Catheterize with a retention catheter.
- Empty the bladder and rinse with sterile saline three times.
- Inject 100 mg creatinine/kg^2
- Draw blood sample for creatinine test 40 minutes after injection.
- Catheterize, rinse bladder, and empty, leave catheter in place for 20 minutes.
- Collect all urine made during the next 20 minutes and the fluid from three rinses. Record the volume.
- Draw second blood sample.

Calculate

$$CrC = \frac{\text{Urine creatinine} \times \text{urine volume/minute}}{\text{Average plasma creatinine} \times \text{wt (kg)}}$$

	Dogs	Cats
Normal	3-5 ml/min/kg	2-4 ml/min/kg

Crystals

↑ urine crystals can indicate metabolic disease or the composition of a urolith

Phosphate, calcium oxalate, and struvite (magnesium ammonium phosphate) crystals are often found in normal urine, but sometimes they are associated with uroliths.

Large numbers of *bilirubin crystals* suggest abnormal bilirubin metabolism.

Calcium oxalate crystals can be seen in acidic urine with oxalate urolithiasis and with ethylene glycol toxicity.

Amorphous and calcium phosphate crystals are seen in alkaline urine. When associated with a urolith, they can suggest the stone's identity.

Cystine crystals are seen in animals with inherited or acquired renal tubular metabolic disorders that interfere with resorption of cystine. Their identification can help characterize a radiolucent urolith.

Magnesium ammonium phosphate (struvite) crystals are normal in small amounts in alkaline urine. Large amounts can indicate impending urolith formation from infection or dietary-induced alkaline conditions.

Ammonium urate crystals are seen in dogs with hepatic portal shunts and ammonium urate uroliths.

Uric acid crystals are rare but signify portal shunts or a possible identity of a urolith.

Cystocentesis

To help determine the significance, cause, and location of bladder lesions, urine samples can be collected by aseptic needle aspiration of the bladder *(cystocentesis)*, rather than by catheterization or free-catch. Even small numbers of bacteria in a urine sample obtained by cystocentesis are significant.

If cytologic abnormalities are detected in free-catch urine samples, but not in those obtained by cystocentesis, the lesion is distal to the bladder. If the cystocentesis sample is abnormal, the lesion is located in the bladder, ureter(s), or kidney(s).

Cytologic Examination

air-dried slides stained with Wright's stain give better cellular detail than wet mounts

Cytologic examination of urine samples can aid in the diagnosis of urinary tract disease. Dried smears of urine sediment provide better cellular detail than wet mounts.

Protocol
1. Centrifuge the urine sample and pour off the supernatant.
2. Using a small artist's brush, paint a thin layer of the sediment on a slide.
3. Dry the slide with a hair dryer.
4. Stain with Wright's stain or Schalm's new methylene blue and microscopically examine for abnormal or neoplastic cells.

Enzymuria

GGT Enzymuria

GGT:Cr ratio is a sensitive test for acute renal tubular damage

Urinary enzymes are a sensitive test for assessing early renal damage. Of these enzymes, urine GGT is the most easily tested. Patients with glomerulonephritis, the induction phase of acute renal failure, and the polyuric phase of acute tubular necrosis have increased excretion of GGT. These increased levels are not seen in cases of pyelonephritis and in the oliguric phase of acute tubular necrosis. Urine GGT reflects brush border damage of the proximal tubules and is often present before formed elements such as casts are seen. Spot tests using the GGT:Cr ratio may be run at any commercial laboratory.

$$GGT:Cr = <0.24$$

NAG Enzymuria

NAG:Cr ratio is a sensitive test for acute renal tubular damage

NAG (N-acetyl-beta-D-glucosaminidase) is a lysosomal enzyme of the kidneys. During the induction phase of acute kidney failure, increases in urinary NAG indicate kidney damage before other abnormalities such as casts or azotemia are present. NAG enzymuria reflects lysosomal dysfunction of both glomerular and proximal tubular epithelial cells and is useful in localizing the site of the kidney lesion. Creatinine ratios are a convenient way of estimating this enzyme without collecting a 24-hour urine sample. The NAG:Cr ratio is not routinely available.

$$NAG:Cr = <0.10$$

Epithelial Cells

↑ epithelial cells suggest a problem in the renal tubules, bladder, or prostate

Small numbers of squamous, transitional or renal tubular epithelial cells can be observed in normal urine. Large numbers of normal or atypical epithelial cells indicate renal tubular, distal urinary tract, or prostate irritation or neoplasia.

Normal   Few epithelial cells

Fractional Excretion

Fractional Excretion of Potassium

↓ fractional excretion of K suggests deficiency

Abnormalities in the renal regulation of external potassium balance may cause potassium excesses or deficits. Kidney disease, increased intake, pharmacologic agents, and electrolyte shifts as a result of acid-base balance increase fractional excretion of potassium. Low fractional excretion suggests a body deficit of this electrolyte. Random tests during renal failure may not correlate well with 72-hour samples.

$$\frac{(Urine\ K/serum\ K)}{(Urine\ Cr/serum\ Cr)} \times 100$$

Dog   15%-20%
Cats   5%-24%

Fractional Excretion of Magnesium

↓ fractional excretion of Mg suggests deficiency

In suspect cases of hypomagnesemia or magnesium containing uroliths, the fractional excretion of magnesium may be useful. In order to avoid dietary interference, a standard diet should be fed for several days before the determination because a 15-hour fast is not effective for controlling external factors of predominantly intracellular electrolytes like magnesium. The major site of magnesium reabsorption is the loop of Henle.

$$\frac{(\text{Urine Mg/serum Mg})}{(\text{Urine Cr/serum Cr})} \times 100$$

Normal value   None reported

My lab   ——————

Fractional Excretion of Sodium

↑ fractional excretion of sodium suggests renal tubular damage

Normally the kidney maintains serum sodium by reabsorption. With early toxicity to the nephron epithelial cells this function is impaired and excess sodium is lost in the urine. Loss of sodium reabsorption occurs before cellular necrosis and is an early sign of kidney damage. This functional change can be estimated by measuring the urine and serum concentrations of sodium and creatinine after a 12-hour fast and calculating the fractional excretion of sodium.

$$\frac{(\text{Urine Na/serum Na})}{(\text{Urine Cr/serum Cr})} \times 100$$

Normal   1%

Fractional Excretion of Phosphorus

↑ fractional excretion of phosphorus suggests excess parathormone

Since phosphorus excretion is under the control of parathyroid hormone, the fractional excretion of phosphorus estimates increased serum levels of parathormone. After a 12-hour fast, the urine and serum levels of phosphorus are measured. The fractional excretion of phosphorus in normal cats and dogs is 10% or less. In management of renal failure, values in dogs <20% and in cats <70% indicate adequate phosphorus restriction and normal parathormone. High values indicate excessive parathormone and the need for calcitrol therapy.

$$\frac{(\text{Urine P/serum P})}{(\text{Urine Cr/serum Cr})} \times 100$$

	Dogs	Cats
Normal	<20%	<70%

Fluorescein Dye Excretion

fluorescein dye in urine suggests antifreeze poisoning

Fluorescein dye excretion may be diagnosed by exposing the urine to ultraviolet light. The dye will produce a green or orange color. This is useful as a rapid screen for antifreeze poisoning because most antifreeze solutions are colored with fluorescein.

This test is also useful to detect urine-spraying in cats. After a cat is fed a small amount of dye, it will be passed in the urine and will fluoresce when exposed to ultraviolet light. This is useful in determining which cat is urinating in a multicat household.

Glucose

hyperglycemia, urinary tract hemorrhage, or renal tubular defects can cause glycosuria

Glucose is normally absent from the urine. *Transient glycosuria* can occur from excitement, corticosteroid administration, and excessive carbohydrate intake.

Pathologic glycosuria occurs in metabolic and urinary tract disease. Hyperglycemia from diabetes mellitus and stress causes *overload glycosuria*. Acquired and congenital renal tubular diseases cause *renal glycosuria*. Hemorrhage into the urine causes *artificial glycosuria*.

False-negative readings can occur when high levels of vitamin C are given and excreted into the urine.

Normal   No glucose in urine

Ketone Bodies

urine ketones are seen with keto-acidotic diabetes mellitus

false-negatives occur because common tests for ketone bodies do not reveal beta-hydroxybutyrate

Ketones are usually absent from the urine and their presence *(ketonuria)* signifies defective carbohydrate metabolism.

The liver, through fatty acid oxidation, produces the ketones beta-hydroxybutyrate, acetoacetate, and acetone when glucose is unavailable. Although beta-hydroxybutyrate is the best indicator of ketoacidosis, the test for this ketone is rarely performed. The usual qualitative tests for ketones detect only acetoacetate and acetone.

Because common tests demonstrate acetoacetate but not beta-hydroxybutyrate, some ketonuria goes undetected. This can give a false impression of worsening ketosis as ketone production switches from beta-hydroxybutyrate to acetoacetate when lactic acidosis is corrected.

A common cause of ketonuria is diabetes mellitus. Starvation usually does not cause detectable ketonuria in dogs and cats.

| Normal | No ketonuria |
| Ketoacidosis | Ketonuria |

Ketones, Modified Urine Test

add three drops of H_2O_2 to convert unde-tectable ketones to acetoacetate

Beta-hydroxybutyrate is commonly present in diabetic ketosis but is not detected by the usual urinary tests for ketone bodies. By adding three drops of H_2O_2 to the urine, the ketones are converted to acetoacetate, which reacts with the nitroprusside reagent strips.

Occult Blood

occult blood in-dicates either myoglobin or hemoglobin

The occult blood test detects hemoglobinuria and myoglobinuria. A positive reaction does not distinguish among hematuria, myoglobinuria, or hemoglobinuria.

Causes of occult blood in the urine include hemolysis (hemoglobin), strenuous exercise (myoglobin), and urinary tract hemorrhage (blood).

| Normal | None |

pH

diet and disease
influence urine
pH; crystal
types vary with
urine pH

The urine of wild *Canidae* and *Felidae* is normally acidic because their diet is usually of animal origin. The urine of domestic dogs and cats consuming a commercial diet is neutral or slightly alkaline. Cystitis, lower urinary tract obstruction, normal digestion, and alkalosis cause alkaline urine. Increased protein catabolism, acidosis, high-meat diets, or medications increase urine acidity. The pH of the urine is important in determining the type of crystals present in the urine and their solubility.

Protein (Albumin)

↑ urine albumin
loss is a sign of
glomerulone-
phritis

The urine dipstick strips detect only albumin. Other urine protein tests, such as acid precipitation and electrophoresis, detect albumin, globulin, and Bence-Jones protein. Protein is normally not detectable in urine unless the urine is *concentrated*. Protein in the urine is termed *albuminuria* or *proteinuria*.

Slight albuminuria can occur with muscular exertion, excessive protein intake, hemorrhage, and estrus. Urinary tract hemorrhage or glomerular lesions cause pathologic albuminuria. To fully evaluate the significance of the urinary albumin (protein) loss, urine can be collected for 24 hours or the daily protein loss estimated with the urine protein:creatinine ratio.

Markedly alkaline urine causes false-positive protein reactions with urine dipsticks.

Normal   Slight or no protein using a dipstick

Protein:Creatinine Ratio

↑ urine Pr:Cr
ratio indicates a
glomerular lesion

The urine protein:creatinine (Pr:Cr) ratio is used to determine the extent of protein loss without the necessity of 24-hour urine collection. A ratio of 0.6 or less indicates normal urine protein loss. A ratio of more than 1 indicates significant urine protein loss. The ratio is calculated with the following equation:

Pr:Cr ratio = urine protein (mg/dl)/urine creatinine (mg/dl)

Proteinuria in a cystocentesis sample without concurrent hemoglobinuria, pyuria, or hematuria suggests increased glomerular permeability.

Normal urine Pr:Cr ratio	<0.6
Glomerular lesion	>1

Nonalbumin Proteinuria

sulfosalicylic acid precipitation demonstrates all urinary proteins

Renal proteinuria can be due to proteins other than albumin. These are not demonstrated by the usual dipstick methods but may be diagnosed with either sulfosalicylic acid precipitation or protein electrophoresis.

Red Blood Cells

↑ RBCs indicate hemorrhage; the lesion may be localized by sampling at different sites

A few RBCs per high-power field can be present in normal urine. Genitourinary tract hemorrhage causes blood in urine (*hematuria*).

Blood apparent only at the onset of voiding indicates a lesion in the urethra, prostate, or vaginal canal.

Blood apparent only at the end of voiding indicates a bladder lesion.

Blood apparent throughout voiding or in a cystocentesis sample indicates a lesion in the bladder, ureter, or kidney.

Normal	0 to few RBCs

Sediment

casts, RBCs, WBCs, or epithelial cells indicate an active urinary tract problem

Sediment in a centrifuged urine sample contains varying amounts of formed elements (RBCs, WBCs, epithelial cells and casts). When these elements exceed normal amounts, the sediment is classified as *active sediment* and indicates acute disease of the urinary tract. Casts indicate an active kidney lesion. To localize the site producing the other elements, sequential urine samples collected by cystocentesis, catheterization, and free-catch are analyzed.

Specific Gravity

specific gravity is altered by disease and hydration status

The specific gravity of urine is a measure of the kidney's ability to concentrate and dilute urine. Specific gravity is an important factor in determining the significance of crystalluria, proteinuria, and cells in the urine.

Chronic renal disease, diabetes insipidus, hyperadrenocorticism, corticosteroid administration, psychogenic polydipsia, and pyometra decrease urine specific gravity.

Fever, dehydration, diabetes mellitus, vomiting, diarrhea, and hemorrhage increase urine specific gravity.

Urine specific gravity varies with hydration and water intake.

Tamm-Horsfall Protein

Cells in the loop of Henle secrete Tamm-Horsfall protein. This protein binds fimbriae on the surface of bacteria and forms netlike aggregates that trap microorganisms and facilitates their elimination.

Tamm-Horsfall protein is excreted in the urine with nephropathy before changes in the BUN or creatinine occur. Acid urine precipitates this protein to form hyalin casts. Erythrocytes coated with this protein are diagnostic for bleeding originating in the kidneys.

Tamm-Horsfall protein may have a role in both upper and lower urinary disease. Its urine concentration is increased in cats with lower urinary tract disease and it has been identified in the matrix of urethral plugs. Incubation of urine with this protein induces crystal formation. It may also be a factor in the progression of pyelonephritis. When tubular injury occurs and this protein enters the interstitium, it can act as an antigen as well as cause interstitial inflammation after phagocytosis by neutrophils.

Urinalysis

urinalysis tests for active kidney lesions, lower urinary tract disease, metabolic diseases

Urinalysis is a profile of tests that detect defects in the urinary tract, as well as some diseases of metabolism and liver failure. This profile offers a rapid, economical method to screen for liver disease, diabetes mellitus, and acidosis, as well as pituitary and adrenal problems. It is an excellent, noninvasive way to evaluate active lesions in the kidney and urinary bladder.

Urinalysis becomes more specific when sequential samples are taken by cystocentesis, catheterization, and voiding or by correlating to water consumption.

Urobilinogen

↓ urobilinogen may indicate bile duct obstruction

Urobilinogen is formed by the action of enteric bacteria on bilirubin. It is absorbed into the portal circulation and eventually excreted by the kidneys into the urine in minute amounts. Absence of urinary urobilinogen in conjunction with signs of obstructive liver disease indicates complete bile duct obstruction. Increased amounts of urobilinogen have no diagnostic significance.

Normal   Positive reaction

White Blood Cells

↑ WBCs indicate inflammation; the lesion may be localized by sampling at different sites

Only a few WBCs are present in the urine of normal animals.

Large numbers of neutrophils in the urine *(pyuria)* indicate inflammation of the genitourinary tract.

Samples should be obtained by catheterization and by cystocentesis to localize the inflammation and differentiate pyuria of genital tract origin from that of urinary tract origin.

Normal   0 to few WBCs

References

Adams LG et al: Comparison of fractional excretion and 24-hour urinary excretion of sodium and potassium in clinically normal cats and cats with induced chronic renal failure, *Am J Vet Res* 52(5):718-722, 1991.

Borjesson DL, Christopher MM, Ling GV: Detection of canine transitional cell carcinoma using a bladder tumor antigen urine dipstick test, *Vet Clin Pathol* 28(1):33-38, 1999.

Buffington CA et al: Effects of Tamm-Horsfall glycoprotein and albumin on struvite crystal growth in urine of cats, *Am J Vet Res* 55(7):965-971, 1994.

Finco DR: Evaluation of renal function. In Osborne CA, Finco DR: *Canine and feline nephrology and urology,* Baltimore, 1995, Williams & Wilkins.

Fukuzaki A et al: Determining the origin of hematuria by immunocytochemical staining of erythrocytes in urine for Tamm-Horsfall protein, *J Urol* 155(1):248-251, 1996.

Gossett KA et al: Evaluation of gamma-glutamyl transpeptidase-to-creatinine ratio from spot samples of urine supernatant, as an indicator of urinary enzyme excretion in dogs, *Am J Vet Res* 48(3):455-457, 1987.

Grauer GF et al: Estimation of quantitative enzymuria in dogs with gentamicin-induced nephrotoxicosis using urine enzyme/creatinine ratios from spot urine samples, *J Vet Int Med* 9:5:324-327, 1995.

Greco DS et al: Urinary gamma-glutamyl transpeptidase activity in dogs with gentamicin-induced nephrotoxicity, *Am J Vet Res* 46(11):2332-2335, 1985.

Jacyszyn K et al: Investigations of the excretion of gamma-glutamyl-transpeptidase into the urine, *Int Urol Nephrol* 7(3):205-214, 1975.

Meyer-Lindenberg A et al: Urine protein analysis with the sodium-dodecyl-sulfate-polyacrylamide gel-electrophoresis (SDS-PAGE) in healthy cats and cats with kidney diseases, *Klinik Zentralbl Veterinarmed A* 44(1):39-54, 1997.

Mikiciuk MG, Thornhill JA: Control of parathyroid hormone in chronic renal failure, *Compend Cont Ed* 11(7):831-834, 836, 1989.

Morgan RV et al: Urine electrolyte excretion. In Morgan RV: *Handbook of small animal practice*, ed 3, Philadelphia, 1997, WB Saunders.

Palacio J, Liste F, Gascon M: Enzymuria as an index of renal damage in canine leishmaniasis, *Vet Rec* 140(18):477-480, 1997.

Uechi M et al: Evaluation of urinary enzymes in dogs with early renal disorder, *Vet Med Sci* 56(3):555-556, 1994.

Section 4
Red Blood Cells

Acanthocytes

acanthocytes are seen in liver disease, splenic tumors, and portacaval shunts

Acanthocytes, also referred to as *spur cells* or *spiculated cells,* are RBCs with irregular surface projections. The projections often have a "budding" enlargement at their terminal end. Marked acanthocytosis can lead to hemolysis and subsequent anemia.

Acanthocytes occur as a result of changes in plasma lipids that induce increased membrane cholesterol without a concurrent change in membrane phospholipids. This results in RBCs with excess membrane, which then forms into projections. Some cells with excess membrane become "floppy," forming a variety of leptocytes, such as target cells. Acanthocytes may be seen in patients with liver disease, portacaval shunts, and splenic hemangiomas or hemangiosarcomas.

Anemia

anemias are classified by response and cause

Anemia occurs when the number of circulating RBCs is below the normal level for the age, sex, and breed of the species concerned. The laboratory identifies anemia by low values for the PCV, hemoglobin, and RBC count. We classify anemias by response and cause.

Anemia, Macrocytic Hypochromic

↑ MCV and ↓ MCHC indicate regenerative anemia

Macrocytic hypochromic anemia is characterized by abnormally large RBCs containing subnormal amounts of hemoglobin. It is seen after acute blood loss or hemolysis. This type of anemia indicates marked RBC regeneration, but several days must elapse before this response is noted. Production of reticulocytes in response to anemia contributes to the pallor, increased MCV, and decreased MCHC.

Anemia, Microcytic Hypochromic

↓ MCV, no reticu-
locytosis, or no
polychromasia
indicates nonre-
generative
anemia

Microcytic hypochromic anemia is characterized by abnormally small RBCs containing subnormal amounts of hemoglobin. It is caused by iron deficiency, impaired iron metabolism, or iron depletion from chronic blood loss. Rarely, portosystemic shunts and chronic inflammation cause this type of anemia.

Anemia, Nonregenerative

↓ reticulocytes
indicates nonre-
generative
anemia

Anemia without reticulocytosis or polychromasia is described as nonregenerative. During the first 2 to 3 days after hemorrhage or hemolysis, anemia may be nonregenerative. The slight anemias of disease may be nonregenerative. When no response is seen for several days, it indicates a primary or a secondary bone marrow disorder.

Anemia, Regenerative

regeneration is
indicated by
polychromasia,
reticulocytes,
and high MCV

Regenerative (or responsive) anemia occurs when the bone marrow is actively responding to anemia by increasing production of RBCs. Findings that indicate regenerative anemia include polychromasia, reticulocytosis, and hypercellular bone marrow with a low myeloid:erythroid ratio.

The presence of regeneration suggests blood loss or RBC destruction. Regenerative anemia also denotes that sufficient time has elapsed for regeneration to occur (2 to 3 days), that there are adequate blood-forming elements (iron, appropriate vitamins, protein) for regeneration, that there are enough erythrocytic colonies in the bone marrow, and that there is adequate kidney function to form erythropoietin.

Anisocytosis

marked anisocytosis may suggest microcytes or macrocytes

Anisocytosis is a variation in RBC size without a change in cell shape. Slight anisocytosis occurs normally in cats and dogs and by itself is not diagnostic. In moderate to marked anisocytosis, RBCs may be macrocytic or microcytic.

Microcytic RBCs occur in immune-mediated hemolytic anemia, microvascular constriction, early Heinz-body anemia, and iron-deficiency anemia. *Macrocytic RBCs* occur with regenerative anemia and rarely with erythrocytic leukemia. Usually macrocytes raise the MCV. If microcytic anemia is also a regenerative anemia, such as occurs with Heinz-body anemia, the MCV is normal and the RDW is increased, but the smear shows marked anisocytosis.

Autoagglutination

Autoagglutination is a clumping of red blood cells into grapelike clusters. It may be seen in tubes of blood or when anticoagulated blood is placed on a cold slide. Microscopic examinations of an unsmeared sample of anticoagulated blood shows active movement of cells into clusters as opposed to linear stacks that form with rouleaux. This reaction is diagnostic for immune-mediated hemolytic anemia.

Basophilic Stippling

↑ basophilic stippling, ↑ nucleated RBCs with ↓ reticulocytes suggests lead poisoning

Basophilic stippling, also called punctate basophilia, is characterized by aggregations of dark blue-staining material (with Wright's stain) in the RBC cytoplasm. Stippling is the result of degenerative changes in cytoplasmic ribonucleic acid (RNA) and occurs with anemia, lead poisoning, and in some healthy dogs.

Basophilic-stippled cells can occur with regenerative anemia, but large numbers of basophilic-stippled RBCs along with nucleated RBCs out of proportion to the anemia suggest lead poisoning. Increased basophilic stippling without reticulocytosis also suggests lead poisoning.

Dacrocytes

dacrocytes are
seen in myelo-
proliferative
disease

Dacrocytes are teardrop-shaped RBCs. They result from the "pitting" function of the spleen on RBCs containing inclusions. They also have been seen in dogs with myeloproliferative disorders.

RBCs deformed as an artifact of blood smear preparation mimic dacrocytes. These deformed cells have their "tail" end consistently pointed in one direction. Dacrocytes have their "tails" oriented randomly.

Echinocytes

crenated cells
are usually an
artifact but may
confuse diagno-
sis of hemobar-
tonellosis

Echinocytes, also called crenated cells or burr cells, are RBCs with several blunt or pointed, evenly spaced surface projections (in contrast to acanthocytes, which have unevenly spaced and differently sized surface projections).

Crenation is a common artifact of blood film preparation. It occurs when cells on the blood film are slowly dried or exposed to salt or acids on a contaminated slide. Echinocytes are also seen in smears made from old blood as RBCs become depleted of ATP. Canine RBCs do not crenate as readily as feline RBCs.

When viewed on a blood smear, the surface projections on crenated RBCs may resemble *Hemobartonella* organisms. Fine focusing under oil immersion should reveal slight refraction of the crenated projections and no refraction of parasites.

Erythrocyte Sedimentation Rate

ESR monitors
patient's re-
sponse to inflam-
mation or tissue
necrosis

The erythrocyte sedimentation rate (ESR) is the speed at which RBCs settle in a tube of anticoagulated blood. Increased ESR is a nonspecific finding that occurs with tissue damage and inflammation. It is caused by increased plasma fibrinogen or other plasma proteins. The ESR may be used to monitor a patient's response to inflammation or tissue necrosis during the course of a disease.

Erythropoietin

erythropoietin stimulates RBC production

Erythropoietin is a hormone secreted by the kidney in adults and the liver in the fetus. It acts on stem cells of the bone marrow to stimulate RBC production (erythropoiesis).

Tissue hypoxia from anemia or inadequate oxygen saturation of hemoglobin is the stimulus for increased erythropoietin production. Erythropoietin stimulates proliferation of rubriblasts and rubricytes, accelerates maturation of rubricytes, and induces release of reticulocytes into the circulation.

Ghost Cells

ghost cells occur in hemolytic anemia

Ghost cells are the empty membranes of hemolyzed RBCs. They may be seen in blood smears from animals with rapid intravascular hemolysis, especially from Heinz-body anemia. They are also seen in blood films prepared from hemolyzed samples.

Heinz Bodies

Heinz bodies indicate a toxic change in RBC hemoglobin

Heinz bodies, also called erythrocyte refractile (ER) bodies or Schmauch's bodies, are small eccentric refractile objects in RBCs. They consist of hemoglobin precipitated by oxidant drugs, plant toxins, or chemicals. Feline RBCs are especially prone to Heinz-body formation and a few feline RBCs may have Heinz bodies as a natural response to cellular aging.

Heinz bodies are easily seen on smears stained with vital stains, such as new methylene blue. With new methylene blue stain they appear as bluish, round refractile bodies near the margin of the cell or protruding from the cell. When using spectrophotometric methods for determining hemoglobin, Heinz bodies lead to erroneously high estimations of hemoglobin.

Causes of Heinz-Body Formation

- Acetaminophen (cats)
- Methylene blue in urinary acidifiers and home aquariums (cats)

- Onions (cats, dogs)
- Long-term prednisolone use (dogs)
- Splenectomy
- Gastrointestinal disease (cats)
- Phenazopyridine
- Other oxidant drugs

Heinz-Body Anemia

Heinz-body anemia is more common in cats than in dogs

Patients with many RBCs containing Heinz bodies often become anemic as a result of splenic removal of RBCs or intravascular hemolysis.

Cats more easily form Heinz bodies than dogs because feline hemoglobin is remarkably unstable, as a result of large numbers of sulfhydryl groups. Cats also tend to form an abundance of methemoglobin because of their low rate of methemoglobin reductase activity as compared with that of other species. It is also possible that Heinz bodies increase in numbers as a result of normal RBC aging in cats.

Heinz-body anemia is typically hemolytic and is followed by a compensatory increase in erythropoiesis. A typical change in the blood is regenerative anemia, indicated by reticulocytosis. The bone marrow is hyperplastic, with a decreased myeloid:erythroid ratio. Large numbers of RBCs containing Heinz bodies may clump together and falsely elevate WBC counts.

Hematocrit

When a blood sample is centrifuged, it separates into three layers: an upper layer of plasma; a middle layer of WBCs and thrombocytes (buffy coat); and a bottom layer of packed RBCs. Technically, the *hematocrit* is a measure of all the cellular elements of blood (WBCs, thrombocytes, RBCs). By common usage, however, it has become synonymous with *packed cell volume* (PCV). See also *Packed Cell Volume*.

Hemoglobin

hemoglobin
value is typically
⅓ the PCV

Hemoglobin (Hb) is the oxygen-carrying pigment formed by developing RBCs in the bone marrow. The hemoglobin value of a blood sample is approximately one third of the PCV. Variations from this indicate a laboratory error, hemolysis, or abnormalities, such as Heinz bodies or lipemia.

Altered hemoglobin may form Heinz bodies or crystals. Determination of hemoglobin provides no clinical advantage over measurement of the PCV other than allowing the determination of MCH and MCHC.

	Hemoglobin
Dogs	12-18 g/dl (avg. 15 g/dl)
Cats	8-15 g/dl (avg. 12 g/dl)

	Mean Corpuscular Hemoglobin (MCH)
Dogs	19.5-24.5 pg (avg. 22.8 pg)
Cats	12.5-17.5 pg (avg. 15.5 pg)

	Mean Corpuscular Hemoglobin Concentration (MCHC)
Normal	31%-36% (avg. 33.2%)

Howell-Jolly Bodies

Howell-Jolly
bodies are
nuclear remnants
seen with
Wright's and new
methylene blue
stains

Howell-Jolly bodies are nuclear remnants in RBCs that occur as small, single or multiple, spherical bodies of varying size. They are seen within immature RBCs and stain dark blue with Wright's and new methylene blue stains.

Howell-Jolly bodies are common in regenerative anemia and in splenectomized patients. Up to 1% of RBCs in normal cats may contain Howell-Jolly bodies. They are occasionally seen in normal canine blood. Increased numbers of RBCs with Howell-Jolly bodies and, less commonly, nucleated RBCs appear in dogs receiving continuous corticosteroid therapy. This is likely a reflection of corticosteroid-induced suppression of splenic function.

Hyperchromasia

Hyperchromasia, or an increased hemoglobin content in RBCs, is a physiologic impossibility because hemoglobin precipitates at a concentration of 37% or more. The MCHC and hemoglobin value may be falsely elevated when the optical density of a blood sample is increased. This occurs with lipemia, Heinz-body anemia, and hemolysis.

Hypochromasia

Hypochromasia is an abnormal decrease in the hemoglobin content of RBCs. On Wright's-stained blood films, hypochromic RBCs are lighter in color than normal cells. They often have only a thin ring of hemoglobin at their periphery, with a large central pale area.

Keratocytes

keratocytes are
damaged RBCs

Keratocytes are RBCs with one or more pointed projections resembling horns and a slightly notched or somewhat flat surface between the projections. Keratocytes form when RBCs are damaged as they circulate through fibrin strands or prosthetic devices within the cardiovascular system.

Leptocytes

leptocytes occur
in regenerative
anemia, chronic
diseases, and
liver disease

Leptocytes are wide, flat RBCs that tend to fold on themselves. These variably shaped cells have been given many descriptive names. They may appear as target cells, folded bowl-shaped cells, dacrocytes, or knizocytes. They vary in size and staining characteristics and may be identified as polychromatic cells (reticulocytes) with Wright's stain. Leptocytes occur in regenerative anemia, chronic diseases, and liver disease.

Macrocytes

Macrocytes are morphologically normal RBCs with an MCV greater than normal for the species. They are found in blood during a regenerative response to anemia. In responsive anemias, these cells are reticulocytes. Some poodles normally exhibit macrocytosis without reticulocytosis.

Microcytes

Microcytes are morphologically normal RBCs with an MCV lower than normal for the species. Microcytic hypochromic anemia is the hallmark of iron deficiency and may be seen in anemias of inflammatory disease. In iron-deficiency anemia, most of the RBCs have marked central pallor because of reduced hemoglobin content. Microcytic hypochromic cells occur in inflammatory disease, immune-mediated anemia, microangiopathic anemia, and Heinz-body anemia.

Japanese Akitas normally have small RBCs with a low MCV but a normal MCHC. A *spherocyte* is a form of microcyte that has retained a normal amount of hemoglobin. See also *Spherocytes*.

New Methylene Blue Stain

New methylene blue stain is commonly used for reticulocyte counts. It selectively stains Heinz bodies, many RBC inclusions, and intracellular and extracellular organisms. Although a water-based product may be used by a commercial laboratory for identifying reticulocytes, the veterinary literature usually refers to a saline-based product proposed by Dr. Oscar Schalm for rapid cytologic staining of blood smears and cytologic slides. It is made according to the following formula and is useful because it is isotonic and does not distort cellular detail the way the water-based product does. Using this saline-based stain avoids confusion in interpreting cat reticulocytes.

Schalm's New Methylene Blue Vital Stain

- 0.5 g of new methylene blue powder
- 99 ml of 0.85% saline
- 1 ml of full-strength formalin

Normochromia

Normochromia is a normal hemoglobin level within RBCs and indicates that the erythrocytic MCHC is within the reference range.

Normocytes

Normocytes are RBCs that fall within the reference range for size (MCV) and hemoglobin content (MCHC) for the species. On a stained blood smear, the feline RBC is a uniformly dense cell approximately 6 μ in diameter. The canine RBC is a biconcave disk approximately 7 μ in diameter, with a central pale area.

Packed Cell Volume

↑ PCV with normal plasma protein suggests polycythemia

↑ PCV with ↑ plasma protein suggests dehydration, hemoconcentration, or hypovolemia

The packed cell volume (PCV) or hematocrit (Hct) is a measure of RBC numbers, expressed as a percentage of the total volume of blood. The PCV, by common usage, has become synonymous with the Hct. Traditionally the PCV is obtained by centrifuging an anticoagulated blood sample; with automated counters this value is calculated from the measured MCV and RBC count. This is the reason that laboratory values may differ slightly from in-clinic values.

The column of packed RBCs (PCV) is measured in millimeters and expressed as a percentage of the total blood volume. Anemia exists when the PCV falls below the reference range for the species. Hemoconcentration may exist when the PCV exceeds the reference range. There is normally a 3:1 ratio of PCV to hemoglobin value.

	Dogs	Cats
Reference range	37%-55%	25%-45%
Mild anemia	30%-37%	20%-25%
Moderate anemia	20%-29%	15%-19%
Severe anemia	13%-20%	10%-14%

Pancytopenia

Pancytopenia is a deficiency of all of the cellular elements of the blood. The blood exhibits neutropenia, lymphopenia, and anemia. Pancytopenia suggests inadequate production of blood cells by the bone marrow and lymphoid cells. Chemotherapeutic drugs, some viruses, or radiation may cause it.

Poikilocytes

poikilocytes occur in chronic blood loss, RBC fragmentation, and lead poisoning

Poikilocytes are abnormally shaped RBCs. Poikilocyte is a general term that encompasses all categories of abnormal RBC shapes, including more specific terms, such as echinocyte, acanthocyte, schizocyte, and crenation. RBC distortion may occur with improperly prepared blood films and should not be confused with poikilocytosis.

Poikilocytosis is a nonspecific change seen in chronic blood loss, iron-deficiency anemia, diseases characterized by RBC fragmentation, and chronic lead poisoning.

Polychromasia

polychromasia in Wright's-stained smears indicates regeneration

Polychromasia describes Wright's-stained RBCs that show various shades of blue, with tinges of pink from varied hemoglobin content. Polychromatic RBCs are immature RBCs that have less hemoglobin than a mature RBC. They retain remnants of the metabolically active endoplasmic reticulum and are equivalent to reticulocytes. The presence of polychromatic RBCs suggests active erythropoiesis and a regenerative response to anemia.

Polycythemia

↑ PCV indicates polycythemia; it may be primary or secondary, absolute or relative

Polycythemia is an increase in the red cell mass of the blood. This is seen as an increase in PCV, hemoglobin concentration, and RBC count. Absolute polycythemia results from increased bone marrow production of RBCs and may be primary, as with polycythemia vera or myeloproliferative disease, or secondary to hypoxia and renal disease.

Absolute polycythemia must be distinguished from relative polycythemia that occurs with dehydration (high plasma protein), hypovolemia (low plasma protein), shock, or splenic contraction (normal plasma protein).

Red Blood Cell Indices

↑ MCV usually indicates responsive anemia

The red blood cell indices consist of the *mean corpuscular volume (MCV), mean corpuscular hemoglobin (MCH)* and *mean corpuscular hemoglobin concentration (MCHC)*. They are used to determine the type of anemia present in the patient.

Red cell indices are estimations of the size and cellular hemoglobin concentration of a population of RBCs. Determining the type of anemia may help select appropriate therapy and monitor the progress of therapy.

Automated blood analyzers often have a built-in function that determines one or more of the indices; the remaining indices are then calculated from determined values. The values can be calculated by knowing the PCV, hemoglobin level, and RBC count. The MCHC and MCH are high at birth but decrease to adult values in 2 months.

	Dogs	Cats	
MCV	60-77 fl	30-45 fl	$\dfrac{PCV \times 10}{RBC\ count}$
MCH	19-24 pg	12-18 pg	$\dfrac{Hemoglobin \times 10}{RBC\ count}$
MCHC	32%-36%	32%-36%	$\dfrac{Hemoglobin \times 100}{PCV}$

Red Blood Cells

↑ RBCs (polycythemia) may be due to fluid loss or increased production

Red blood cells (RBCs) transport oxygen from the lungs to body tissues. Their production is stimulated by erythropoietin, secretion of which is controlled by the blood-oxygen tension. Erythropoietin stimulates maturation of RBC precursors in bone marrow into mature RBCs.

↓ RBCs (anemia) is classified by response and by cause

Blood loss, parasitism, renal failure, RBC damage, chronic inflammatory disease, hematopoietic malignancies, and insufficient dietary iron, copper, or vitamin B_{12} cause a deficiency of RBCs (*anemia*).

Shock, fluid loss, or increased RBC production can cause increased RBC numbers (*polycythemia*). Dehydration or protein fluid extravasation causes a relative decrease in the fluid portion of the blood and a relative increase in the cellular portion. Carbon monoxide, lung disease, heart disease, and high altitude cause excessive RBC production by stimulating erythropoietin secretion. Erythrocytic malignancies and polycythemia vera cause excessive RBC production without normal stimulation.

	Dogs	Cats
PCV at <6 months	22%-42%	26%-45%
PCV of adults	37%-55%	30%-45%

Red Cell Distribution Width (RDW)

The red cell distribution width is an electronic measure of anisocytosis. It increases where the degree of anisocytosis is increased. In regenerative anemia, it increases when large cells are produced even before the MCV exceeds the reference range. It also increases when small cells are produced, as in iron-deficiency anemia.

Red Blood Cells, Nucleated

↑ nRBCs with reticulocytosis is a normal response to anemia; if no reticulocytes, erythropoiesis is abnormal

Nucleated RBCs (nRBCs) are larger and more immature than reticulocytes and mature RBCs. These immature, nucleated stages of the erythrocyte generally occur within the bone marrow and are rarely observed in the peripheral blood of normal dogs and cats. They appear as metarubricytes in small numbers in response to acute blood loss or anemia.

Nucleated RBCs without concurrent anemia or reticulocytosis are a sign of disease. They are found in splenic disease, extramedullary hemopoiesis, lead poisoning, hyperadrenocorticism, leukemia, and bone marrow disease. Circulating nucleated RBCs can be metarubricytes or younger cells, such as rubricytes. See also *Reticulocyte:Nucleated Red Blood Cell Ratio*.

Normal	None to few

Reticulocyte:Nucleated Red Blood Cell Ratio

nRBC numbers should be less than reticulocyte numbers

In anemic dogs and cats, we sometimes count both the reticulocytes and nucleated red blood cells (nRBCs) to confirm an adequate bone marrow response. To be sure that these values are synchronous, the reticulocyte:nRBC ratio should be greater than 1. Nucleated RBCs outnumber reticulocytes in such conditions as peracute profound anemia, lead poisoning, and bone marrow myelophthisis with extramedullary hemopoiesis.

Normal response	>1
Abnormal response	≤1

Reticulocyte Percentage

↑ RP indicates adequate reticulocyte response in regenerative anemia

The absolute reticulocyte percentage corrects the reticulocyte count for the degree of anemia. It gives a slightly more accurate assessment of erythropoiesis than reticulocyte numbers alone.

$$RP = \frac{\% \text{ Reticulocytes} \times PCV}{\text{Normal PCV}}$$

Use 45% as normal PCV for dogs, 37% for cats.

	Dogs	Cats
No response	<1%	<1%
Slight response	1%-4%	1%-2%
Good response	>4%	>2%

Reticulocyte Production Index

↑ RPI indicates adequate reticulocyte response in regenerative anemia

The reticulocyte production index (RPI) adjusts the reticulocyte count for the degree of anemia and for the increased life span of very young reticulocytes. Because they are released early, reticulocytes persist for longer periods in the blood of anemic animals. After 4 days of anemia, the following equation is useful in evaluating the reticulocyte response in dogs:

$$RPI = \frac{(\% \text{ Reticulocytes} \times PCV) \div 45}{\text{Correction factor}}$$

Use the following correction factors:

PCV	<15%	2.5
PCV	15%-25%	2
PCV	26%-35%	1.5
PCV	>35%	1

	RPI
No response (no increase over normal release)	1
Poor response	<2
Responsive (hemorrhage or hemolysis)	2
Responsive (always from hemolysis)	>3

Reticulocytes

↑ reticulocytes indicate regenerative anemia

↓ reticulocytes indicate bone marrow depression or nonregenerative anemia

Reticulocytes are immature RBCs without a nucleus. They retain a fine network of endoplasmic reticulum that stains with reticulocyte stains, such as Schalm's new methylene blue stain. With Wright's stain, reticulocytes are polychromatic.

These immature cells are slightly larger than mature RBCs and normally circulate in small numbers. Elevated numbers of circulating reticulocytes (*reticulocytosis*) occur in chronic hemorrhagic or hemolytic anemia with increased erythropoiesis. A lack of circulating reticulocytes in chronic anemia indicates bone marrow depression.

In cats, punctate and aggregate forms are evident with certain reticulocyte stains. The punctate forms should be ignored in most evaluations. They are not prominent enough to be a problem with the wet-mount method using Schalm's new methylene blue stain.

The time required for release of newly formed reticulocytes in large numbers into the peripheral blood following hypoxia is 3 to 4 days, with peak numbers attained by days 5 to 7.

Reticulocytosis without evidence of anemia may indicate reduced oxygenation of blood. This leads to increased erythropoietin levels, which in turn stimulate erythropoiesis and release of reticulocytes from the bone marrow.

Usually an estimation is made by counting the number of reticulocytes per 100 RBCs.

Reticulocyte Count		
	Dogs	Cats
No response to anemia	<1%	<1%
Slight response	2%-4%	1%-2%
Moderate response	5%-20%	3%-4%
Marked response	>20%	>5%

Rouleaux

rouleaux are differentiated from agglutination by mixing blood with saline

Rouleaux is a term describing grouping of RBCs in stacks resembling piles of coins. Formation of rouleaux parallels the erythrocyte sedimentation rate (ESR) and increases with increased plasma proteins. Some rouleaux may occur in normal dogs and cats, but increased rouleaux formation suggests increased total plasma protein or fibrinogen concentration secondary to inflammation.

Rouleaux must be differentiated from agglutination that occurs in immune-mediated anemias. Agglutinated cells form clusters, rather than stacks. Another way to distinguish rouleaux from agglutination is to mix equal parts of blood and physiologic saline and observe on a wet-mount slide. Rouleaux disappear after mixing; true immune-mediated agglutination appears as grapelike clusters of cells that remain after mixing with saline.

Schizocytes

schizocytes are fragments of damaged RBCs

Schizocytes or schistocytes are irregular fragments of RBCs that have been damaged during circulation. They may resemble triangles, rods, half-moons, or other bizarre forms.

They are commonly seen with disseminated intravascular coagulation (DIC), microangiopathic hemolytic anemia, congestive heart failure, glomerulonephritis, myelofibrosis, and splenic hemangiosarcoma.

Siderocytes

siderocytes indicate abnormal erythropoiesis

Siderocytes are abnormal RBCs containing basophilic focal hemosiderin (iron) granules called *Pappenheimer bodies*. Nucleated RBCs containing hemosiderin are called *sideroblasts*. On Wright's-stained smears, the granules resemble basophilic stipples, but the granules are larger, darker, and more focal.

Siderocytes and sideroblasts indicate abnormal erythropoiesis. These cells occur in some nonresponsive anemias, severe lead poisoning, and chloramphenicol therapy.

Spherocytes

spherocytes in dogs suggest immune-mediated hemolytic anemia

Spherocytes are intensely red-staining, small, spherical RBCs with a reduced ratio of cell surface area to cytoplasmic volume. Spherocytes are formed when antibody or complement coats the RBC and macrophages in the spleen and liver remove portions of the damaged RBC. Excessive loss of the surface membrane in relation to the contents results in a small cell with decreased deformability and increased osmotic fragility.

Spherocytes are characteristically found in dogs with autoimmune hemolytic anemia. They are difficult to recognize on smears of feline blood because normal feline RBCs are small and do not have central pallor.

Normal RBCs may appear to be spherocytes if the thick portion of a blood smear is examined.

Spherocytosis suggests immune-mediated hemolytic anemia. Spherocyte numbers can be estimated as low to high by examining a blood smear under oil immersion (1000×). The following estimates assume a monolayer of cells, with 250 RBCs per oil-immersion field.

Spherocytes Per Field	Estimated Percentage
5-10	2%-4%
11-50	4%-20%
51-150	20%-60%
>150	>60%

Target Cells

target cells form with excessive RBC membrane and low hemoglobin

Target cells, also known as codocytes, are thin, cup-shaped RBCs with a dense central area of hemoglobin that is separated from the peripheral hemoglobinized region by a pale zone. Target cells develop when hemoglobin is redistributed within the cell. This is a result of excessive cell membrane in proportion to decreased hemoglobin concentration.

Target cells are found in patients with hypochromic anemia, cholestatic liver disease, bone marrow suppression, and after splenectomy. They may also be seen as an artifact in hypertonic solutions.

Torocytes

torocytes are seen in iron-deficiency anemia

Torocytes are RBCs with a well-defined central area of pallor and a thickened peripheral rim of hemoglobin. Torocytes are seen in hypochromic anemias (iron deficiency) and may occur as an artifact of smear preparation.

Section 5
White Blood Cells

Barr Bodies

Barr bodies can be used to screen tricolor or white tomcats for infertility

The Barr body is a drumstick-shaped nuclear projection occasionally (approximately 5%) found on neutrophils and rarely on eosinophils. It represents an accumulation of female (X) chromatin. Tricolor (or white) tomcats can be screened for seminiferous tubule dysgenesis that causes sterility by looking for Barr bodies in epithelial cell scrapings or in neutrophils on blood smears.

Basket Cells

Basket cells (also known as smudge cells) are ruptured WBCs. On blood smears, the nuclear chromatin spreads out into a lacelike pattern and stains eosinophilic. Basket cells may be the result of trauma during blood film preparation, or they may indicate increased fragility of immature cells, as in acute leukemia. Numerous basket cells make differential WBC counts inaccurate.

Basophils

↑ basophils occur with heart-worm thrombi, hyperlipidemia

Basophils and tissue mast cells contain granules of histamine and heparin. These substances initiate inflammation, prevent coagulation, and activate lipoprotein lipase. Basophils may be seen with a variety of diseases, while the presence of many mast cells on a blood smear signifies mast-cell neoplasia.

Mast cells and basophils are similar in appearance because both contain purple metachromatic granules. Mast-cell granules usually stain intensely and are often numerous enough to obscure the nucleus. Canine and feline basophils contain fewer dark granules. The granules in feline basophils stain light blue and are often missing from the cytoplasm, making them difficult to identify on blood films.

Basophils have a tri-lobed nucleus, similar to that of neutrophils; mast cells have a single, round nucleus.

Basophilia   >100/μl

Chediak-Higashi Syndrome

neutrophils contain giant cytoplasmic granules

Chediak-Higashi syndrome is a hereditary disease of cats that is characterized by gigantic cytoplasmic granules in neutrophils and abnormal neutrophil and platelet function. This is an autosomal recessive disorder. The neutrophils in affected animals can phagocytize bacteria, but they have defective chemotactic, degranulation, and bactericidal abilities. Abnormal platelet function results in poor hemostasis.

Döhle Bodies

Döhle bodies indicate a toxic change of neutrophils, most commonly seen in cats

Döhle bodies are angular cytoplasmic structures seen in neutrophils. They are remnants of the rough endoplasmic reticulum and are the result of defective maturation of the cytoplasm. Döhle bodies occur as a result of toxic change to the neutrophils during granulopoiesis within the bone marrow.

Eosinopenia

↓ eosinophils occur with stress, corticosteroid use, hyperadrenocorticism

Decreased numbers of circulating eosinophils (*eosinopenia*) occur with hyperadrenocorticism, stress, and administration of exogenous corticosteroids. Eosinopenia usually develops in acute disease.

	Dogs	Cats
Eosinopenia	<100/μl	0/μl

Eosinophilia

↑ eosinophils occur with allergy, parasitism, eosinophilic inflammation, hypoadrenocorticism

Increased numbers of circulating eosinophils (*eosinophilia*) occur in allergic disease, parasitism, eosinophilic gastroenteritis, eosinophilic granuloma, eosinophilic myositis, feline eosinophilic granuloma, and hypoadrenocorticism. Persistent eosinophilia may indicate skin, heart, lung, intestinal, or neoplastic problems.

	Dogs	Cats
Eosinophilia	>1500/μl	>1500/μl

Eosinophils

eosinophils de-
toxify histamine
and kill parasites

Eosinophils are WBCs with numerous functions. They are parasiticidal, help regulate allergic and inflammatory responses by inhibiting mast cell release of histamine and serotonin, detoxify histamine at the site of antigen-antibody reactions, regulate the intensity of IgE reactions, and have some phagocytic activity against invading bacteria. Their granules contain potent cytotoxic proteins and lipids that are active in almost all types of inflammation and tissue injury.

Eosinophils are easily recognized on stained blood smears by their large yellow-orange granules. They normally occur in small numbers in peripheral blood.

	Dogs	Cats
	Dogs	Cats
Normal	100-1000/μl	100-1000/μl

Granulocytes

granulocytes
consist of neu-
trophils, eosino-
phils, and
basophils

Granulocytes are WBCs that contain cytoplasmic granules. These include neutrophils, eosinophils, and basophils. These cells are produced in the bone marrow.

Hemogram

the hemogram
evaluates RBCs
and WBCs with
total and differ-
ential counts

The hemogram estimates the number of the circulating RBCs and WBCs. The hemogram usually includes the total RBC count, RBC morphology, estimation of platelet numbers, and a leukogram (see below).

Numbers of RBCs are estimated by counts, centrifugation (PCV), and hemoglobin content.

Numbers of the various WBCs, called a *leukogram*, can be determined by counts, differential centrifugation, and staining characteristics. The standard leukogram gives a five-part WBC differentiation (neutrophils, lymphocytes, monocytes, eosinophils, and basophils). The quantitative buffy coat (QBC) leukogram gives a two-part WBC differentiation (granulocytes, monocytes), which can be further evaluated with a stained blood smear. Many small automatic counters give a three part differential (granulocytes, lymphocytes, and monocytes).

Left Shift

a regenerative left shift indicates a good response; band cells do not exceed 10% of mature cells

The term *left shift* indicates increased numbers of circulating immature neutrophils (band cells, metamyelocytes, and myelocytes).

A *regenerative left shift* is characterized by band cells and increased numbers of mature neutrophils. The number of immature neutrophils does not exceed 10% of the mature neutrophils, and no young cells, such as metamyelocytes, are present.

a degenerative left shift indicates a poor response; band cells >10% of neutrophils, or metamyelocytes or myelocytes are present

A *degenerative left shift* is characterized by circulating band cells that exceed 10% of the segmented neutrophils, in conjunction with decreased numbers of neutrophils or the presence of very young cells, such as metamyelocytes or myelocytes. In a degenerative left shift, the total WBC count may vary from below normal to slightly elevated. A degenerative left shift is an unfavorable prognostic sign.

Leukemia

aleukemic leukemia: no ↑ WBCs, rare abnormal cells, tumor in tissue phase

Leukemia comprises a group of neoplastic diseases of the hematopoietic system. Leukemias are classified on the basis of the type of cell involved (lymphocytic, monocytic, myelogenous, erythremic) or the number of abnormal cells in the peripheral blood (aleukemic, subleukemic, leukemic).

Aleukemic leukemia indicates normal numbers of WBCs with no or only rare abnormal cells. Bone marrow evaluation is necessary.

subleukemic leukemia: slight ↑ WBCs, with a few abnormal cells

Subleukemic leukemia indicates a few abnormal WBC types, with a normal or only slightly increased total WBC count.

leukemic leukemia: ↑ WBCs with many abnormal or immature cells

Leukemic leukemia indicates a marked increase in total WBC numbers, with many abnormal and immature hematopoietic cells.

Leukocytes

A leukocyte is any WBC: neutrophils, eosinophils, monocytes, lymphocytes, or basophils. These include both the granulocytes and the mononuclear cells of the lymphoid system. A total WBC count is the sum of all leukocytes.

	Dogs	Cats
Normal	6000-15,000/μl	5500-19,000/μl

Leukocytosis

↑ in WBCs is called leukocytosis

physiologic causes include exercise, fear, digestion

pathologic causes include infection, hemolysis, hemorrhage, intoxication, leukemia, trauma

Leukocytosis is characterized by increased numbers of WBCs. It is generally caused by an increase in the number of circulating neutrophils (*neutrophilia*), although lymphocytosis (especially with leukemia) occasionally produces leukocytosis. Absolute values of individual WBC types provide much more diagnostic specificity than a simple WBC count.

Exercise, fear, and digestion cause *physiologic leukocytosis.*

Infection, rapidly growing neoplasms, acute hemolysis, hemorrhage, intoxication, leukemia, and trauma cause *pathologic leukocytosis.*

	Dogs	Cats
Leukocytosis	>15,000/μl	>19,000/μl

Leukopenia

↓ WBCs is called leukopenia

pathologic causes include severe inflammation, bone marrow disease

Leukopenia (decreased total WBC) is usually characterized by decreased numbers of circulating neutrophils. The most common causes of leukopenia are excessive consumption in an inflammatory process and primary bone marrow disease. Persistent leukopenia is a poor prognostic sign.

	Dogs	Cats
Leukopenia	<6000/μl	<5500/μl

Lupus Erythematosus Cell

LE cells may be seen with systemic lupus erythematosus

Lupus erythematosus (LE) cells are occasionally seen in dogs with systemic lupus erythematosus. LE cells are WBCs that have phagocytized the nuclear mass of other, nonviable WBCs. This phagocytosis is initiated by binding of IgG antibody to the WBC nuclei.

distinguish LE cells from tart cells

LE cells are differentiated from "tart" cells by the appearance of the ingested nuclear material. LE cells contain a round homogeneous mass that is about the size of a lymphocyte nucleus. Tart cells represent *nucleophagocytosis*, in which the phagocytized nucleus retains its normal nuclear chromatin pattern.

Lymphocytes

Lymphocytes in the blood are a mixed population of B cells and T cells. They are the major cellular component of immunity in the body. B lymphocytes synthesize antibodies that are responsible for humoral immunity. T lymphocytes are the principal component of cellular immunity. Lymphocytes also participate in immune regulation and surveillance, and some are cytotoxic.

	Dogs	Cats
Normal	1500-5000/μl	1500-7000/μl

Lymphocytes, B Cells

B cells cannot be differentiated from other lymphocytes on routine blood smears

B cells are lymphocytes involved with formation of humoral antibody. Relative proportions of B cells and T cells may be altered with inherited defects of the immune system, lymphosarcoma, and with some viral infections (FeLV).

B cells account for a small percentage of circulating lymphocytes. Special diagnostic procedures are required to accurately identify B cells; they cannot be differentiated from other lymphocytes on routine blood smears.

Lymphocytes, T Cells

T cells are the main circulating lymphocyte

T cells or T lymphocytes are the main type of circulating lymphocyte. They may be accurately identified by special tests. T cells function in cell-mediated immunity, including defense against intracellular organisms, defense against neoplasia, delayed hypersensitivity, and graft injection. Relative proportions of B cells and T cells may be altered with inherited defects of the immune system, lymphosarcoma, and some viral infections (FeLV, FIV).

Lymphocytosis

↑ lymphocytes occur with chronic inflammation, infection, hypoadrenocorticism, lymphocytic leukemia

Lymphocytosis is characterized by increased numbers of circulating lymphocytes. Pathologic lymphocytosis occurs in chronic inflammation, recovery from acute infection, lymphocytic leukemia, and hypoadrenocorticism. Lymphocytosis usually indicates a strong immune stimulus of some chronic duration from a bacterial infection, viremia or immune-mediated disease. Lymphocytic leukemia may or may not be accompanied by lymphocytosis.

Lymphocytosis not associated with disease occurs with physiologic leukocytosis, in healthy cats from excitement, immature age-related responses in young puppies and kittens, and sometimes following vaccination.

	Dogs	Cats
Lymphocytosis	>5000/µl	>7000/µl

Lymphopenia

↓ lymphocytes occur with stress, corticosteroids, lymphotoxic viruses, loss of lymph

Lymphopenia is characterized by decreased numbers of circulating lymphocytes. It may occur with acute severe disease, some viral diseases (canine distemper, hepatitis, parvovirus and coronavirus infections, feline panleukopenia, FeLV infection), stress-related corticosteroid response, and loss of lymph (chylothorax, lymphangiectasia).

	Dogs	Cats
Lymphopenia	<1000/µl	<1500/µl

Macrophages

Macrophages develop from bone marrow precursors that mature and enter the bloodstream as monocytes. These monocytes are recruited into different tissues where they differentiate into tissue resident macrophages that perform important functions in tissue homeostasis and the immune response.

Macrophages have a variety of functions
1. Engulf large particles such as bacteria, yeast, and dying cells by a process called *phagocytosis.*
2. Secrete signaling molecules called *cytokines* and *chemokines,* which orchestrate the immune response.
3. Play a central role in acute and chronic inflammation.
4. Secrete proteases and growth factors that are important in tissue remodeling and in wound repair after injury.
5. Present processed foreign antigens to T lymphocytes, allowing the development of a specific immune response.

Mast Cells

mast cells are rare cells seen with stress, shock, parvovirus infection, mast-cell tumors

buffy coat smears are used to screen for mastocytoma

Mast cells cause an immediate hypersensitivity reaction by releasing their stored vasoactive chemicals. They are normally absent from the blood and are rare in bone marrow.

Occasional mast cells may be found in a blood smear from a severely stressed animal or an animal in shock. Mastocytemia or mastocytosis may occur in dogs with parvovirus infection or possibly from other nonspecific causes. Many mast cells on a blood smear suggests mast-cell neoplasia. Because these cells are rare even with metastatic mastocytoma, buffy coat smears are used to screen for mast cells in suspected mastocytoma.

Mast cells and basophils are similar in appearance. The basophil nucleus is trilobed, similar to that of neutrophils, while mast cells have a single, round nucleus.

The granules in mast cells usually stain more intensely and are more numerous than those of basophils. However, granular staining characteristics of both mast cells and basophils vary, depending on the staining technique and the stage of mast-cell neoplasia.

Monocytes

monocytes are often misidentified as band neutrophils or lymphocytes

Monocytes are the immature blood stage of tissue macrophages. Their main function is phagocytosis of foreign material, cellular debris, and pathogens that are not effectively controlled by neutrophils. They engulf intracellular organisms and those causing a granulomatous inflammatory response. They are effective scavengers, removing tissue debris, cellular remnants, and foreign material. Monocytes are also active in regulating the immune response, processing antigen, and activating killer cells and macrophages.

Decreased numbers of circulating monocytes (*monocytopenia*) are rare and have no diagnostic significance.

Monocytes are the most commonly misidentified leukocyte in blood smears, often being placed into either band cell or lymphocyte categories.

	Dogs	Cats
Normal	<2000/μl	<1000/μl

Monocytosis

↑ monocytes occur with stress, granulomas, necrosis, chronic inflammation

Increased numbers of circulating monocytes (*monocytosis*) occur in chronic suppurative, pyogranulomatous, necrotic, malignant, hemolytic, hemorrhagic, or immune-mediated diseases. Monocytosis also occurs in dogs as a corticosteroid-induced response from stress, adrenal hyperfunction, or exogenous corticosteroids. Some animals with chronic disease have persistent monocytosis.

	Dogs	Cats
Monocytosis	>2000/μl	>1000/μl

Neutropenia

↓ neutrophils occur in toxemia, viral infection, bone marrow depression, overwhelming infection

Neutropenia is characterized by a decreased number of circulating neutrophils. It may be due to insufficient production or increased destruction of neutrophils. Conditions that cause neutropenia include endotoxemia, viral infections, overwhelming bacterial infections, and administration of drugs that cause bone marrow suppression.

	Dogs	Cats
Neutropenia	<3000/μl	<2500/μl

Neutrophilia

↑ neutrophils occur in stress, inflammation, bacterial infection, tissue necrosis

Neutrophilia is characterized by an increased number of circulating neutrophils. It can be physiologically induced by exercise and corticosteroids or pathologically induced by infections and tissue destruction. The primary differential diagnoses for neutrophilia are inflammation (both septic and nonseptic), stress, exercise, or excitement.

	Dogs	Cats
Neutrophilia	>12,000/μl	>13,000/μl

Neutrophils

↑ neutrophils often indicate infection

Neutrophils phagocytize and kill microorganisms. They also initiate and modify the acute inflammatory process, cause tissue damage, and are cytotoxic.

Production and storage in the bone marrow, margination of cells in the capillary beds, and the demands of peripheral tissues affect the numbers of circulating neutrophils.

	Dogs	Cats
Normal	3000-11,500/μl	2500-12,000/μl

Neutrophils, Band

↑ band cells are
called a left shift

The band cell is an immature neutrophil occasionally found circulating in peripheral blood. An increase in the absolute number of bands indicates increased demand resulting from inflammation. Increased numbers are termed a "left shift."

Slight increases in bands (300 to 1000/µl) may occur in nonsuppurative diseases, such as hemorrhagic or granulomatous disease. Bands in excess of 1000/µl indicate an intense purulent exudative process. Human laboratory tests often refer to band cells as "stab" cells and often misdiagnose canine neutrophils as band cells because the canine neutrophil is less lobulated than the human neutrophil.

Neutrophils, Hypersegmentation

hypersegmented
neutrophils are
seen with
delayed blood
film preparation
and vitamin B_{12}
or folate defi-
ciency

Neutrophils with five or more nuclear lobes are *hypersegmented.* Cellular aging from prolonged circulation or delayed blood slide preparation usually causes this hypersegmentation. Occasionally this condition occurs in poodles with RBC macrocytosis, simulating vitamin B_{12} or folate deficiency. When large numbers are present, check for a malignancy (see Right Shift on p. 122).

Pelger-Huet Anomaly

The Pelger-Huet anomaly is a hereditary disease characterized by hyposegmentation of neutrophil nuclei. Pelger-Huet neutrophils contain nonsegmented nuclei, with a mature nuclear chromatin pattern. Pelger-Huet anomaly is generally an incidental finding, and the animal's defense mechanisms are not compromised.

Plasma Cells

Plasma cells are derived from B lymphocytes in response to antigenic stimulation. Plasma cells are rarely found in peripheral blood but are often seen in antigen-stimulated lymphoid tissues, such as lymph nodes, spleen, and bone marrow. These cells may also be called circulating plasmacytoid cells or immunocytes. They may be found in the blood during chronic antigenic stimulation.

Quantitative Buffy Coat Analysis

The quantitative buffy coat analysis (QBC) system is an in-office hematology analyzer. It measures the hematocrit, total WBC count, granulocyte count, nongranulocyte count, and platelet count. The QBC leukogram gives a two-part WBC differentiation (granulocytes, monocytes). If more detail is needed, WBCs on a stained blood smear may be counted and a differential count calculated using the estimated total WBC count.

Right Shift

The term *right shift* indicates increased numbers of circulating hypermature neutrophils in neutrophilic blood samples. These are cells showing hypersegmentation. This is usually seen in noninfectious inflammatory processes such as inflammation secondary to a malignancy.

Thorn Test

the Thorn test screens for adrenal insufficiency

The Thorn test, an indirect cortisol assay, is used to evaluate adrenal function in animals with eosinophilia. A test dose of ACTH is administered and circulating eosinophil numbers are evaluated before and after administration. A positive Thorn test, as indicated by a decrease in eosinophil and lymphocyte numbers, suggests normal adrenal function.

Although the Thorn test has been replaced by more definitive laboratory tests, it provides an economical screen for adrenal insufficiency (hypoadrenocorticism).

Toxic Granules

blue neutrophil granules are seen in severe toxemic conditions

In severe toxemic states, neutrophil morphology is altered during granulopoiesis. The cytoplasm of "toxic" neutrophils stains bluish because of persistent ribosomal RNA. The cytoplasm of toxic neutrophils is often vacuolated, and azurophilic primary cytoplasmic granules may be evident.

White Blood Cell Count, Absolute

absolute WBC counts are more useful than relative counts

The absolute white blood cell (WBC) count represents the number of each leukocytic cell type per 1 µl of blood. The absolute count is calculated by multiplying the differential count (percent of each type of leukocyte) by the total WBC count. Errors of interpretation are much less likely with absolute values than with percentages (relative counts).

White Blood Cell Count, Adjusted

↑ nucleated RBCs artificially raise the WBC count

In animals with severe regenerative anemia, many nucleated red blood cells are released into the circulating blood and artificially raise the white cell count.

To adjust the total WBC count for large numbers of nucleated RBCs, use the following equation:

$$\text{Adjusted WBC count} = \text{WBC} + \frac{100}{100 + \text{nRBCs}}$$

White Blood Cell Count, Differential

the differential count screens for viral infections, bacterial infections, stress, and inflammation

In a differential WBC count, the number of each leukocytic cell type is reported as a percentage of the total WBC count. To determine absolute numbers of each cell type, individual (100 to 200) WBCs are identified and reported as a percentage of the total WBC count. This percentage is then multiplied by the total WBC count to obtain absolute numbers of each cell type.

The five-part traditional system classifies the cells into neutrophils, lymphocytes, monocytes, eosinophils, and basophils. Immature forms are classified separately. The three part differential classifies the cells as granulocytes (neutrophils, eosinophils, and basophils), lymphocytes, and monocytes.

The two-part quantitative buffy coat (QBC) system classifies the cells into granulocytes or mononuclear cells. The QBC system provides abbreviated CBC type information within 7 minutes of blood collection. It gives a total WBC count and screens for infection.

White Blood Cell Count, Total

total WBC count screens for viral infection, bacterial infection, allergy, cortisol levels

↑ in WBCs is called *leukocytosis*, ↓ in WBCs is called *leukopenia*

The total WBC count combines circulating numbers of neutrophils, lymphocytes, monocytes, eosinophils, and basophils.

Because neutrophils are the predominant leukocytic cell type, a high total WBC count (*leukocytosis*) is generally a result of an increase in this cell line. However, absolute values of individual leukocytic cell lines (found by performing a differential count and multiplying each cell line percentage by the total WBC count) often provide more diagnostic specificity. Leukopenia (decreased WBCs) is generally evident only with a decrease in neutrophils.

Leukocytosis and leukopenia occur with a variety of diseases.

	Dogs	Cats
Normal	6000-15,000/μl	6000-18,000/μl
Leukocytosis	>15,000/μl	>18,000/μl
Leukopenia	<6000/μl	<6000/μl

Section 6
Simple Coagulation Tests

Activated Clotting Time

↑ ACT screens for multiple clotting defects, anticoagulant poisoning

The activated clotting time (ACT), a simplified version of APTT, is used to screen for anticoagulant poisoning, which reduces Factors II, VII, IX, and X.

ACT tests for Factor X, which must be decreased to less than 5% of normal to prolong the ACT. This test is inexpensive and can be done quickly in your hospital. It is less sensitive than the APTT or PT.

	Dogs	Cats
ACT	<120 seconds	<90 seconds

Activated Partial Thromboplastin Time

↑ APTT with normal PT indicates a problem with Factors VIII, IX, XI, or XII

Activated partial thromboplastin time (APTT) is a test of the intrinsic coagulation pathway (Factors VIII, IX, XI, XII) plus the common pathway (Factors V, X, prothrombin, fibrinogen). It is used to screen for all coagulation factors except Factor VII. This test can also be used to monitor the response to heparin therapy and to diagnose anticoagulant poisoning (Factors IX and X).

Normal APTT	4-18 seconds (>75% of control APTT)
My lab	_____

Bleeding Time

bleeding time tests platelets and clotting factors

Bleeding time is a sensitive way of assessing platelet function and clotting problems.

Protocol
1. Clip a toenail short enough to bleed.
2. Allow the clipped nail to bleed freely.
3. Determine the time for bleeding to stop.

Interpretation
A normal animal stops bleeding within 3 to 6 minutes. Coagulation defects, thrombocytopenia, toxic platelet dysfunction, and von Willebrand's disease cause prolonged bleeding.

	Dogs	Cats
Normal bleeding time	<6 minutes	<3 minutes

Antiplatelet Antibody Test

Platelet factor 3 (PF-3) is an indirect assay for serum antiplatelet antibodies. If present, they shorten the coagulation time when compared with the test performed with normal serum. This test has been replaced with direct tests.

Megakaryocyte fluorescence is an IFA test for antibodies attached to megakaryocytes in the bone marrow. This test may be useful with nonresponsive thrombocytopenia that also shows decreased bone marrow megakaryocytes.

Platelet bound immunoglobulins are the preferred test for determining immune thrombocytopenia. Flow cell techniques currently are the most accurate tests but these are done at limited institutions. The antibody is stable enough to allow samples to be shipped. A negative test rules out immune destruction, but a positive test does not differentiate between primary and secondary immune-mediated thrombocytopenia (IMT). Secondary IMT is caused by live virus vaccines, drugs, *rickettsia*, and viruses.

Requires 3 to 5 ml of EDTA-anticoagulated blood, and samples need to be sent on ice by overnight mail to:

Clinical Pathology
College of Veterinary Medicine
Kansas State University
1800 Denison Avenue
Manhattan, KS 66506

Antithrombin III (AT III)

AT III is a globulin produced in the liver, which interacts with heparin to inhibit factors (II, X, XI, XII). Decreased AT III is an early screen for a hypercoagulable (i.e., DIC, glomerulonephritis, and protein-losing enteropathies). Increased levels occur in patients with estrogen administration, obstructive jaundice, and vitamin K_1 deficiency. Assay methods vary.

	Normal
Immunologic	17-30 mg/dl
Functional	80%-120%

Clot Lysis Test

↑ rate of clot lysis suggests fibrin degradation from DIC

The clot lysis test is an indirect screen for fibrin degradation products. Premature lysis of a blood clot suggests increased activity of the fibrinolytic system.

Protocol
1. After performing a dilute whole-blood clot retraction test, incubate the blood and check for clot lysis.
2. Record the time required for clot lysis.

Interpretation
Clots normally lyse in 8 to 20 hours. More rapid lysis indicates increased fibrin degradation, such as with disseminated intravascular coagulation (DIC).

Normal clot lysis	>8 hours
Abnormally rapid lysis	<8 hours

Clot Retraction

↑ time for clot retraction indicates platelet dysfunction

The dilute whole-blood clot retraction test is a rapid screen of platelet function.

Protocol
1. Do a platelet count to be sure that they number greater than 100,000/μl.

2. Collect 0.5 ml of blood into a syringe containing 4.5 ml of cold normal saline to make a 1:10 dilution of the platelets.
3. Place the diluted blood in a tube containing 1 unit of bovine thrombin to form the clot.
4. Incubate the clot for 1 hour at 37° F.

Interpretation
The clot contracts to one-third of its original size when there are adequate numbers of normally functioning platelets. Lack of clot contraction indicates platelet dysfunction if the platelet count is normal.

Platelet dysfunction is seen most commonly in uremia or after ingestion of aspirin.

Normal clot retraction	<1 hour

D-dimers Screen

D-dimers are a marker for intravascular coagulation and occur earlier than fibrin degradation products (FDPs). They are derived from cross-linked fibrin following the enzymatic action of plasmin, and they differ from FDPs, which are derived from fibrinogen or fibrin following action by thrombin or plasmin.

Normal (SU)	<0.5 μg/ml
Normal (IU)	<0.5 mg/L

Coagulation Tests

Major hemostatic abnormalities may be tested rapidly in the veterinary hospital with a few screening tests for coagulation and platelet abnormalities.

These screening tests can miss mild hemostatic abnormalities. If the history suggests a hemorrhagic problem in a patient with normal screening tests, a blood reference laboratory should perform specialized coagulation tests.

Factor VIII-Related Antigen

↓ factor VIII:RAg indicates von Willebrand's disease

Factor VIII-related antigen (Factor VIII:RAg) is used to diagnose von Willebrand's disease. When levels of Factor VIII-RAg fall below 30% of normal, bleeding occurs despite normal platelet counts. Carriers of this bleeding tendency can be detected by quantitative analysis for this factor.

Increased bleeding risk	<30% of normal
Carrier	<50% of normal

Fibrin Degradation Products

Fibrin degradation products (FDPs) are derived from breakdown of fibrin clots during excessive coagulation in the body. This test is used to document disseminated intravascular coagulation (DIC).

Normal animals have no FDPs

Platelet Count

bleeding occurs when platelet numbers are <50,000/μl

A platelet *(thrombocyte)* count below 100,000/μl is significant. Platelets can be counted directly, or numbers can be estimated from the blood smear (>5 per oil-immersion field) or by a quantitative buffy coat (QBC) method.

Decreased platelet numbers *(thrombocytopenia)* occur with disseminated intravascular coagulation (DIC), bone marrow depression, autoimmune hemolytic anemia, systemic lupus erythematosus, and severe hemorrhage. Normal platelet numbers in dogs and cats are 150,000 to 500,000/μl. Their life span is approximately 10 days.

Normal	150,000-500,000/μl
Thrombocytopenia	<150,000/μl
Bleeding risk	<50,000/μl
My lab	_____

Platelet Morphology

Microscopic examination of platelet morphology on stained blood smears can reveal abnormalities. Normal canine platelets are smaller than RBCs, stain blue, and contain azurophilic granules. Normal feline platelets are small, spherical bodies. Numerous large platelets suggest thrombopoiesis.

Mean Platelet Volume (MPV)

The MPV is a machine calculation of platelet size. In thrombocytopenic dogs, increased mean platelet volume gives indirect evidence of adequate megakaryocyte response. Mean volume $>12 \ \mu^3$ indicates adequate response, but decreased volume $<12 \ \mu^3$ is not accurate in predicting lack of bone marrow megakaryocyte production.

$<12 \ \mu^3$	No indication of response
$>12 \ \mu^3$	Good megakaryocyte response

Prothrombin Time

↑ PT is commonly seen with vitamin K$_1$ deficiency; PT is more sensitive than ACT

Prothrombin time (PT) evaluates the common coagulation pathways (Factors V, X, prothrombin, fibrinogen). It is a sensitive test in diagnosing anticoagulant (vitamin K$_1$ deficiency) poisoning and is more sensitive than the activated clotting time (ACT) for diagnosis of this problem.

Normal PT	5-9 seconds ($>75\%$ of control PT)
My lab	_____

Thrombin Time

↑ TT screens for DIC and monitors the response to heparin

Thrombin time (TT) is a test for fibrinogen and is used to monitor the effects of heparin therapy. In animals with clotting problems, a prolonged TT suggests disseminated intravascular coagulation (DIC).

Normal TT	15-20 seconds
My lab	_____

Thrombotest (PIVKA Test)

thrombotest is sensitive to proteins involved in vitamin K absence (PIVKA)

Thrombotest is a combined prothrombin time reagent consisting of lyophilized bovine brain thromboplastin and adsorbed bovine plasma. It is sensitive to the depression of the clotting Factors II, VII, and X. Because it monitors three of the vitamin K-dependent factors (II, VII, IX, and X), it is more sensitive than the ACT, APTT, or PT tests.

Normal   <25 seconds

References

Lewis DC et al: Detection of platelet-bound and serum platelet-bindable antibodies for diagnosis of idiopathic thrombocytopenic purpura in dogs, *J Am Vet Med Assoc* 206(1):47-52, 1995 (clinical study).

Lewis DC et al: Development and characterization of a flow cytometric assay for detection of platelet-bound immunoglobulin G in dogs, *Am J Vet Res* 56(12):1555-1558, 1995.

Sullivan PS, Manning KL, McDonald TP: Association of mean platelet volume and bone marrow megakaryocytopoiesis in thrombocytopenic dogs, *J Am Vet Med Assoc* 206(3):332-334, 1995.

Williamson LH: Antithrombin III: a natural anticoagulant, *Compend Contin Educ Pract Vet* 13(1):100-107, 1991.

Section 7
Bone Marrow Tests

Aspiration and Biopsy

The simplest and most clinically useful method for assessing bone marrow is by aspiration or core biopsy. Aspiration permits identification of marrow cell lines and their stages of differentiation, and estimates iron stores. Core biopsy or spicule examination permits estimations of marrow cellularity.

Cellularity

bone marrow cellularity is estimated from solid flecks

Bone marrow cellularity is estimated by comparing the proportion of fat cells to blood cells in a solid core biopsy or a squashed fleck of aspirated bone marrow. The ratio of blood cells to fat cells varies with age. *Hypocellular marrow* yields few flecks. Marrow of *normal cellularity* usually yields many flecks with an appropriate blood cell:fat cell ratio for the age of the patient. *Hypercellular marrow* usually yields many marrow flecks with an increased blood cell:fat cell ratio.

	Blood Cells:Fat Cells
Immature animal	3:1
Young adult animal	1:1
Old animal	1:3

Erythrocyte Maturation Index

↓ EMI in an anemic animal indicates ineffective erythropoiesis

The erythrocyte maturation index (EMI) is the sum of erythroid cells in the maturation phase (polychromatophilic rubricytes, orthochromatophilic rubricytes, metarubricytes) divided by the sum of erythroid cells in the proliferation phase (rubriblasts, prorubricytes, basophilic rubricytes).

EMI= maturing erythroid cells/proliferating erythroid cells

Normal	3.6
Abnormal	<3

Examination of Bone Marrow

bone marrow examination determines the cause of ↓ RBCs, ↓ WBCs, hypercalcemia, lymphosarcoma

Bone marrow examination answers questions arising from the complete blood count. Unexplained decreases in the numbers of platelets, RBCs, or WBCs can be evaluated by a bone marrow aspirate and core biopsy. Hyperglobulinemia (myeloma), hypercalcemia (lymphosarcoma), iron-storage problems, and occasionally infections with fungi, *Toxoplasma,* or *rickettsiae* warrant bone marrow examination.

Bone marrow can be rapidly assessed by evaluating the cellularity, the myeloid to erythroid (M:E) ratio, the myeloid maturation index (MMI) and the erythroid maturation index (EMI).

Hemosiderin

Hemosiderin is the intracellular storage form of iron. The granules consist of an ill-defined complex of ferric hydroxides, polysaccharides, and proteins. Hemosiderin is found in bone marrow, the spleen, and sites of old hemorrhage.

Iron Stores

↓ hemosiderin in marrow indicates iron deficiency

Because serum iron levels do not correspond to total body iron, bone marrow smears are often used to assess iron stores. *Hemosiderin* appears as gold to black granules in Wright's stained cells and as blue-black particles with Prussian blue stain.

In normal dogs and cats, a few hemosiderin deposits are seen in each marrow particle. Numerous deposits are seen with increased RBC destruction or old age. If no deposits are seen, iron deficiency should be suspected. Normal or increased iron deposits are seen in the depression anemia of chronic inflammation.

| Normal | Few hemosiderin deposits per marrow particle |

Maturation Stages of Marrow Cells

proliferating RBCs: rubriblasts, prorubricytes, basophilic rubricytes

The cells of bone marrow are classified into developmental stages by their nucleus. Younger cells are capable of proliferation, whereas older cells are functionally mature and do not proliferate.

proliferating WBCs: myeloblasts, progranulocytes, myelocytes

For diagnostic purposes, the erythrocytic and granulocytic cells can be classified into proliferating or maturing stages.

Limiting the classification to proliferating and maturing pools makes bone marrow evaluation rapid and practical.

Resting cells	Stem cells
Proliferating RBCs	Rubriblasts, prorubricytes, basophilic rubricytes
Maturing RBCs	Metachromatic rubricytes, rubricytes, metarubricytes
Proliferating WBCs	Myeloblasts, progranulocytes, myelocytes
Maturing WBCs	Metamyelocytes, bands

Megakaryocytes

normal megakaryocytes have >4 nuclei

Megakaryocytes are the bone marrow precursor cells for thrombocytes (platelets). Adequate numbers of megakaryocytes in a bone marrow preparation assure the examiner that the aspirate was obtained from bone marrow. Absence of megakaryocytes with abundant RBCs alerts the examiner to the possibility that the aspirate is mostly or totally peripheral blood.

The megakaryocyte is evaluated in cases of thrombocytopenia. Relative numbers, progressive maturation, and cytologic characteristics are qualitatively evaluated.

The most immature recognizable megakaryocyte is the *promegakaryocyte*. It has deep blue cytoplasm and contains two to four nuclei linked by thin strands. It is much larger than WBC and RBC precursors. The *megakaryocyte* is the next stage. These large cells (50 to 200 μ) contain more than four nuclei. Usually >50% are mature. Numerous promegakaryocytes indicate a maturation defect or active regeneration.

The normal megakaryocyte should have more than four nuclei and a granular appearance. These large cells are usually found at the edges of the marrow smear or are associated with marrow particles. If no megakaryocytes are seen, the prognosis is grave. If only a few are seen, megakaryocyte numbers are probably decreased.

Normal	3-50 megakaryocytes per fleck
Hypoplasia	<3 per large fleck
Hyperplasia	>50 per large fleck

Myeloid:Erythroid Ratio

M:E ratio only has meaning when considered with the CBC

↓ M:E normal with ↑ WBCs, ↓ M:E normal with responding anemia

The myeloid:erythroid (M:E) ratio can be used to screen for precursor-cell abnormalities. The M:E ratio is derived by counting several hundred nucleated cells, determining whether they are of myeloid (granulocytic) or erythroid (RBC) origin, and calculating the relative percentage of each population for the M:E ratio.

The M:E ratio should correspond to the response in the peripheral blood sample. Normal dogs have approximately a 1:1 ratio and cats have a ratio >2:1. An increased M:E ratio occurs in bacterial infections, leukemoid reactions, myeloid leukemias, and red cell aplasia. A decreased M:E ratio occurs in agranulocytosis and erythroid hyperplasia. Usually a three-fold deviation is necessary to diagnose an abnormality.

Anemia without a decreased M:E ratio suggests red cell hypoplasia. Leukopenia without an increased M:E ratio suggests myeloid hypoplasia.

	Dogs	Cats
Normal M:E ratio	1	≥1.5

Myeloid Maturation Index

↓ MMI in a neu-
tropenic animal
indicates ineffec-
tive granulopoi-
esis

The myeloid maturation index (MMI) is the sum of myeloid cells in the maturation phase (metamyelocytes, bands, segmenters) divided by the sum of the myeloid cells in the proliferation phase (myeloblasts, progranulocytes, myelocytes).

$$MMI = \frac{\text{Maturing myeloid cells}}{\text{Proliferating myeloid cells}}$$

| Normal | 9 |
| Abnormal | <8 |

References

Feldman BF, Thomason KJ: Useful indexes, formulas, and ratios in veterinary laboratory diagnostics, *Comp on Cont Educ* 11(2):169-172, 174-178, 180, 1989.

Section 8
Serologic and Special Tests

Acetylcholine Receptor Antibody

AChR antibodies indicate myasthenia gravis

Animals with acquired myasthenia gravis develop antibodies to acetylcholine receptors (AChR). Clinical signs include weakness induced by exercise, megaesophagus, and dysphagia. Antibodies to AChR indicate immune-mediated myasthenia gravis.

Normal	No AChR titer
Myasthenia gravis	Positive AChR titer

Acute Phase Proteins

Acute phase proteins (APPs) are glycoproteins unrelated to immunoglobulin. They are synthesized by the liver and released into the bloodstream in response to stressors such as inflammation, bacterial infection, endotoxins, neoplasia, and thermal or mechanical injury. The synthesis of APPs is stimulated by monokines such as interleukins (I1-1, I1-6) and tumor necrosis factor.

The biologic functions of APPs vary. Some act as proteinase inhibitors, enzymes, transport proteins, coagulation proteins, and modulators of the immune response. However, all APPs appear to play a role in the restoration of homeostasis after injury, tissue necrosis, infection, or cancer.

Since changes in plasma concentrations of APPs such as alpha acid glycoprotein (AGP) are sensitive, nonspecific indicators of inflammation, AGP is used to detect and monitor infection, inflammatory disease, and cancer therapy.

Alpha-Fetoprotein (AFP)

Embryonic antigens such as alpha-fetoprotein are usually found in very low levels in normal animals. Because malignant cells in the liver produce this fetal protein, it can be used as a marker for malignancy.

A high percent of dogs with hepatocellular carcinoma and cholangiocarcinoma and some dogs with metastatic liver tumors produce high levels of AFP. This marker has a high specificity and positive predictive value with values over 225 ng/ml but has low negative predictive value. In cases where primary or metastatic liver tumors are suggested by radiographs, ultrasound or other tests, markedly elevated AFP confirms a liver tumor but a low level does not rule out a malignancy.

Normal	<100 ng/ml
Metastatic liver tumor	100-225 ng/ml
Primary liver tumor	>250 ng/ml

Antinuclear Antibody Test (ANA)

The ANA test detects antibodies against DNA. In some immune-mediated disease, autoantibodies form against nuclear DNA or cell-surface DNA. Since the ANA test detects these autoantibodies, it is one criterion for the diagnosis of systemic lupus erythematosus (SLE). Because chronic inflammation can cause the release of single strands of DNA and generate antibodies, a better test detects ANA against double-stranded DNA.

Because of this overlap, the ANA test is only one criterion for the diagnosis of SLE. Low titers also occur with polymyositis in aged animals, rheumatoid arthritis, and drug allergies.

	Dog	Cat
Normal	<1:10	<1:40
My lab	_____	_____

Borreliosis (Lyme Disease) Tests

Antibodies may be detected in serum by IFA, ELISA, or Western immunoblot techniques. Titers are difficult to interpret and levels vary in different laboratories. Cross-reactions with other spirochetes occur with ELISA and IFA methods. Increasing antibody titers suggest recent exposure. Culture, histopathology, or polymerase chain reactions are needed for a definitive diagnosis. Rising titers confirm active *Borrelia* infection. In enzootic areas, immune animals can have high titers. A fourfold increase in titer, in two samples collected several weeks apart, is necessary to confirm active infection.

In nonenzootic areas, a titer >1:64 suggests borreliosis.

Brucellosis Tests

ELISA tests are specific but not a sensitive screening test

Rapid slide agglutination test (RSAT) may be positive 2 weeks after inoculation. Although there are few false-negatives, there are many false-positives because of cross-reactions with other infections. A positive test should be confirmed. The mercaptoethane slide agglutination test ME-SAT becomes positive around 4 weeks but is more specific that RSAT.

Tube agglutination test (TAT) becomes positive in 3 to 6 weeks. Titers greater than 1:200 indicate an active infection. Titers below 1:100 are not diagnostic of an active infection. False-positives may occur. The mercaptoethane tube agglutination test (ME-TAT) may become positive after 5 to 8 weeks and produce less false-positives. Titers greater than 1:100 indicate active infection.

Agar gel immunodiffusion (AGID) takes 5 to 10 weeks to become positive. It may be run on cell wall antigen or cytoplasmic antigen. This is a complex procedure but is the most sensitive test. Results are reported as positive, suspicious, or negative.

Catecholamines (Epinephrine, Norepinephrine, Dopamine)

catecholamines may be used to assess cardiac hypertrophy and heart failure

Stress, heart failure, and tumors of the sympathoadrenal system can increase serum levels of catecholamines (epinephrine, norepinephrine, and dopamine). Pheochromocytomas cause increases to 2000 pg/ml. Progressive cardiac hypertrophy and heart failure also increase norepinephrine levels. In the future, assays for catecholamines could be used to monitor the response to treatment of heart disease.

Normal	<1000 pg/ml

Coombs' Test

a positive Coombs' test indicates autoimmune hemolytic anemia

The Coombs' test identifies antibody or complement on the RBC. The test serum must be species specific (antidog or anticat) and polyvalent (to detect IgG, IgM, and complement).

IgG, IgM, and complement attach to RBCs that have been altered by a virus, chemical, or parasite. The antibody coats the RBC, causing autoagglutination, spherocytosis, or hemolysis.

The Coombs' test should not be requested unless the patient shows regenerative anemia without evidence of extravascular hemorrhage.

Enzyme-Linked Immunosorbent Assay (ELISA)

This test may be run for either antibodies or antigens. In the antibody test system, purified antigens are precoated onto an ELISA plate. The patient's serum, which contains antibodies, is incubated on the plate so it reacts with the fixed antigen. Then antidog or anticat immunoglobulin coupled to an enzyme is applied. The chromagen or substrate changes color when cleaved by the enzyme attached to the second antibody. This test is highly sensitive, easily run, and usually accurate. In the antigen test system, the plate is coated with antibodies and the antigen in the test system is bound. The test is read following a second application of antibody to the antigen, which is also bound to an enzyme.

Feline Immunodeficiency Virus Tests (FIV Tests)

FIV Antibody Test

This is an ELISA test that detects serum antibodies. When positive, this test discloses exposure to the FIV virus but can be negative in 30% of FIV infected cats. An infected cat can have a negative test because the antibodies may not be detected for 9 weeks after infection or because of poor antibody response resulting from illness. Sick suspect cats with a negative FIV antibody test should be retested in 1 to 2 months.

FIV Western Blot Test

This is an immunologic test that checks for multiple viral antigen following gel electrophoresis. Although accurate, this test is labor-intensive and expensive.

FIV-PCR

This antigen test is highly specific but may be falsely negative in animals with only small numbers of infected cells in the peripheral blood. For accuracy experienced technicians should perform it; it is currently done mainly in research laboratories.

Altered T Cell Subsets

Changes in the ratio between T cell subsets CD4 and CD8 may be measured histologically in lymph nodes or by Flow cell methods. Individuals with FIV, will decrease the number of CD4 cells. This indicates the state of the immune system. A decreasing ratio indicates a poor prognosis. This test is not routine, but it may be available from research laboratories. The CD4 cells tend to drop with any illness and do not make the dramatic drop seen in human AIDS cases. This test may be valuable in assessing the effect of immune-stimulating drugs.

Feline Infectious Peritonitis Tests (FIP Test)

A positive FIP test with clinical signs is highly suggestive of FIP but a negative test does not rule out this viral disease. A positive test in an animal showing no signs of disease suggests that the cat may be a carrier and should not be introduced to a new colony of cats, but it is not a definitive sign that the cat will develop clinical feline infectious peritonitis disease.

Feline Corona Virus Antibody Tests (FeCV ELISA, FeCV-IFA)

These are nonspecific serum antibody tests that screen for exposure to any feline corona virus. Cats exposed to enteric corona virus, vaccine virus, or the actual FIP virus will be positive. This test has no predictive value and should only be used as presumptive evidence that a cat with clinical signs has feline infectious peritonitis (FIP). The tendency to shed virus cannot be determined by this test alone in healthy cats, even if they have a high FeCV titer.

FIP-Specific ELISA

This serologic test detects antibodies directed against a protein (called 7b), which is secreted by some pathogenic FIP-causing coronaviruses and not by other coronaviruses that infect cats. Cats with antibodies to this protein have been exposed to pathogenic FIPV but many cats with FIP have no antibodies because other mutations can also occur in the FeCV and result in FIP. Thus this test is not specific enough to confirm all cases of FIP.

Titers range from negative (<1:40) to 1:640.

FeCV-PCR

The FeCV-PCR test may be done on the blood or feces, and provides a clinically available tool for identifying FeCV shedders before they are introduced into a new home or cattery. A single fecal RT-PCR result on its own, however, is meaningless. If the cat is intermittently shedding FcoV, the day following sampling the cat may have changed from being a shedder to a non-shedder or vice versa. Fecal testing has to be part of a series of tests and is best accompanied by (IFA) testing because RT-PCR can be prone to both false positive results and false negative results.

FIPVs appear to be mutants of FeCV that occur in immunocompromised cats. In catteries, risk factors for FIP included the immune status of an individual cat, coronavirus titer, overall frequency of fecal coronavirus shedding, and the proportion of cats in the cattery that were chronic coronavirus shedders.

FIP-Specific PCR

The FIP specific PCR is able to detect some modified corona virus in exudative fluids and in feces. Because FIP develops from different mutations of FeCV, testing for this one mutation will miss many virus variants. When a cat is positive, a diagnosis can be confirmed, but if a cat with clinical signs is negative, the FIP virus may still be the cause.

Feline Leukemia Virus Tests

Early detection of feline leukemia virus (FeLV) infection is desirable to prevent transmission of the virus to susceptible cats and to formulate a prognosis. Diagnostic assays are based on detection of viral antigens or viral DNA.

Fluorescent Antibody Test

The fluorescent antibody (FA) test detects FeLV antigens in circulating platelets and WBCs. Infected cats show a positive FA test at a later stage of FeLV infection than with enzyme-linked immunosorbent assay, but the FA test can help monitor the progression of FeLV infection in a patient.

Enzyme-Linked Immunosorbent Assay

Enzyme-linked immunosorbent assay (ELISA) detects viral antigen in serum, effusions, tears, and saliva. This test can detect FeLV infection before the FA test.

Polymerase Chain Reaction Test

The polymerase chain reaction (PCR) test is a sensitive, rapid way to detect viral DNA in an FeLV-infected cat's blood and bone marrow cells.

Feline Leukemia Virus Test Patterns

interpret positive
FeLV tests in
low-risk cats
with great
caution; persis-
tent viremia
usually causes
death in 3 years

Although enzyme-linked immunosorbent assay (ELISA) is a sensitive test for the carrier state of feline leukemia virus (FeLV) infection, it should not be used alone to predict a fatal outcome of FeLV infection. ELISA procedures detect soluble p27 viral antigen and can diagnose infection 5 weeks earlier than the indirect fluorescent antibody (FA) procedure. It can also detect localized infection. These subclinical infections can later progress to viremia or can be eliminated by body defenses.

Results of ELISA are occasionally falsely positive. To prevent misinterpretation, a positive test in a healthy low-risk animal should be rechecked a few weeks later or confirmed with an FA test or polymerase chain reaction (PCR).

The FA detects FeLV particles within circulating cells, indicating a more serious infection involving the bone marrow. A persistently positive FA result indicates an active FeLV infection.

The likely outcome of FeLV infection can be more accurately predicted when the general health of the cat is considered and multiple tests are performed over several weeks.

Interpretation of FeLV Tests
- FA negative, ELISA negative: The cat is not a carrier of FeLV, the infection is too early to detect, or the cat has become infected and is immune to the virus.
- FA positive, ELISA positive: The cat is viremic. If an FA test done 4 weeks later is also positive, the cat is persistently viremic and has an 80% chance of death from FeLV-related disease within 3 years.
- FA positive, ELISA negative, then FA negative, ELISA negative: These cats have been infected with FeLV but have become immune.
- FA negative, ELISA positive: These results are called discordant and suggest a sequestered site of infection. Cats with persistently discordant results have a 50% chance of dying from FeLV-related disease within 3 years.

Flow Cytometry

This technique objectively examines, quantifies, and separates single cells on the basis of one or more parameters. The procedure channels individual cells in a narrow fluid stream past a laser beam. Optical sensors detect signals generated as the cells pass through the laser beam. Cells can be identified based on their light scatter.

Antibodies coupled to fluorochromes can be used to label the cells so that each cell can be identified by its immune characteristics. A computer collects the fluorescence signature of each cell and displays the pattern of fluorescence for the user to analyze.

Fungal Titers

rising titers indicate infection

Serologic titers can confirm infections of *Blastomyces, Histoplasma, Cryptococcus, Coccidioides,* and *Aspergillus*. A positive test gives presumptive confirmation of a fungal disease, but a rising titer in samples collected 2 to 3 weeks apart provide definitive diagnosis.

Aspergillosis Tests

Antibodies are detected in serum by agar gel immunodiffusion (AGID) and ELISA techniques. Although positive results correlate with active infection many animals may be falsely negative and others may be falsely positive as a result of cross-reaction with *Penicillium* spp. Nasal biopsy that shows invasion of the turbinates helps confirm a diagnosis.

Babesiosis Tests

IFA assays can detect serum antibodies to various species of *Babesia*. Because response to treatment varies, it is important to determine which species is involved. Demonstration of organisms in a Giemsa's stained blood smear gives a definitive diagnosis. This is best done on capillary blood. In chronic cases organisms are hard to find so a presumptive diagnosis is made on the basis of clinical signs and a positive titer.

Blastomycosis Tests

Agar gel immunodiffusion and ELISA tests are used to screen animals for circulating antibodies. If no antibodies are detected the animal has >90% chance of not having an infection. False-negative results occur in animals with peracute or advanced infections. If antibodies are present, the animal has >90% chance of being infected. Antibody titers may remain positive after successful treatment. Identifying the yeast by cytology, histopathology, or fungal culture gives a definitive diagnosis.

Coccidioidomycosis *(Coccidioides immitis)* Test

Antibodies may be detected by complement fixation (CF), tube precipitation (TP), and agar gel immunodiffusion (AGID). False-negative results may occur with TP tests in early infection, per acute infection, chronic infections, or primary cutaneous infections. False-positive results of the CF test occur in anticomplementary serum, or cross-reactions with histoplasmosis and blastomycosis. A decreasing titer over several months suggests successful treatment but a low CF titer (<1:32) may remain. A rising titer indicates active infection.

Cryptococcosis Tests

The latex agglutination test may be used on blood, urine, or CSF. Positive titers usually indicate exposure but cross-reactions occur with toxoplasmosis. Titers >1:10 usually indicate an active infection. A fourfold decrease in serum titer indicates successful response to therapy. Identifying a thick-coated budding yeast by cytology, histopathology, or fungal culture gives a definitive diagnosis.

Histoplasmosis Test

Circulating antibodies are detected by complement fixation (CF) and agar gel immunodiffusion (AGID). A positive test confirms exposure but not clinical disease unless a significant rise (fourfold) in titer is seen after several weeks. The CF test cross-reacts with other fungal antibodies. AGID titers may persist >1 year after resolution of the disease. Thus neither test is reliable in dogs nor cats for definitive diagnosis. Identifying the yeast by cytology, histopathology, or fungal culture gives a definitive diagnosis. Rectal scrapings are often diagnostic with colonic histoplasmosis. Fine needle aspiration or bone marrow aspiration may demonstrate the organism.

Heartworm Testing

Heartworm Microfilaria Tests

Microfilaria of the heartworm *Dirofilaria immitis* can be observed by microscopic examination of filters through which anticoagulated blood has been passed, by centrifuged blood samples, or by smears of the buffy coat of centrifuged blood. The microfilaria of *Dirofilaria immitis* can be differentiated from those of *Dipetalonema reconditum* by morphologic characteristics.

Microfilaria may not be evident in dogs recently treated with a filaricidal drug, infected only with male heartworms, or infected with immature heartworms. The small numbers of heartworms in cats produce few microfilaria.

Heartworm Antigen Tests

Antigen tests can be used in both dogs and cats. These tests are highly specific (i.e., very low rate of false-positives), but they lack the sensitivity to detect many infections in cats and often provide false-negative test results. Antigen tests detect antigens from adult female heartworms. These tests therefore fail to detect infections with immature heartworms, male heartworms, and some infections with only one to two adult female worms. Given the potential for immature heartworms to cause clinical disease and the propensity for cats to have single-sex heartworm infections (approximately one third of infections), antigen tests are not useful as screening tests and their utility is restricted to detecting infections with mature adult female heartworms.

Heartworm Antibody Test

Heartworm antibody tests are available for both dogs and cats. The specific antigen varies with the manufacturer, but the test systems are calibrated to pick up infection with immature worms as well as infections when only male worms are present. Low titers may indicate exposure but no active infections, while high titers suggest active disease. Following infection, the titer will remain high for several months. The exact titer for diagnosis will vary with the test system.

Immunoblot Tests

Blot tests are a combination of protein electrophoresis separation plus an immune reaction.

Western Blot (WB)

This test allows visualization of antibodies directed against multiple protein of an infective agent. Proteins from a lysate of infected cells are electrophoresed in a gel and separated based on size and charge.

These protein bands are reacted with a specific antibody and developed with a second antibody conjugated to an enzyme that gives a visible reaction. This is more accurate than a single antigen test system because usually several sites on the organism give positive results and produce a fingerprint.

Southern Blot (SB)

This test detects gene sequences of a test sample following electrophoreses. Currently it is primarily a research tool.

Immunofluorescence Antibody Test

Antibodies deposited in tissues can be detected by direct immunofluorescence. Samples are usually fixed in Michelle's media and treated with anticanine or antifeline reagent labeled with fluorescein. This test is commonly used for diagnosis of autoimmune skin diseases, glomerulonephritis, and occasionally for immune-mediated thrombocytopenia.

Immune Antibody Tests, Direct

Fluorescein-labeled antibody and immunoperoxidase methods can be used to diagnose immune-mediated disease and specific infectious agents. Immune globulins, complement, and organisms can be detected in specially fixed tissues.

Antibody directed against somatic antigens or immune complexes deposited in tissues are used to diagnose systemic lupus erythematosus, discoid lupus, pemphigus, and immune-mediated thrombocytopenia. Antibody directed against infectious agents is used to diagnose FIP, FeLV, canine distemper, and others.

Leptospirosis Tests

Serologic tests do not differentiate between active infection, previous infection, or vaccination. Antibodies may be detected by the microscopic agglutination test (MAT), ELISA (IgM and IgG), and microscopic microcapsular agglutination test (MCAT). A definitive diagnosis requires either a rising titer over 2 to 4 weeks or observation of organisms in the urine by darkfield microscopy.

Lupus Erythematosus Test

the LE cell test can provide a rapid in-hospital screen for SLE

Neutrophils or macrophages that have ingested nuclear debris from tissue cells damaged by antinuclear antibody are known as *lupus erythematosus (LE) cells*. These cells occur in the blood of patients with systemic lupus erythematosus (SLE).

Although this test has been replaced by the antinuclear antibody (ANA) test, it may be done in your hospital for a rapid SLE screen.

Corticosteroids can inhibit LE cell formation.

Protocol
1. Collect blood in a heparinized blood tube containing glass beads (special tube available from diagnostic laboratories).
2. Incubate for 2 hours at 37° F.
3. Remove fibrinogen from the sample by shaking the sample.
4. Fill a capillary tube and centrifuge.
5. Make a smear of the buffy coat.
6. Examine the smear for phagocytes containing large particles of homogeneous nuclear material in their cytoplasm.

Polymerase Chain Reaction (PCR)

The polymerase chain reaction (PCR) is a method for amplifying and detecting specific DNA sequences. In applied medicine, PCR technology is primarily used in diagnostic tests to detect viral or bacterial sequences in blood, fluid, or tissue specimens. For the test to be accurate, a specific DNA sequence, unique to the organism under study, must be identified and molecularly sequenced. Because of its specificity and ability to amplify (theoretically) as few as one specific DNA sequence in a large sample, the PCR test is particularly useful for detecting covert or low-grade infections.

The PCR technology must be modified to detect some organisms. For RNA viruses (such as coronaviruses), the viral RNA must be converted to DNA by using a reverse transcriptase enzyme before being subjected to PCR testing. Some DNA sequences found in pathogens of interest are very similar to sequences in harmless but ubiquitous organisms. In this instance, false-positive results can occur with routine PCR because of the similarity of the proteins. Nested set PCR using several different sets of primers during the amplification sequence is used to overcome this problem. Unfortunately, while nested set PCR increases the specificity of the test, the sensitivity of the test is decreased.

Rheumatoid Factors

↑ RF is not suffi-
cient for a diag-
nosis of
rheumatoid
arthritis

Rheumatoid factors (RF) are antibodies against autologous altered IgG or IgM. They are often found in patients with immune-mediated erosive (rheumatoid) arthritis. They also occur in old patients and in those with systemic lupus erythematosus.

The presence of rheumatoid factor alone is not sufficient for diagnosis of rheumatoid arthritis. Typical radiographic signs and joint changes are needed to support this diagnosis.

Rickettsial Tests

Ehrlichiosis (*Ehrlichia canis*) Test

Indirect immunofluorescence, western immunoblotting, or PCR may detect antibodies. Titers >1:20 are positive in endemic areas. In nonendemic areas any measurable titer (>1:10) is suspicious. Retest in 2 weeks if a suspected animal is negative. A definitive diagnosis can be made if morulae (a cluster of organisms) are seen in leukocytes. Positive titer may persist in treated dogs for over 2 years.

Hemobartonella PCR Test

The PCR test is the most accurate method of diagnosis of active and carrier states of feline infectious anemia. It can detect *H. felis* in blood samples obtained from cats during peak parasitemia, during most of the carrier phase, and after challenge with immunosuppressive drugs. During and immediately after antibiotic treatment, this test may fail to detect the organisms.

Rocky Mountain Spotted Fever Tests

IFA and ELISA procedures can be used to detect both IgM and IgG antibodies. Normal values may vary between laboratories and areas of the country. Increased titers in samples submitted 2 to 4 weeks apart are suggestive of an active infection. The presence of antibodies only suggests exposure but not necessarily an active infection. Following treatment, titers have remained elevated for 10 months.

Normal titer <1:28

Toxoplasmosis Tests

Serum ELISA, IFA, Western blot immunoassays, Sabin-Feldman dye tests and agglutination tests can detect *T. gondii* antibodies. IgM titers appear within the first 2 weeks but usually decrease after 12 weeks. IgG titers appear after 4 weeks and last for years. A rising IgG titer suggests active disease but a single positive test denotes exposure only, not active disease.

Serum ELISA tests can detect *T. gondii* specific antigens as the organisms are intermittently released from tissue cysts. A positive test indicates active infection. PCR assays on the aqueous humor can confirm the presence of organisms.

Antibodies in the aqueous humor and CSF can be used to determine previous infection in the central nervous system or the eye but does not confirm active disease.

Fecal flotation using a solution with a specific gravity of 1.15-1.18 that shows small oocytes (10×12 μm) indicates a potential shedder.

+ Antigen or antibody test	Exposure
Recent or active toxoplasmosis	IgM >1:64
Recent or active toxoplasmosis	Rising titer IgG
+ Fecal test	Zoonotic risk

Tumor Necrosis Factor (TNF)

TNF levels may indicate the prognosis in heart failure

Tumor necrosis factor (TNF), also called cachectin, is a cytokine produced by endotoxin-activated macrophages. It causes necrosis of certain tumors, stimulates catabolism, activates the renin-angiotensin system, and inhibits beta-adrenergic responsiveness. It may cause the weight loss seen in patients with "cardiac cachexia."

Increased TNF levels have been found in people and animals with heart failure. Although assays for TNF are very expensive, it may be used as a prognostic test before treatment of severe heart failure.

Normal	<30 pg/ml (human values)
Abnormal	>70 pg/ml (human values)

References

Addie DD, Jarrett O: Use of a reverse-transcriptase polymerase chain reaction for monitoring the shedding of feline coronavirus by health cats, *Veterinary Record* 148(21):649-652, 2001.

Berent LM , Messick JB , Cooper SK: *Am J Vet Res* 59(10):1215-1220, 1998.

Bjorneby J: Antech Literature, Irvine, CA, 1998, Antech Diagnostics.

Cardiotech Services, Inc, 3027 Sherbrooke Road, Louisville, Ky, 40205, 502-473-7066; Development Technologies International Inc, 203 Broadway Street, Frederick, MD 21701, 301-694-0089, Fax: 301-694-5752.

Concannon PW et al: Postimplantation increase in plasma fibrinogen concentration with increase in relaxin concentration in pregnant dogs, *Am J Vet Res* 57(9):1382-1385, 1996.

Endo Y et al: Alteration of T-cell subsets in the lymph nodes from cats infected with feline immunodeficiency virus, *J Vet Med Sci* 59(9):739-746, 1997.

Foley JE et al: Risk factors for feline infectious peritonitis among cats in multiple-cat environments with endemic feline enteric coronavirus, *J Am Vet Med Assoc* 210(9):1313-1318, 1997.

Gamble DA, Lobbiani A, Gramegna M, Moore LE, Colucci G: Development of a nested PCR assay for detection of feline infectious peritonitis virus in clinical specimens, *J Clin Microbiol* 35(3):673-675, 1997.

Hahn KA, Richardson RC: Detection of serum alpha-fetoprotein in dogs with naturally occurring malignant neoplasia, *Vet Clin Pathol* 24(1):18-21, 1995 (clinical study).

Herrewegh AA et al: Detection of feline coronavirus RNA in feces, tissues, and body fluids of naturally infected cats by reverse transcriptase PCR, *J Clin Microbiol* 33(3):684-689, 1995.

Hoffmann-Fezer G et al: Comparison of T-cell subpopulations in cats naturally infected with feline leukemia virus or feline immunodeficiency virus, *Res Vet Sci* 61(3):222-226, 1996.

Inoshima Y et al: Quantification of feline immunodeficiency virus (FIV) proviral DNA in peripheral blood mononuclear cells of cats infected with Japanese strains of FIV, *J Vet Med Sci* 57(3):487-492, 1995.

Lowseth LA et al: Detection of serum alpha-fetoprotein in dogs with hepatic tumors, *J Am Vet Med Assoc* 199(6):735-741, 1991.

McReynolds C, Macy D: Feline infectious peritonitis. Part I. Etiology and diagnosis, *Compend Contin Educ Pract Vet* 19(9):1007-1016, 1065, 1997.

Steele K: Personal communication, San Diego, 1998, Engene Biotechnologies. Vennema H, Polland A, Folley J, Pedersen NC: Feline infectious peritonitis viruses arise by mutation from endemic feline entericcoronaviruses, *Virology* 243(1):150-157, 1998.

Vennema H, Poland A, Foley J, Pedersen NC: Feline infectious peritonitis viruses arise by mutation from endemic feline entericcoronaviruses, *Virology* 243(1):150-157, 1998.

Wolf A: What is PCR? *Feline Medicine Symposium,* North American Veterinary Conference, 1996.

Yamada T et al: Purification of canine alpha-fetoprotein and alpha-fetoprotein values in dogs, *Vet Immunol Immunopathol* 47(1-2):25-33, 1995.

Section 9
Diagnosis by Laboratory Findings

Hypocalcemia

Hypocalcemia is a total corrected serum calcium concentration of less than 6.5 mg/dl. Since blood calcium is bound to serum albumin, abnormal levels of blood calcium must be corrected to avoid a false diagnosis of hypocalcemia.

Tetany from hypocalcemia is seen only if the blood pH is alkalotic. Acidosis ionizes more calcium and protects against tetany, whereas alkalosis decreases the ionized calcium and predisposes to eclampsia.

Serum phosphorus levels and secretion of parathyroid hormone control serum calcium. High serum phosphorus levels form insoluble calcium-phosphorus mineral deposits, which lower serum calcium levels. This is seen with phosphorus retention of uremia and with the high-meat diets of young animals. Because some dogs with severe renal secondary hyperparathyroidism have high ionized calcium, this test is helpful when treating secondary hyperparathyroidism with vitamin D therapy.

Pancreatitis lowers serum calcium because of formation of insoluble saponified calcium deposits in digested mesenteric fat. Hypoparathyroidism decreases calcium resorption and mobilization from bone stores. Lactation rarely lowers measurable calcium but causes alkalosis that decreases ionized calcium.

Differential Diagnoses
- Acute pancreatitis
- Anuric renal failure
- Chronic renal failure
- Distal renal tubular acidosis
- Glomerulonephritis
- Hypoparathyroidism
- Nephrotoxicosis
- Nutritional secondary hyperparathyroidism
- Postrenal uremia
- Protein-losing enteropathy
- Renal secondary hyperparathyroidism

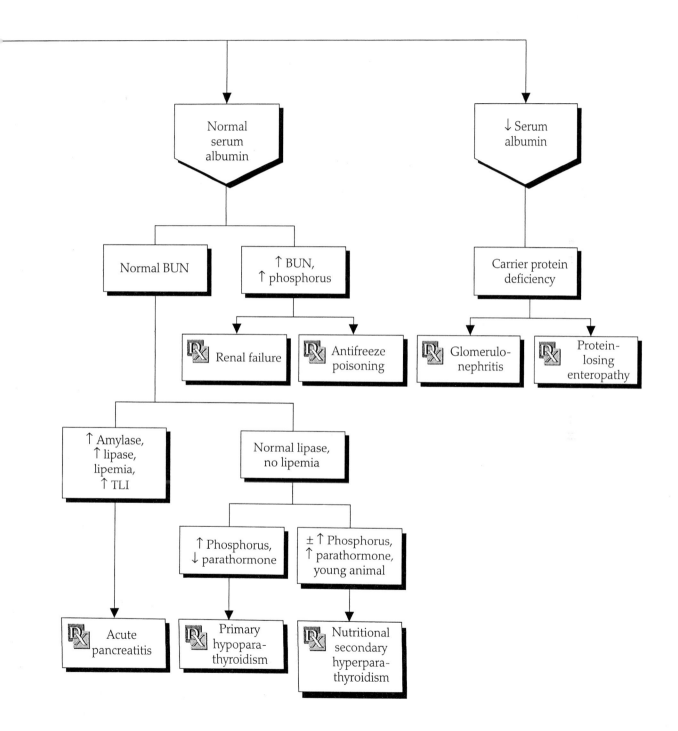

Hypercalcemia

Hypercalcemia is a total corrected serum calcium concentration greater than 12 mg/dl. A high corrected serum calcium level is dangerous because of cardiotoxicity and dystrophic calcification. Because blood calcium is bound to serum albumin, the blood calcium level must be corrected for albumin levels to avoid a false diagnosis of hypercalcemia. Dehydration and hemoconcentration give an impression of hypercalcemia because they raise serum albumin.

Animals with hypercalcemia should be checked radiographically for osteolytic bone lesions. If bone lesions are not detected, the blood panel can disclose hypercalcemic diseases such as Addison's disease and renal failure. Other causes of hypercalcemia can be inferred from the relationship of calcium, phosphorus, and chloride levels. Vitamin D toxicity can cause hypercalcemia with concurrent hyperphosphatemia. A parathormone-like hormone abnormality, such as hyperparathyroidism or pseudohyperparathyroidism (hypercalcemia of malignancy), causes hypercalcemia with normal or low phosphorus. A high Cl:P ratio (>33) suggests hyperparathyroidism. A low Cl:P ratio (<33) suggests pseudohyperparathyroidism and can be an early sign of lymphosarcoma or perianal carcinoma. Serum ionized calcium does not provide a diagnostic advantage over total calcium in the detection of hypercalcemia of malignancy.

Differential Diagnoses
- Dehydration
- Hypoadrenocorticism
- Maintenance renal failure
- Osteomyelitis and bone tumors
- Primary hyperparathyroidism
- Pseudohyperparathyroidism

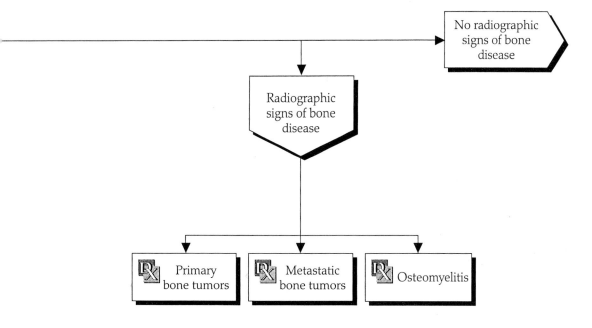

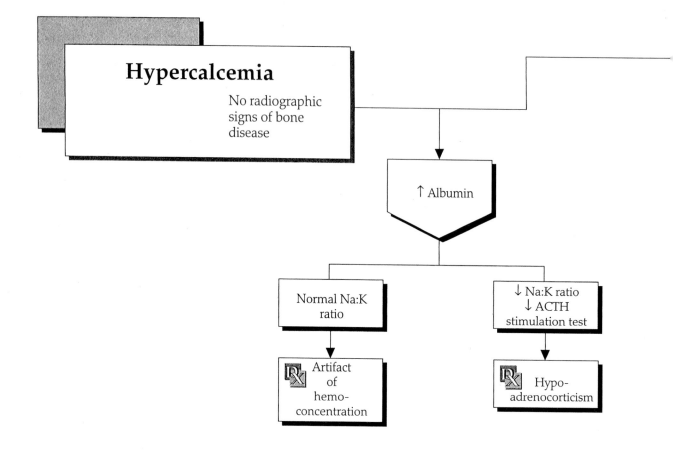

Hypercalcemia

No radiographic
signs of bone
disease

↑ Albumin

Normal Na:K
ratio

↓ Na:K ratio
↓ ACTH
stimulation test

℞ Artifact
of
hemo-
concentration

℞ Hypo-
adrenocorticism

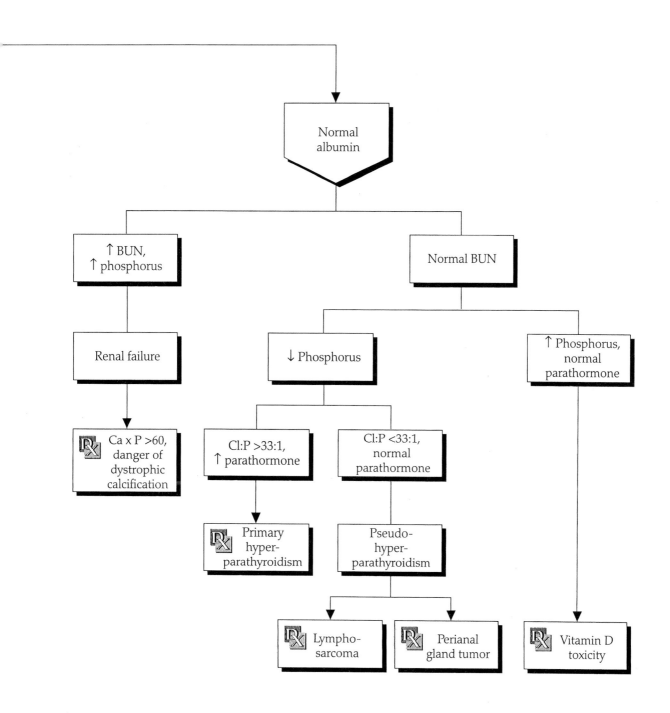

Hypercholesterolemia

Hypercholesterolemia is not a definitive sign of any disease but can occur in obstructive biliary disease, diabetes mellitus, hypothyroidism, hyperadrenocorticism, acute nephritis, nephrotic syndrome, acute pancreatitis, and primary dyslipoproteinemias. In the early induction stage of acute renal failure it may be the only indication of a systemic problem.

Differential Diagnoses
- Hypothyroidism
- Hyperadrenocorticism
- Diabetes mellitus
- Nephrotic syndrome
- Obstructive biliary disease
- Acute renal failure induction stage

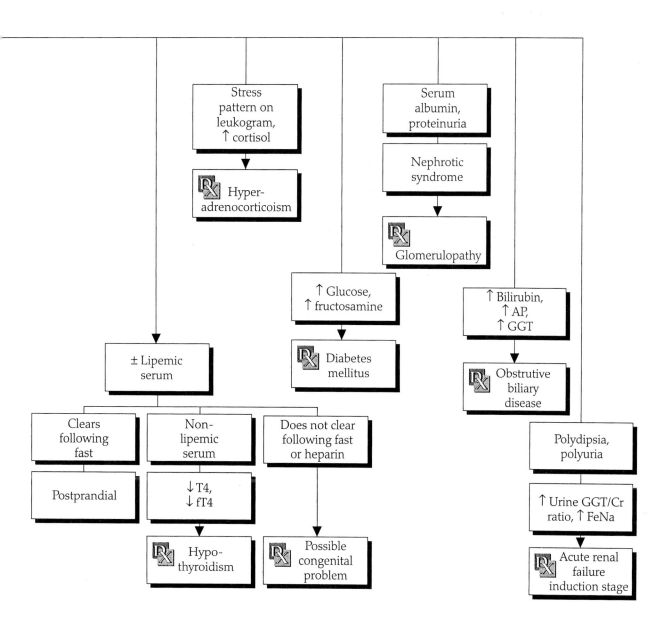

Decreased Bicarbonate

Plasma bicarbonate, measured as CO_2 or HCO_3, is a crude indication of acid-base disorders. Because the blood pH is rarely measured in clinical situations, evaluation of respiration is needed to differentiate metabolic from respiratory-induced changes.

In cases of hyperventilation, decreased bicarbonate suggests respiratory alkalosis. When there is no hyperventilation, decreased bicarbonate usually indicates metabolic acidosis resulting from concurrent disease, such as uremia or diabetes mellitus.

An anion gap greater than 20 indicates metabolic acidosis resulting from retention of organic acids. This is seen with lactic acidosis and ketoacidosis. An anion gap less than 20 suggests that acidosis is due to bicarbonate loss from renal disease or diarrhea.

Differential Diagnoses
- Chronic renal failure
- Diabetic ketoacidosis
- Distal renal tubule acidosis
- Fanconi's syndrome
- Feline urologic syndrome
- Juvenile renal disease
- Lactic acidosis
- NSAID-induced renal disease
- Nephrotoxicosis
- Postrenal uremia

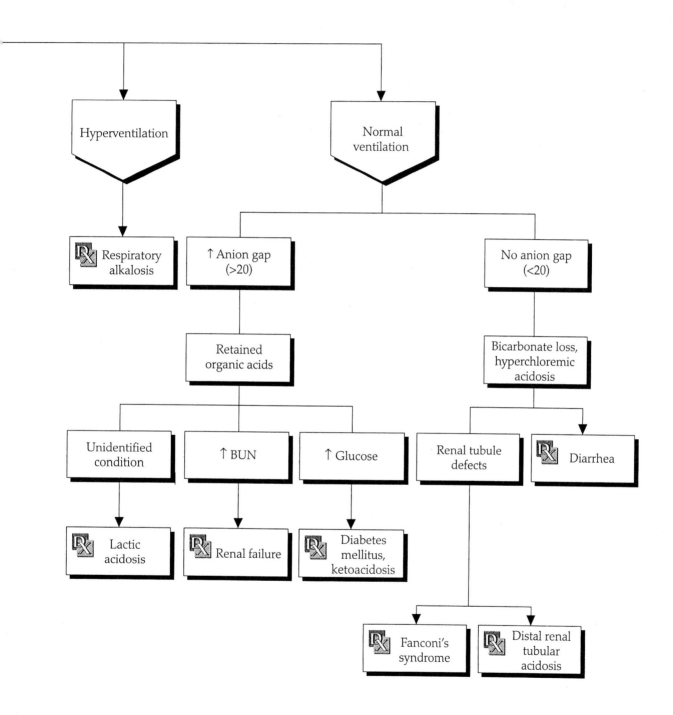

Hypoglycemia

Hypoglycemia is a decrease in blood glucose concentration below 70 mg/dl. The most common cause of decreased blood glucose levels is improper handling of the blood sample before it reaches the laboratory.

If the blood sample was submitted properly and hypoglycemia is persistent, a glucagon stimulation test can differentiate among decreased glucose production, glycogen storage problems, and high insulin levels. If insulin levels are excessive following glucagon stimulation, an insulinoma is probable. If the insulin level is normal in a debilitated animal, adrenal insufficiency and shock are frequent causes.

Differential Diagnoses
- Glycogen storage disease
- Hepatic cirrhosis
- Hypoadrenocorticism
- Pancreatic islet-cell tumor
- Shock

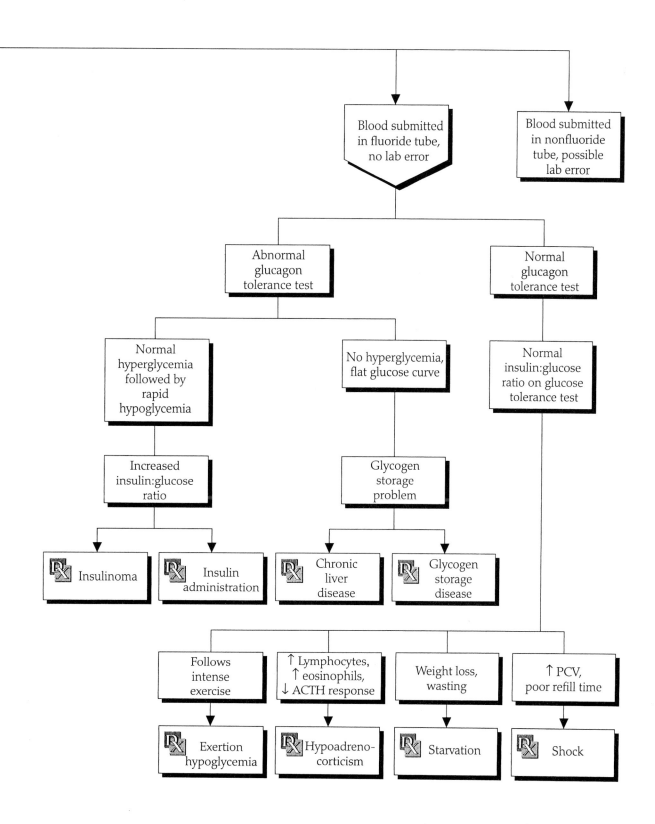

Hyperglycemia

Hyperglycemia is an increased blood glucose concentration above 120 mg/dl. A blood glucose level above 170 mg/dl exceeds the resorptive capacity of the kidney tubules and causes glucosuria. Mild physiologic hyperglycemia is caused by fear and struggling during blood collection. Increased glucose production or decreased glucose utilization causes pathologic hyperglycemia.

Polycythemia and physiologic leukocytosis suggest fear-induced epinephrine release. This type of hyperglycemia is caused by hepatic glycogenolysis. Leukocytosis, lymphopenia, and eosinopenia suggest stress or adrenal hyperfunction. The resulting hyperglycemia is caused by hepatic gluconeogenesis.

Lipemia sometimes accompanies hyperglycemia. Hyperglycemia with lipemia that clears with heparin injection suggests postprandial hyperglycemia. Hyperglycemia with lipemia that does not clear with heparin suggests cortisol excess or pancreatitis.

Marked persistent hyperglycemia suggests diabetes mellitus. In screening for diabetes mellitus, normal levels of fructosamine in a hyperglycemic animal rule out a diagnosis of diabetes mellitus. Deficient insulin levels indicate insulin-dependent diabetes. Adequate insulin levels with an abnormal glucose tolerance curve suggests Type II or Type III diabetes mellitus.

Differential Diagnoses
- Diabetic ketoacidosis
- Excitement
- Iatrogenic cortisol excess
- Pituitary-dependent hyperadrenocorticism
- Primary hyperadrenocorticism
- Sick cat syndrome
- Stress
- Type I diabetes mellitus
- Type II diabetes mellitus
- Type III diabetes mellitus

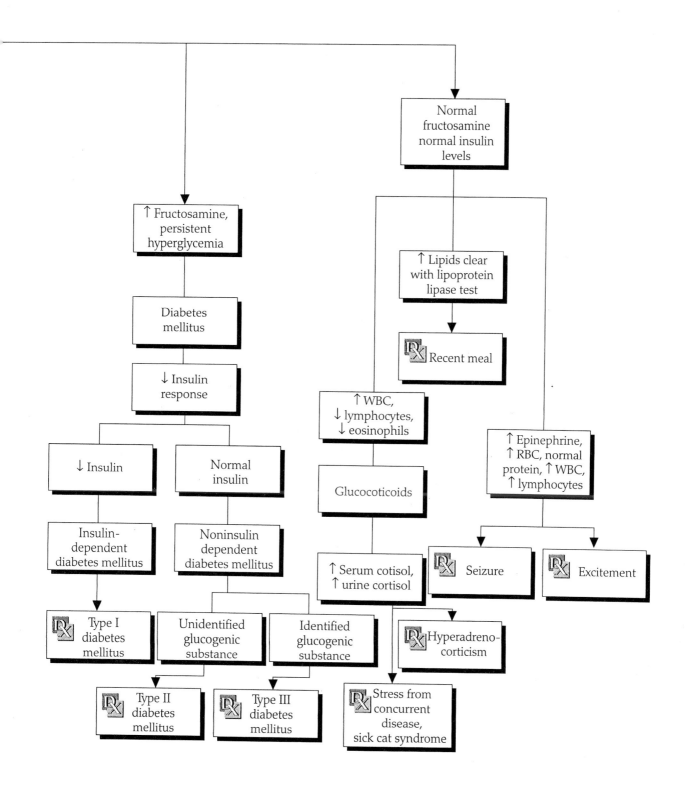

Hyponatremia

Hyponatremia is a low serum sodium concentration below 140 mEq/L. Many diseases can lower serum sodium. Conditions that decrease intake, increase excretion, and cause overhydration decrease the concentration of serum sodium. For diagnostic purposes, the Na:K ratio is the key test.

Aldosterone from the adrenal cortex controls sodium resorption and potassium excretion in the renal tubules. Deficiencies cause a markedly low (<23) Na:K ratio and suggest adrenal failure.

When sodium is low but the Na:K ratio is normal, changes in fluid movement or substances that dilute the blood are probable causes. Fluid moves to the third compartment space with edema, ascites, or exudation. Body fluid containing sodium is lost with diarrhea, vomiting, polyuria, or burns. Serum sodium levels are diluted with excessive water, glucose, or fat in the blood.

Differential Diagnoses
- Chronic renal failure
- Diabetes mellitus
- Glomerulonephritis
- Hepatic cirrhosis
- Hyperlipidemia
- Primary hypoadrenocorticism
- Psychogenic polydipsia

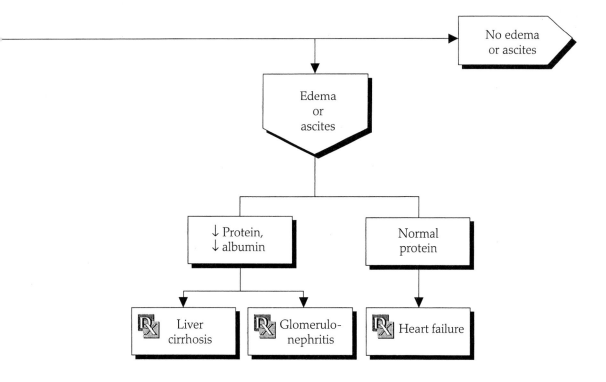

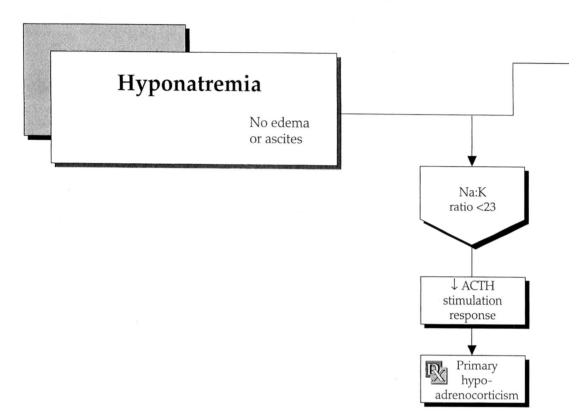

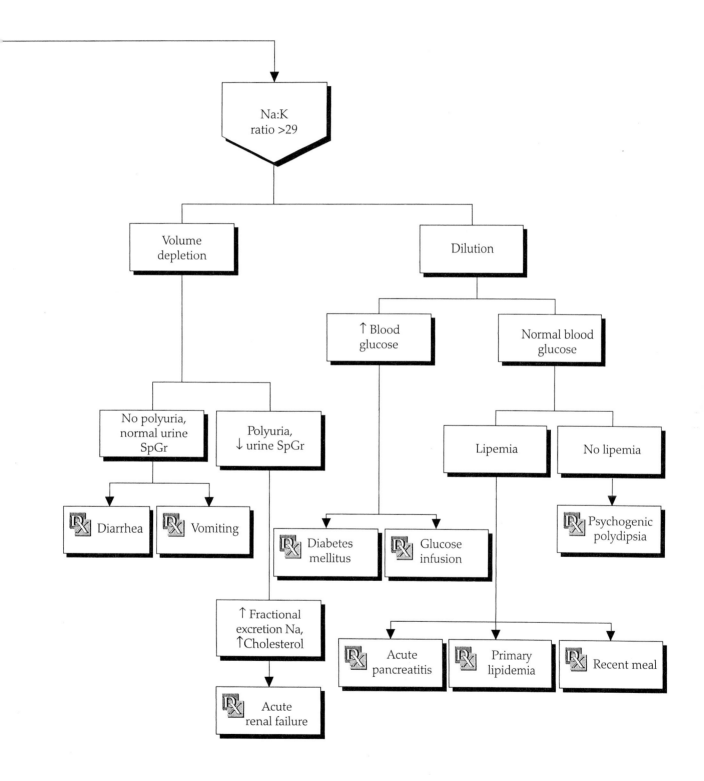

Hypophosphatemia

Mild hypophosphatemia (2 to 3 mg/dl) without hypercalcemia or hyperglycemia can usually be ignored. Significant hypophosphatemia is seen with hyperparathyroidism, pseudohyperparathyroidism, and diabetes mellitus that is overtreated with insulin and bicarbonate.

The kidneys regulate the serum phosphorus level. Conditions that elevate the serum calcium level or blood pH (alkalosis) reduce serum phosphorus levels by forming insoluble phosphates in tissues.

To determine the underlying cause of hypophosphatemia with hypercalcemia, calculate the serum chloride to phosphorus (Cl:P) ratio. Hyperchloremic acidosis with a small anion gap occurs with primary hyperparathyroidism and produces a high Cl:P ratio (>33). Alkalosis with a low Cl:P ratio (<33) occurs with pseudohyperparathyroidism.

Differential Diagnoses
- Diabetic ketoacidosis
- Primary hyperparathyroidism
- Pseudohyperparathyroidism

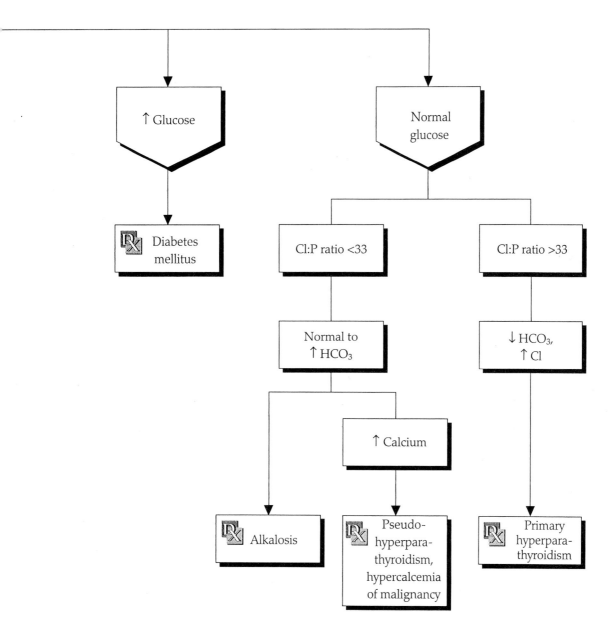

Hyperphosphatemia

Hyperphosphatemia is a serum phosphorus level above 6 mg/dl in an adult dog, above 7 mg/dl in an adult cat, and above 9 mg/dl in an immature animal. Because RBCs contain large amounts of phosphorus, the phosphorus value of hemolyzed blood samples is falsely elevated. If the blood is hemolyzed, another sample must be collected for testing.

The most common cause of severe hyperphosphatemia is uremia. If the animal is uremic, the serum calcium $\times$ phosphorus product can be calculated to determine the likelihood of dystrophic calcification.

If the BUN level is normal, a serum calcium assay helps determine possible causes of hyperphosphatemia. Low serum calcium suggests hypoparathyroidism. The serum calcium level is normal in young animals fed a high-meat diet and in hyperthyroid cats, but the ionized calcium may be decreased. Concurrent high calcium levels are seen with hypoadrenocorticism and vitamin D excess.

Differential Diagnoses
- Hyperthyroidism
- Hypoparathyroidism
- Laboratory error
- Nutritional secondary hyperparathyroidism
- Vitamin D toxicity

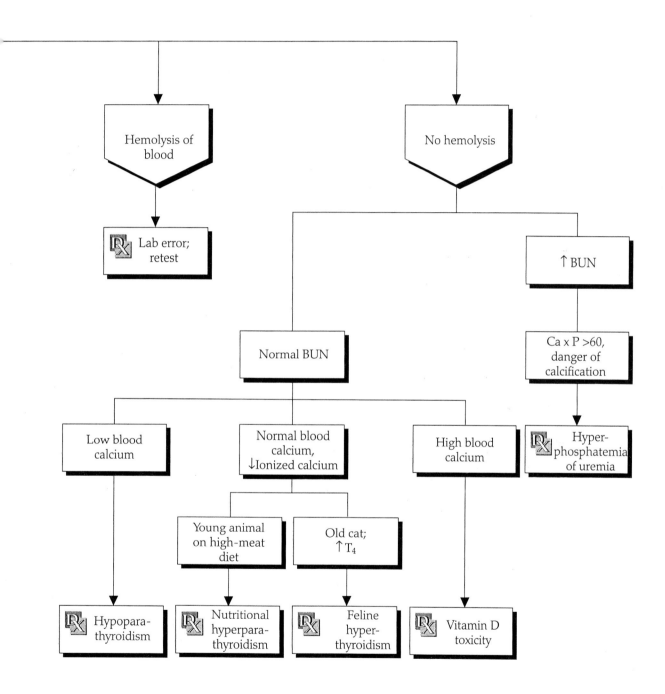

Hypoproteinemia

Plasma protein levels below 5.5 g/dl are pathologic and may be due to deficiencies of albumin, globulin, or both. If albumin levels are normal, the low plasma proteins are due to deficiencies in globulin. This may indicate immunodeficiency or serum loss.

When both albumin and globulin are low, the serum is either diluted (see hyponatremia) or protein has been lost through hemorrhage or exudation. The site of occult loss is often the intestine. This can be confirmed by testing for fecal alpha-1 protease inhibitor.

If only albumin is low, the urine should be checked for protein loss. If protein is not being passed in the urine, liver function may be checked by biopsy and bile acid or ammonia assays.

The duration of the protein loss can be estimated by checking fructosamine levels. Hypoalbuminemia and normal serum fructosamine indicate hypoalbuminemia of less than 1 week. Hypoalbuminemia and hypofructosaminemia indicate persistent hypoalbuminemia of more than 1 week, and normal albumin and hypofructosaminemia indicate recovery from either hypoalbuminemia or hypoglycemia.

Differential Diagnoses
- Bacterial enteritis
- Hepatic cirrhosis
- Hyperproteinemia
- Intestinal histoplasmosis
- Intestinal parasitism
- Maldigestion/malabsorption
- Protein-losing enteropathy
- Small bowel diarrhea

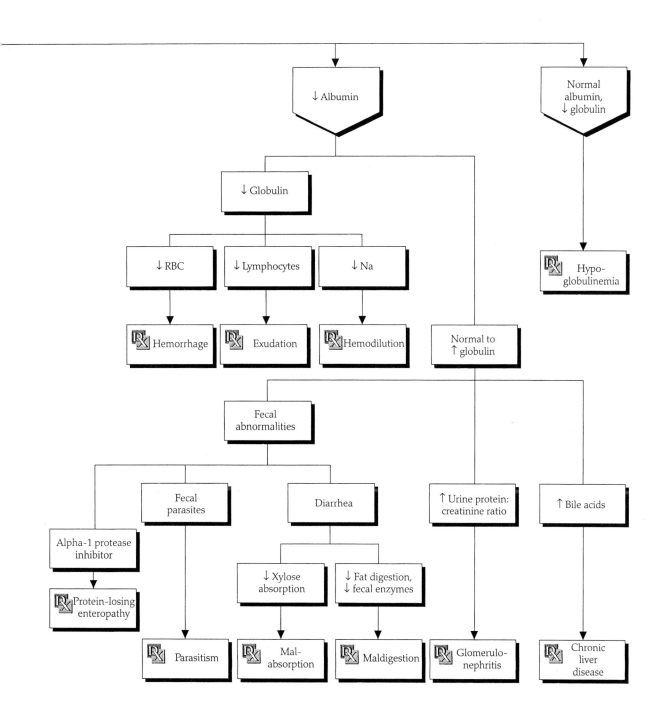

Hyperproteinemia

Total plasma protein levels above 8 g/dl indicate significant hyperproteinemia. An increased albumin level usually indicates dehydration. When albumin is normal or decreased, a high total plasma protein is usually due to increased serum globulin caused by neoplasia or an immune response.

Inflammatory hyperglobulinemia produces a polyclonal electrophoretic pattern. This pattern is seen in feline infectious peritonitis, heartworm disease, and many chronic infections. In contrast, a single peak or monoclonal pattern is characteristic of lymphosarcoma, multiple myeloma, and ehrlichiosis.

Differential Diagnoses
- Chronic inflammation
- Dehydration
- Ehrlichiosis
- Feline infectious peritonitis
- Heartworm disease
- Lymphocytic cholangitis
- Lymphosarcoma
- Myeloma
- Suppurative cholangitis

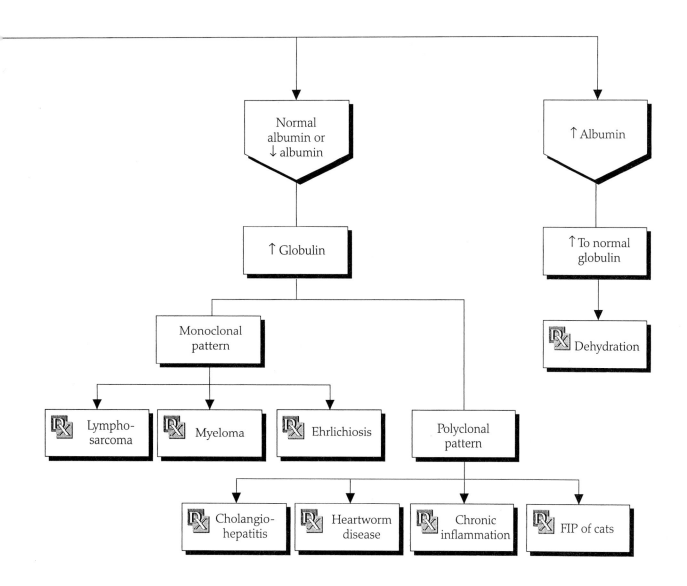

Elevated Bile Acids and Ammonia

Increased serum bile acid and ammonia levels are primarily used to diagnose seizures resulting from portosystemic vascular shunts. In young animals with seizures but no obvious liver disease, bile acids are used to check for congenital macroscopic and microscopic vascular shunts.

Bile acid levels are also increased in animals with vascular shunts secondary to hepatic disease. Temporary increases occur in acute injury. Decreasing levels suggest healing, whereas persistent levels suggest the formation of shunts secondary to hepatic fibrosis.

Animals with elevated serum bile acid or ammonia levels should be tested for active liver disease. Young animals with a congenital problem do not show laboratory signs of active liver disease. Mature animals with acquired shunts are likely to have increased serum AST activity, which indicates active liver parenchymal disease, or they may have increased serum alkaline phosphatase, GGT, and bilirubin values, which indicate portal disease.

Low levels of bile acids with high alkaline phosphatase levels would suggest steroid hepatopathy rather than cholangitis.

Differential Diagnoses
- Corticosteroid-induced hepatopathy
- Hepatic cirrhosis
- Lymphocytic cholangitis
- Portosystemic shunts
- Suppurative cholangitis

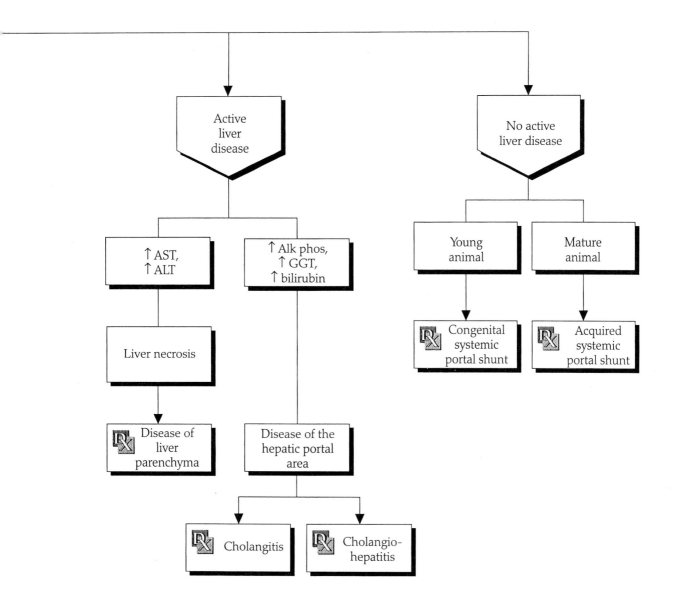

Elevated BUN and Creatinine

The BUN level is increased when the serum level is greater than 30 mg/dl. The creatinine level is increased when the serum level is greater than 2 mg/dl. Signs of uremia usually occur when the BUN exceeds 100 mg/dl. Persistently increased values of twice the normal range of the BUN and creatinine indicate significant loss of functional renal tissue.

Urinalysis can indicate whether the increased BUN and creatinine levels are due to prerenal, renal, or postrenal conditions. Urine volume is markedly decreased with kidney shutdown, a ruptured urinary bladder, or urethral obstruction.

Normal quantities of urine with a high specific gravity and normal sediment occur with prerenal problems, such as heart failure and dehydration. These prerenal problems usually cause no marked protein loss or casts in the urine.

Normal quantities of urine with a high specific gravity and active sediment occur with such renal problems as glomerulonephritis or pyelonephritis. Casts in the urine indicate active renal disease.

An increased volume of urine with a low specific gravity without casts suggests chronic renal failure. An increased volume of urine with a low specific gravity with casts suggests the diuretic phase of acute renal failure.

Differential Diagnoses
- Anuric renal failure
- Chronic renal failure
- Diuretic renal failure
- Feline urologic syndrome
- Glomerulonephritis
- Heartworm infection
- Hypoadrenocorticism
- Juvenile renal disease
- Maintenance renal failure
- Nephrotoxicosis
- NSAID-induced renal disease
- Postrenal obstruction
- Pyelonephritis
- Renal ischemia
- Uroabdomen

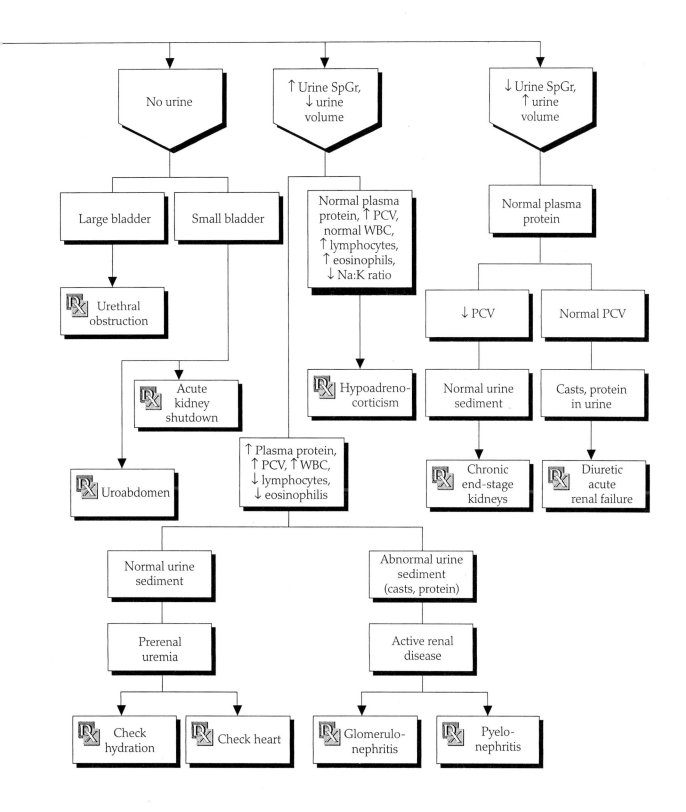

Elevated Lipase, Amylase, and Trypsin-Like Immunoreactivity

Increased serum lipase, amylase, and trypsin-like immunoreactivity (TLI) indicate pancreatitis. Activity of the enzymes also can be increased with kidney failure and upper GI inflammation, in addition to acute pancreatitis.

In some animals with pancreatitis, serum activity of lipase and amylase is normal because the enzymes have already been cleared from the blood by the time of testing. In these animals, serum alkaline phosphatase and GGT activities can be increased because of secondary cholangitis. If lipemia is present, this could indicate autodigestion of pancreatic fat by the lipase, or it could be a sign of impending pancreatitis.

Persistent elevated lipase and amylase after pancreatic disease is controlled may be due to macroenzymes. Macroenzymes can cause diagnostic errors and the performance of unnecessary tests or invasive procedures.

Serum amylase and lipase levels are of limited diagnostic value in cats. Feline specific TLI is a better test in the cat.

Differential Diagnoses
- Acute pancreatitis
- Acute renal failure
- Chronic renal failure
- Secondary hyperlipidemia

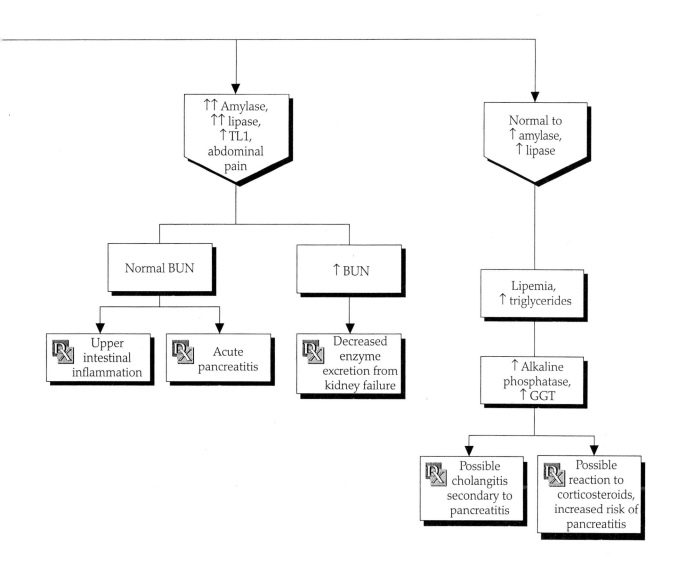

Elevated Liver Enzymes

Increased activity of liver-specific enzymes indicates acute, active liver disease. Damage to hepatic parenchymal cells is reflected by increased serum ALT and AST activities. Damage or abnormal function of the biliary system is reflected by increased serum alkaline phosphatase and GGT activities.

Primary pathogens, such as canine hepatitis virus, or secondary agents, such as parasites, intestinal bacteria, and toxins, can cause necrosis. These ascend the bile ducts or enter the liver sinusoids through the blood. Immune-mediated disease or internal disturbances that interfere with lipid, glycogen, and fluid metabolism can also damage liver cells.

Chronic liver disease causing fibrosis and vascular shunts may lead to liver failure without leakage of liver enzymes. Other tests, such as blood ammonia, bile acids, bilirubin, plasma protein, glucagon response, BSP clearance, and liver biopsy, may give more information in these cases of liver failure.

Persistent elevated ALT and AST after a liver insult may be due to macroenzymes. Macroenzymes can cause diagnostic errors and the performance of unnecessary tests or invasive procedures.

Differential Diagnoses
- Acute pancreatitis
- Acute toxic hepatitis
- Cholangitis/cholangiohepatitis
- Chronic toxic hepatitis
- Copper toxicosis
- Corticosteroid-induced hepatopathy
- Hepatic lipidosis
- Hepatic tumors
- Hyperadrenocorticism
- Septicemia, endotoxemia

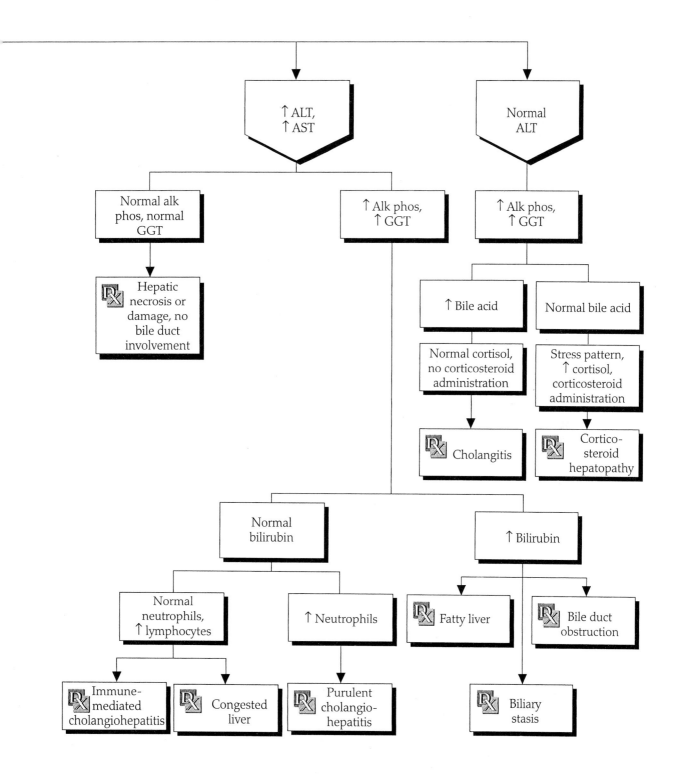

Hypokalemia

Hypokalemia is a serum potassium concentration below 3.6 mEq/L. Potassium depletion is usually due to excessive loss of potassium in the urine or stool. Potassium is lost in the urine with cortisol excess, diuretic administration, osmotic diuresis, and renal tubular disease. This may be confirmed by demonstrating increased fractional excretion of potassium despite low serum levels. Gastrointestinal losses are due to diarrhea or vomiting.

Transfer of extracellular potassium into cells may also cause hypokalemia, as in the administration of insulin to patients with diabetes mellitus and in animals with acute alkalosis.

Hypokalemia can be caused by decreased potassium intake during periods of anorexia or by ingestion of acidified potassium-deficient foods. In sick animals, this is likely to occur when potassium-poor fluids, such as saline or glucose, are administered. In healthy cats, this is likely to occur when acidified potassium-deficient foods are fed to decrease urolithiasis.

Differential Diagnoses
- Diabetes mellitus
- Diarrhea
- Diuretic renal failure
- Fluid administration
- Insulin administration
- Vomiting
- Hypokalemic nephropathy

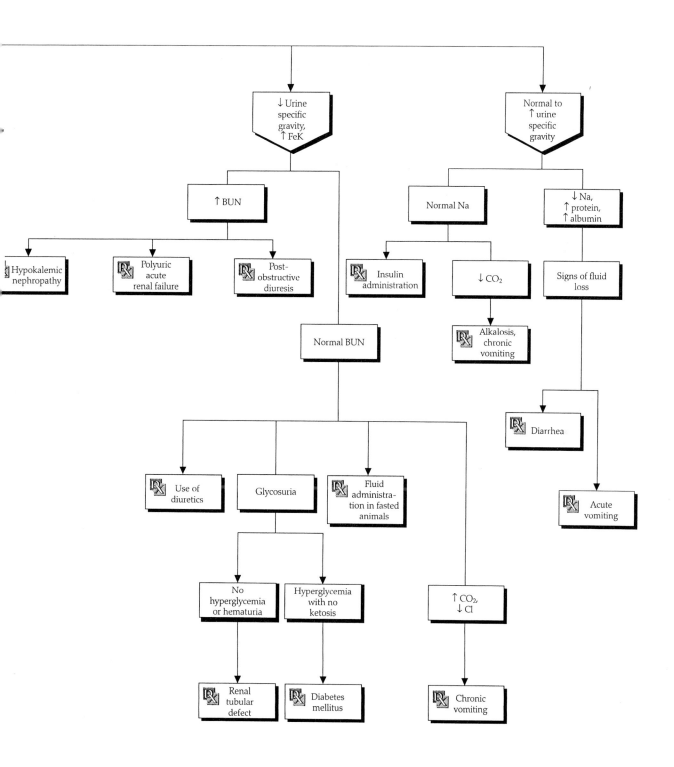

Hyperkalemia

Hyperkalemia is a serum potassium concentration greater than 5.6 mEq/L. Increased serum potassium is usually caused by decreased urinary excretion of potassium. It is occasionally caused by excessive administration of drugs (potassium chloride or potassium penicillin) in a hospitalized animal or by translocation from the intracellular space.

Renal elimination of potassium is usually decreased with oliguric renal failure, terminal chronic renal failure, urethral obstruction and uroabdomen. Potassium excretion is also decreased with hypoadrenocorticism and the administration of aldosterone inhibitors, such as spironolactone. Potassium is redistributed from cells to the serum in acidosis, massive crushing injuries, or thrombocytosis.

Differential Diagnoses
- Acidosis
- Anuric renal failure
- Dehydration
- Hypoadrenocorticism
- Postrenal obstruction
- Uroabdomen

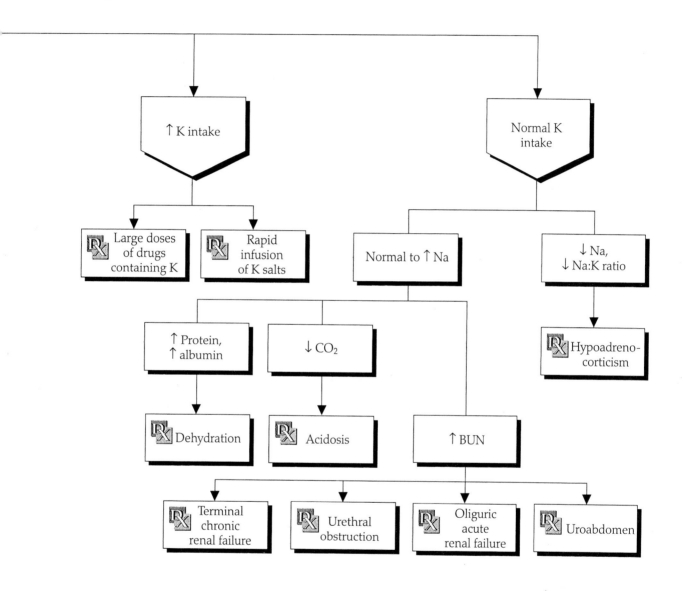

Section 10
Diagnosis by Clinical Signs

Weakness

Weakness may be continuous or episodic. *Continuous weakness* refers to generalized lack of energy, with muscle fatigue or fainting. *Episodic weakness* occurs with exercise and lessens with rest. Signs include ataxia, paresis, panting, reluctance to rise or walk, and collapse.

The blood panel and special laboratory tests can reveal the five broad categories of disease that cause weakness. Blood tests may disclose inflammatory conditions, nutritional disorders, some causes of hypoxemia, some muscle diseases, and many metabolic diseases. Special tests are required to diagnose cardiovascular and neuromuscular diseases.

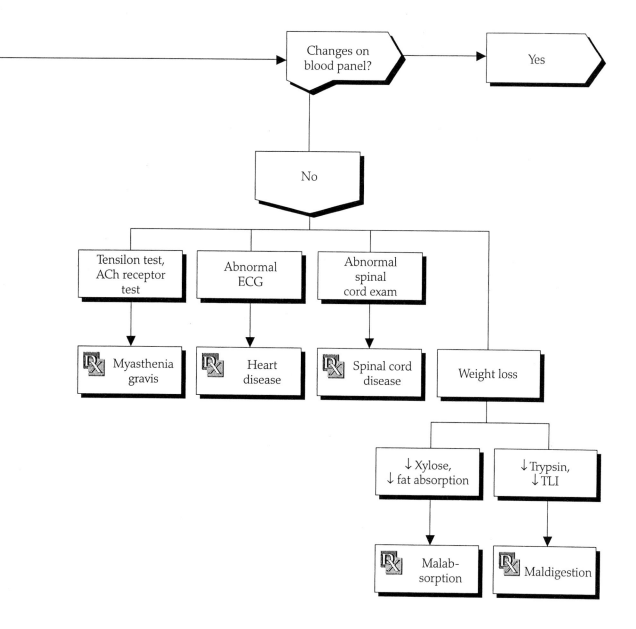

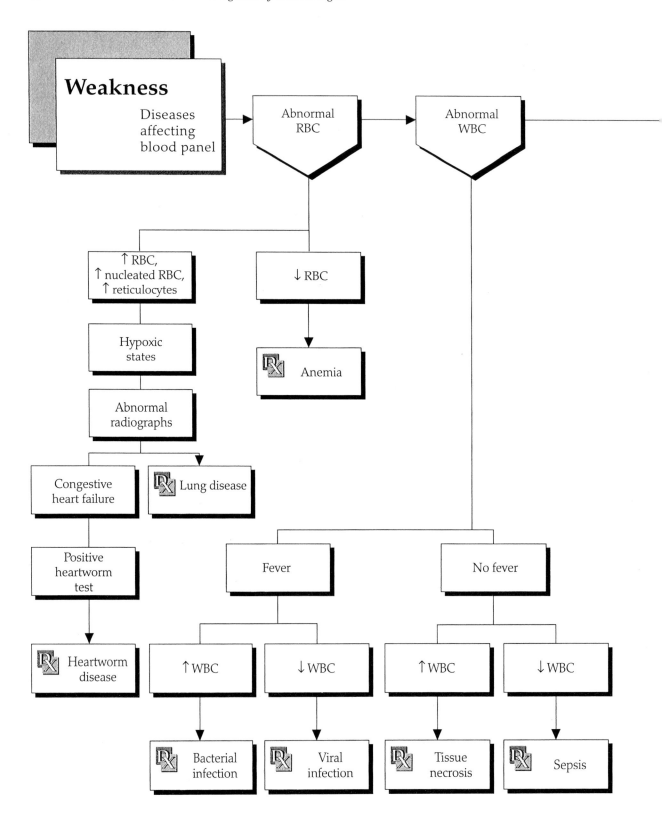

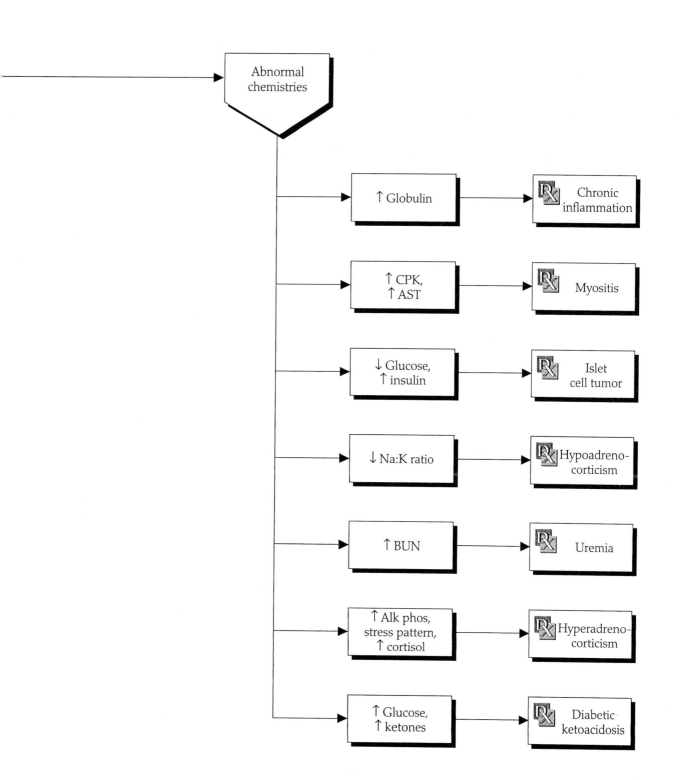

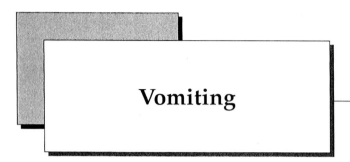

Vomiting

Vomiting is a complex reflex that ejects gastric contents back up the esophagus and out of the mouth. It is regulated by the emetic center in the medulla via pathways from the viscera, vestibular apparatus, higher CNS centers, and the chemoreceptor trigger zone.

The serum chemistry panel and hemogram can disclose some of the diseases that cause vomiting, but many causes of vomiting do not cause blood abnormalities. The serum chemistry panel and hemogram screen for diseases of the pancreas, kidneys, liver, and adrenal glands, as well as concurrent inflammation or infection.

For best results, blood studies should be combined with survey radiographs. New tests, such as the sucrose absorption/excretion test, provide a noninvasive way of evaluating stomach erosion or ulceration.

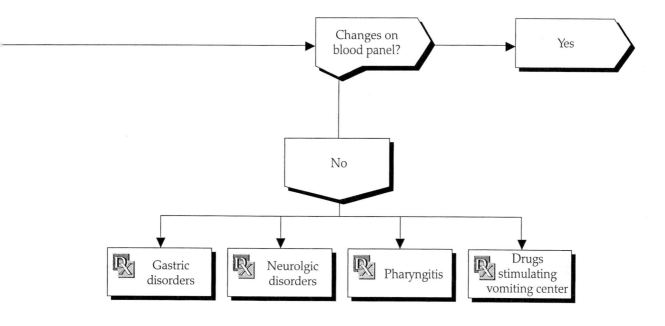

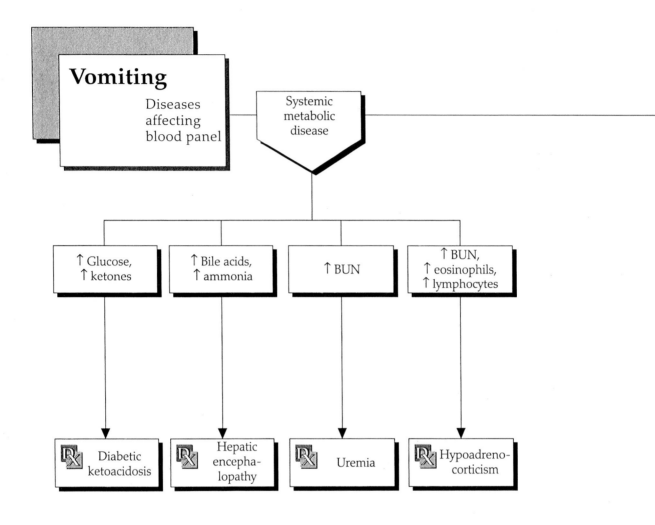

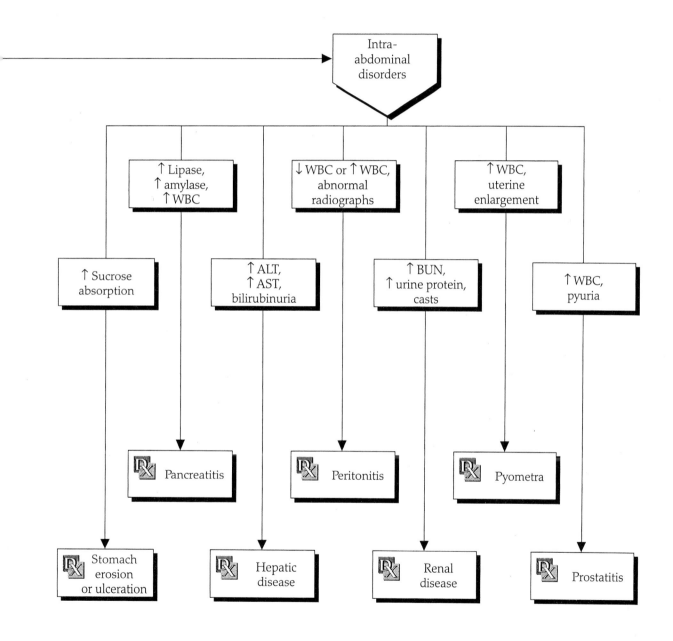

Seizures

Seizures are episodes of excessive neuronal discharge that produce uncontrolled muscular activity.

Epilepsy refers to recurrent episodes of loss of consciousness, abnormal motor signs, or convulsions.

Grand mal seizures are characterized by generalized tonic-clonic muscular activity.

Focal seizures involving limited areas of the brain can cause behavioral changes, such as aggression, fly biting, tail chasing, or movements of a limited muscle group.

Seizures can be caused by intracranial disease, extracranial disease, or unknown factors (idiopathic). Of these categories, extracranial metabolic diseases are best disclosed by the blood panel.

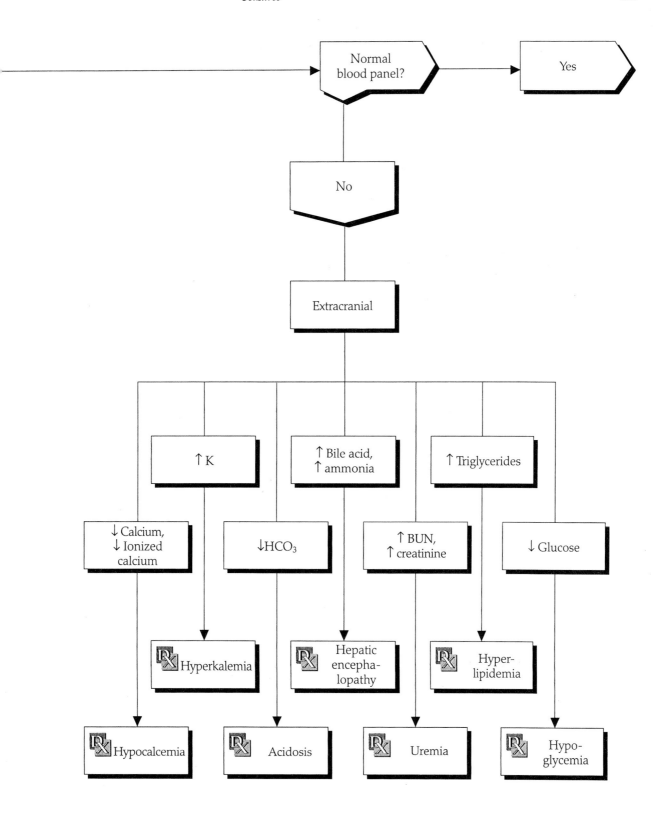

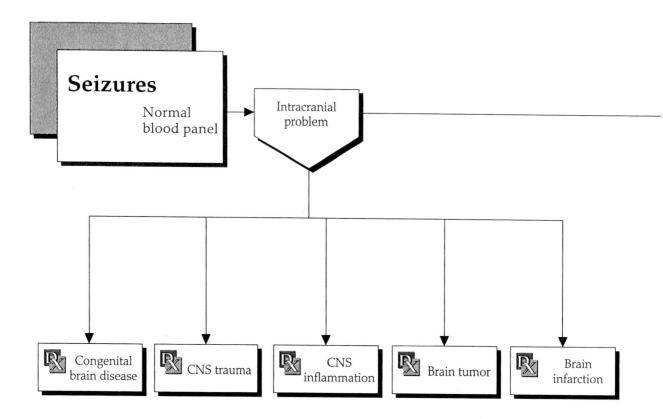

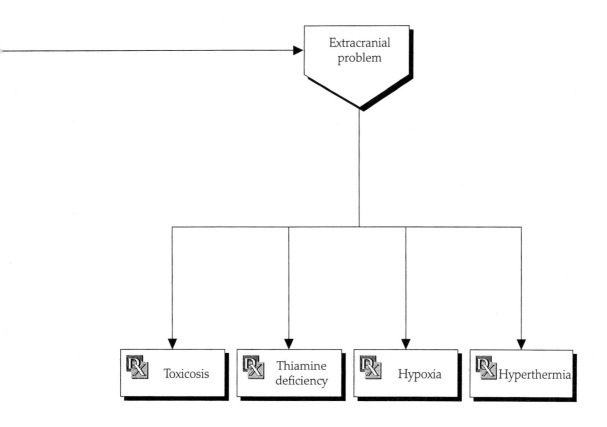

Polyuria, Polydipsia

Polyuria is the excretion of large volumes of urine. *Polydipsia* is the intake of large volumes of water.

Normal daily water intake in dogs is less than 50 ml/lb (110 ml/kg). Normal daily urine production is 25 ml/lb (55 ml/kg).

Variation of antidiuretic hormone (ADH, vasopressin) secretion and regulation of water intake maintain water balance in the body. ADH release is governed by change in extracellular fluid osmolality and blood volume, whereas thirst is regulated by plasma osmolality and blood volume.

Many diseases affect water intake. The blood panel and urinalysis screen for abnormalities in the kidney, liver, adrenal gland, and glucose metabolism.

Very early kidney damage causes polyuria. This is suggested by lipid abnormalities and special urine tests such as urine GGT and increased urine fractional excretion of sodium.

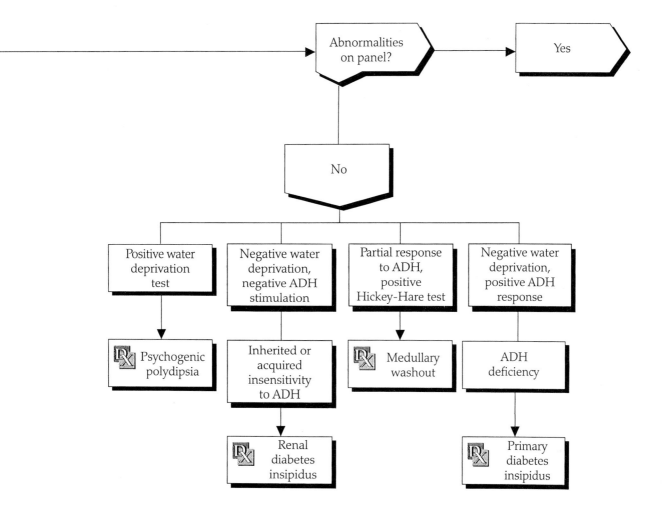

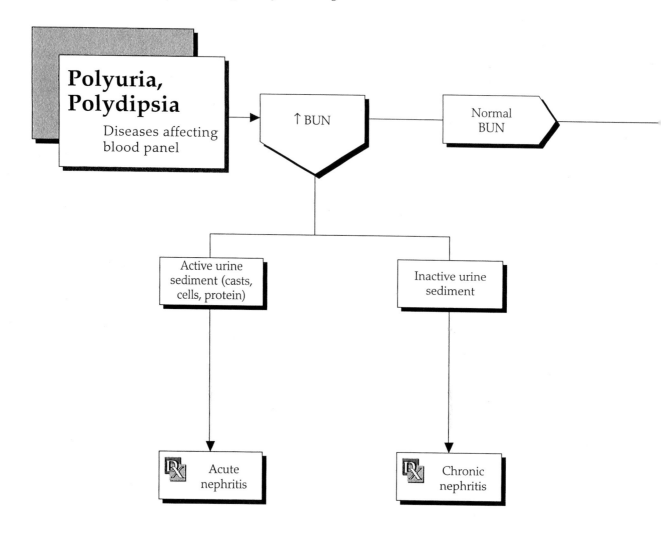

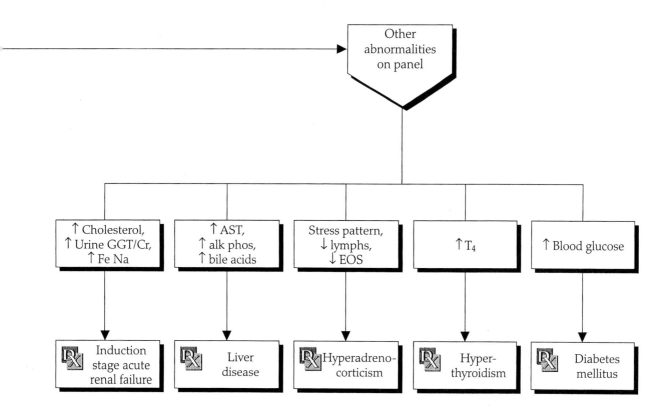

Jaundice

Jaundice (icterus) is a yellow discoloration of tissues or plasma caused by increased levels of bilirubin. *Hyperbilirubinemia* does not cause jaundice until bilirubin values reach 2 mg/dl.

Bilirubin occurs in *unconjugated* (prehepatic) or *conjugated* (hepatic) forms. The skin and urine are discolored by water-soluble conjugated bilirubin. Fatty tissue is stained by lipid-soluble unconjugated bilirubin.

Elevated bilirubin levels can be detected before jaundice becomes evident using chemical tests on blood and urine. Bilirubinuria is a sensitive sign of liver disease in cats.

Hemolysis, extrahepatic biliary obstruction, and hepatic disease can produce hyperbilirubinemia.

Hemolytic anemia increases levels of unconjugated (indirect) bilirubin. Unconjugated bilirubin is not passed in the urine but the dog conjugates bilirubin in its renal tubules and may have bilirubinuria.

Cholestasis is an intrahepatic cause of hyperbilirubinemia. Bilirubin enters the circulation directly from the hepatocytes and bile canaliculi. Extrahepatic biliary obstruction may be transient or chronic. Pancreatitis or enteritis can transiently obstruct the bile duct. Tumors, strictures, trauma, or foreign objects also may occlude the bile duct.

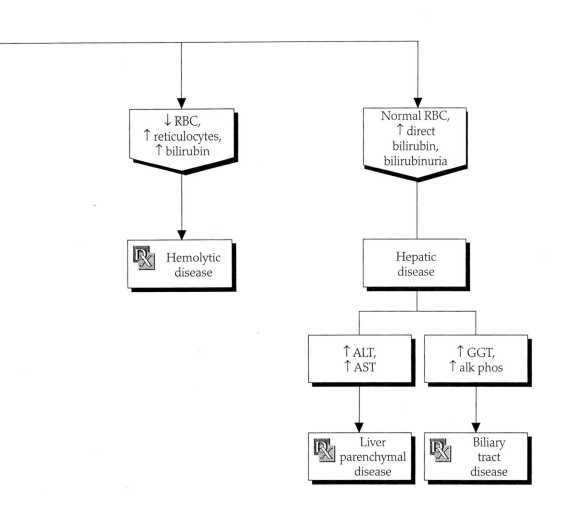

Elevated Body Temperature

Fever is an elevation of body temperature (102° F to 106° F) caused by pyogens produced by disease. Vasoconstriction, shivering, and heat seeking increase the body temperature.

Hyperthermia is an increase in body temperature (>106° F) caused by dysfunction of physiologic mechanisms of heat loss or a lesion of the thermoregulatory center in the hypothalamus. Hyperthermia is not caused by chemical mediators.

The blood panel is used to screen for infection, thyroid disease, tissue necrosis, or alterations in serum proteins. Serologic tests can be used to screen for autoantibodies or antibodies against infectious agents. Neoplasia is suggested by a leukocytosis with a right shift (hypersegmented neutrophils).

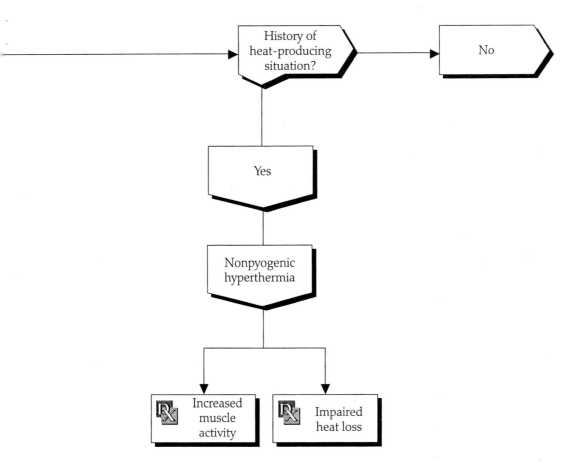

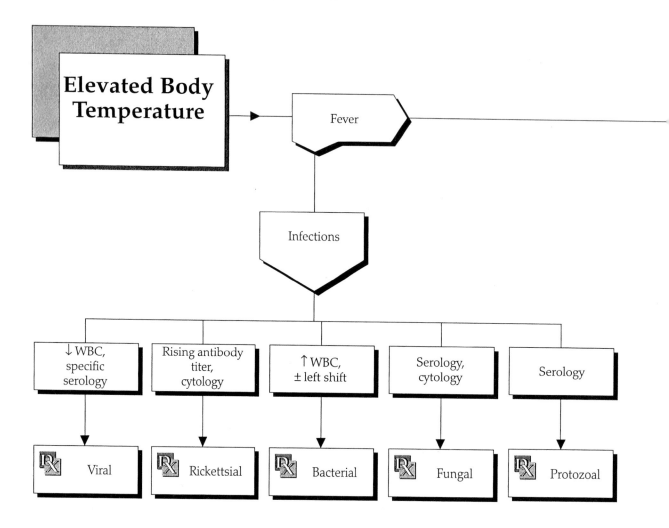

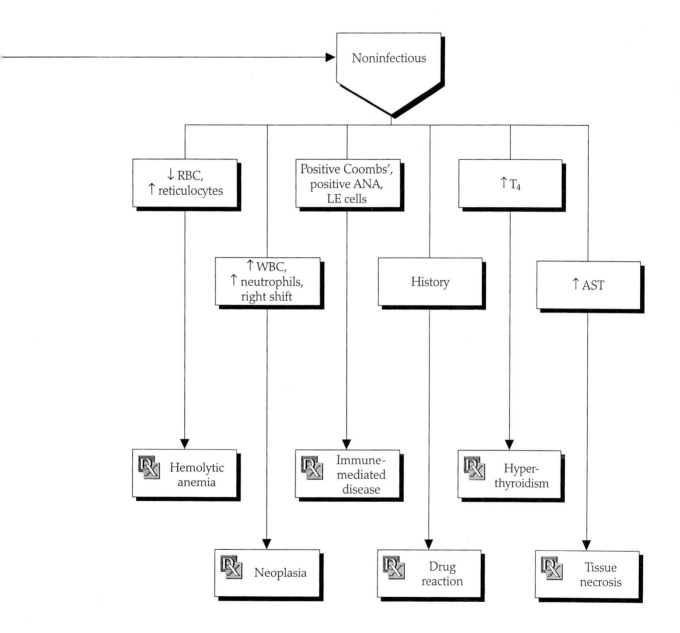

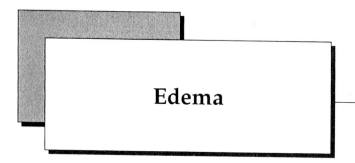

Edema

Edema is an abnormal volume of fluid in the extracellular space. It usually refers to subcutaneous fluid, unless the organ is identified, as in pulmonary edema.

Effusion of fluid into body cavities has specific names. *Ascites* is accumulation of serous fluid within the peritoneal cavity. *Pericardial* or *pleural effusions* refer to fluid accumulation within the pericardial sac or thoracic cavity.

Edema can be caused by increased capillary hydrostatic pressure, decreased plasma oncotic pressure, increased capillary permeability, or decreased lymphatic flow. The blood panel only demonstrates decreased plasma oncotic pressure related to hypoproteinemia.

Common causes of edema with hypoproteinemia are glomerular disease, intestinal parasitism, hepatic cirrhosis, protein-losing enteropathy, and starvation.

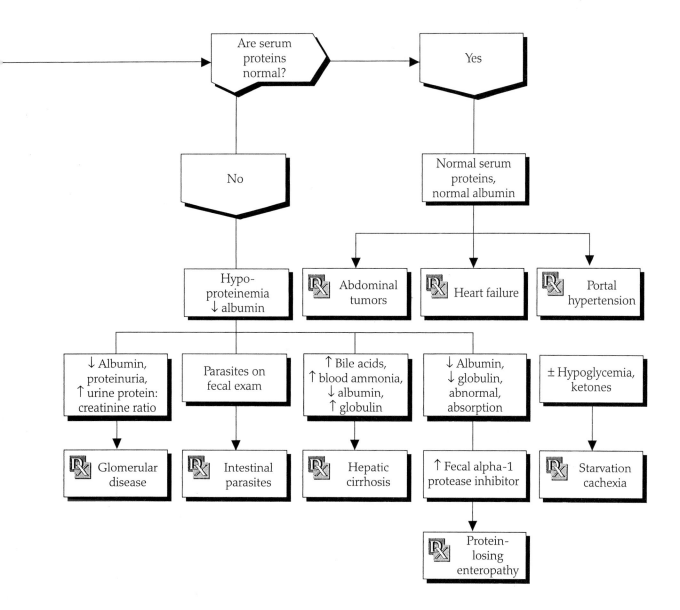

Abdominal Effusions

Abdominal fluids can be blood, chyle, a transudate, a modified exudate, or an exudate. Hemorrhage into a body cavity has a similar consistency to circulating blood but does not clot. RBCs secondary to inflammation usually has a PCV <8%. Blood secondary to traumatic sampling usually clots.

Chyle is rarely found in the abdomen. When present it is pink to white with a triglyceride content greater than the serum and cholesterol less than serum.

Transudates contain <1000 cells/μl, protein <2.5 g/dl, and a specific gravity <1.017. Exudates have protein >3g/dl, a specific gravity >1.025, and often a high WBC count. Modified transudates have a protein content between 2 to 3 g with more mononuclear cells and sometimes RBCs.

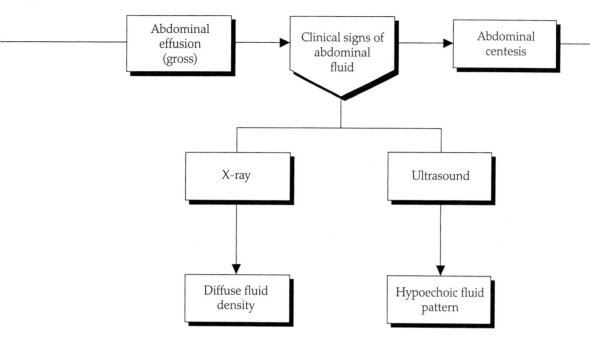

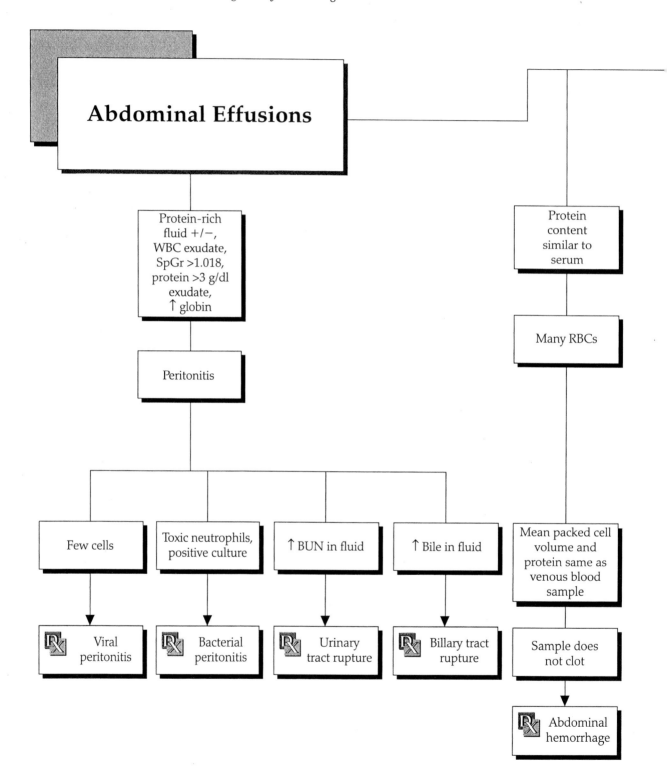

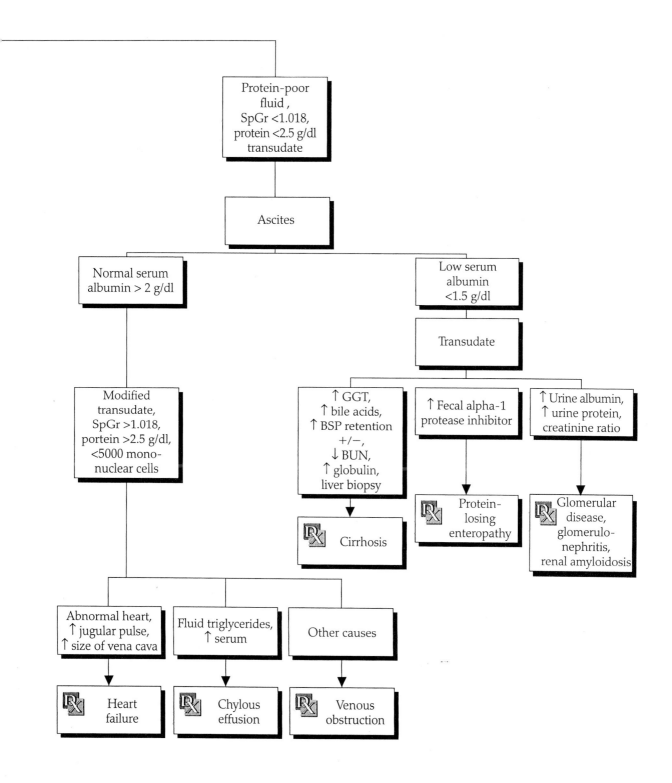

Small Intestine Diarrhea

High-Volume

Diarrhea is a common sign of intestinal disease. The feces become more fluid and voluminous and are passed more frequently. Small bowel diarrhea is characterized by a slight increase in frequency of defecation and a marked increase in volume, flatulence, and borborygmi. Acute diarrhea caused by dietary indiscretions, infectious disease, intoxications, and intestinal obstructions resolves within 4 weeks. It is usually self-limiting or responsive to standard treatment. Chronic diarrhea persists longer than 4 weeks.

The mechanisms producing diarrhea are osmotic, exudative, secretory, or hypermotility. Because the cause of diarrhea is often unknown, identifying the underlying mechanism may help guide treatment.

Dietary overload and malabsorption cause *osmotic diarrhea.*

Mucosal inflammation or erosions and lymphatic hypertension cause *exudative diarrhea.* These increase the gut mucosa's permeability to water, proteins, and electrolytes.

Many agents, such as bacterial endotoxins and deconjugated bile salts, cause *secretory diarrhea.* These agents activate cyclic AMP, increase secretion of chloride, and decrease absorption of sodium to produce watery stools.

Diseases or agents that diminish segmental contractions cause *hypermotility diarrhea.*

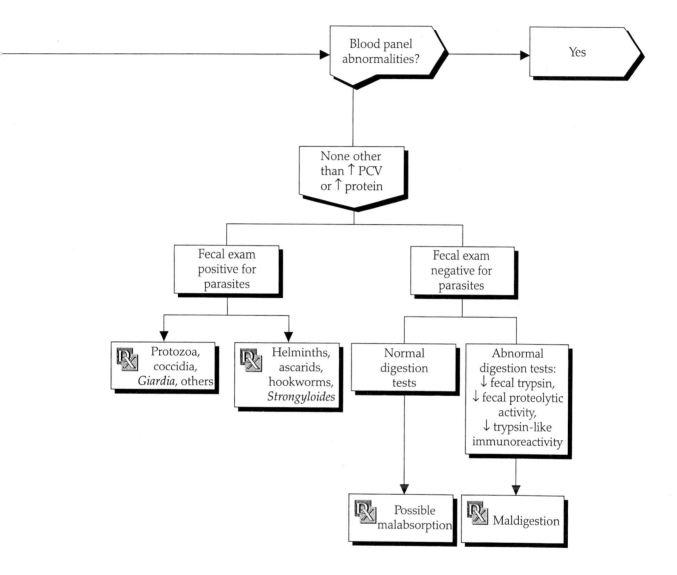

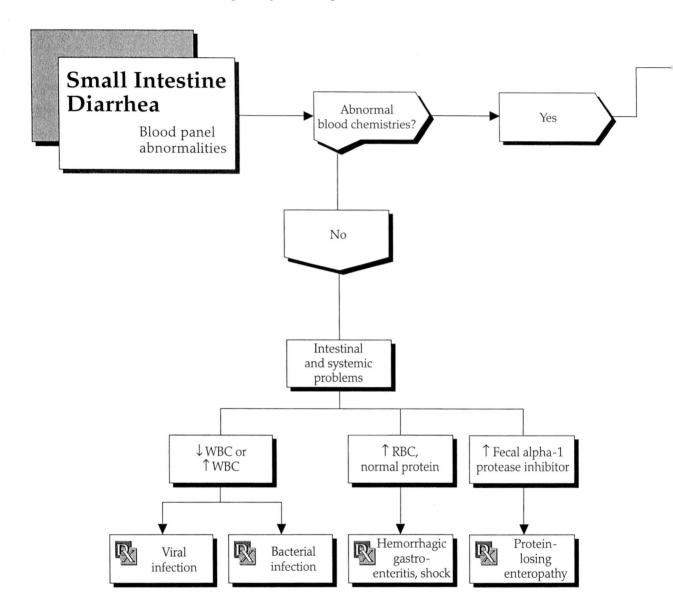

Small Intestine Diarrhea

Blood panel abnormalities

Abnormal blood chemistries?

Yes

No

Intestinal and systemic problems

↓ WBC or ↑ WBC

↑ RBC, normal protein

↑ Fecal alpha-1 protease inhibitor

Viral infection

Bacterial infection

Hemorrhagic gastro-enteritis, shock

Protein-losing enteropathy

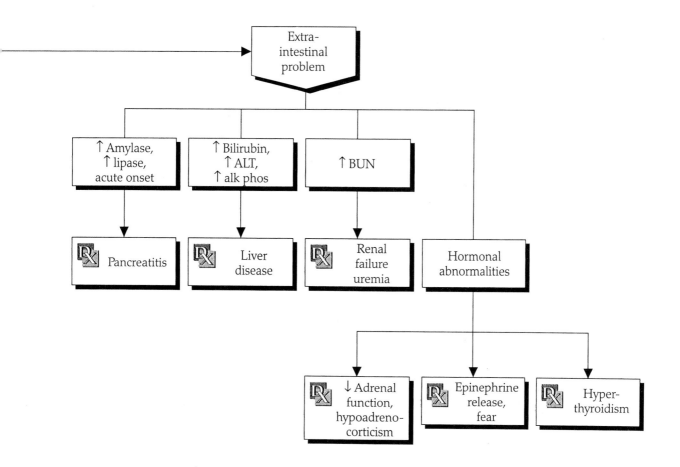

Large Intestine Diarrhea

High-Frequency, Low-Volume

Diseases of the cecum, colon, and rectum cause *large intestine diarrhea*. The principal signs are tenesmus and frequent passage of small amounts of feces with mucus and blood.

The blood panel is used to look for concurrent disease, such as infection, liver disease, kidney failure, and dehydration, but the panel rarely discloses the cause.

The cause of large intestine diarrhea is more likely to be found by direct examination of the feces for inflammation, infection, digestive enzymes, and parasites, or by evaluation of the intestinal wall by radiography, endoscopy, or biopsy.

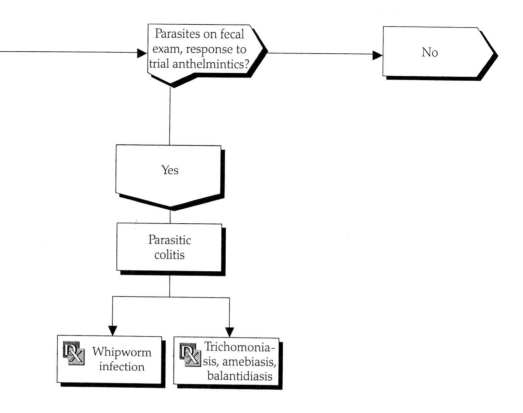

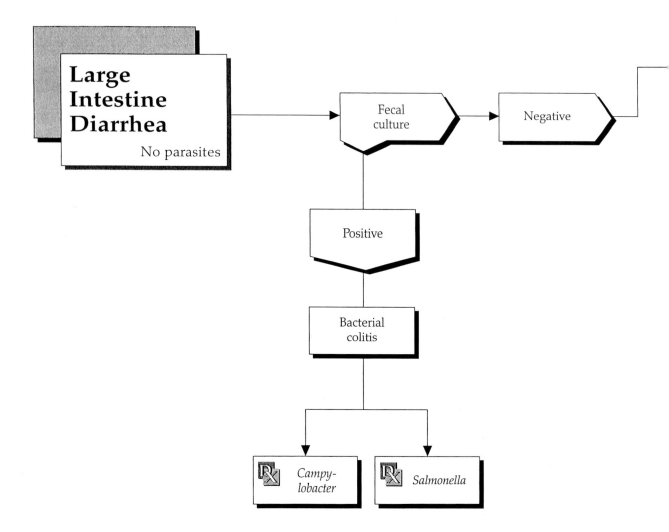

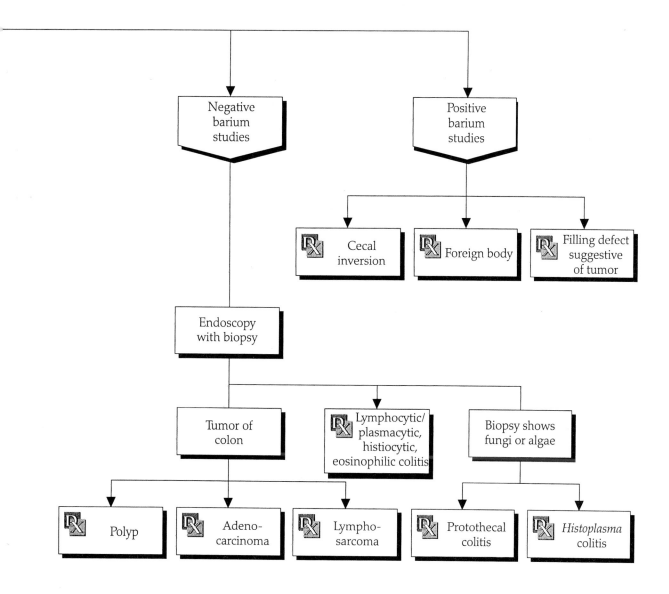

Abnormal Bleeding

Spontaneous bleeding occurs when the vascular system is damaged or when hemostatic mechanisms fail. Toenail bleeding time, activated clotting time, platelet counts, and platelet function tests can be used in the veterinary hospital to screen for coagulation defects. PIVKA clotting time is a more sensitive in-hospital test for detection of bleeding tendencies. Other sensitive tests, such as one-step prothrombin time and partial thromboplastin time, can be performed by reference laboratories. If these are negative, tests for individual coagulation factors are necessary. Deficiencies have been reported for factors VII, VIII, IX, X, XI, and XIII.

Thrombocytopenia can be due to increased platelet destruction, which is indicated by increased platelet factor 3 and increased platelet bound immunoglobulins. A bone marrow examination may show increased megakaryocytes indicating an active response to increased platelet consumption or decreased megakaryocytes. Immune megakaryocyte destruction is confirmed by IFA testing that shows increased megakaryocyte fluorescence.

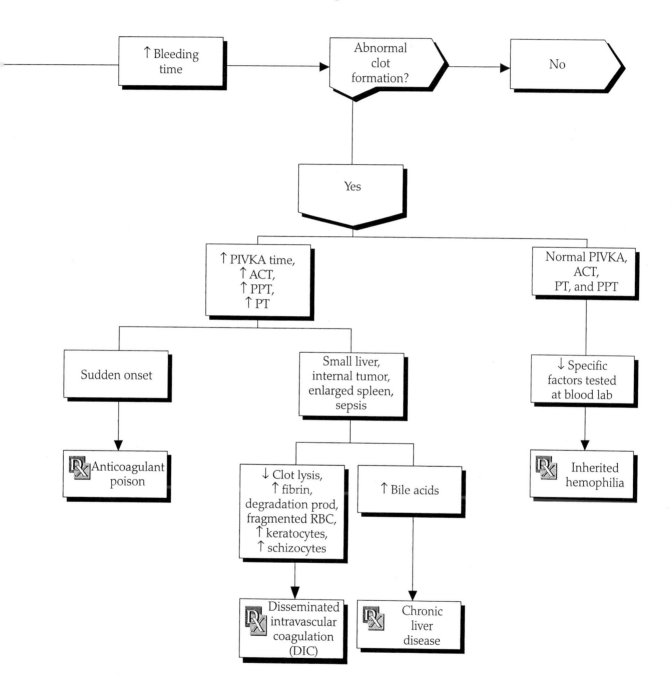

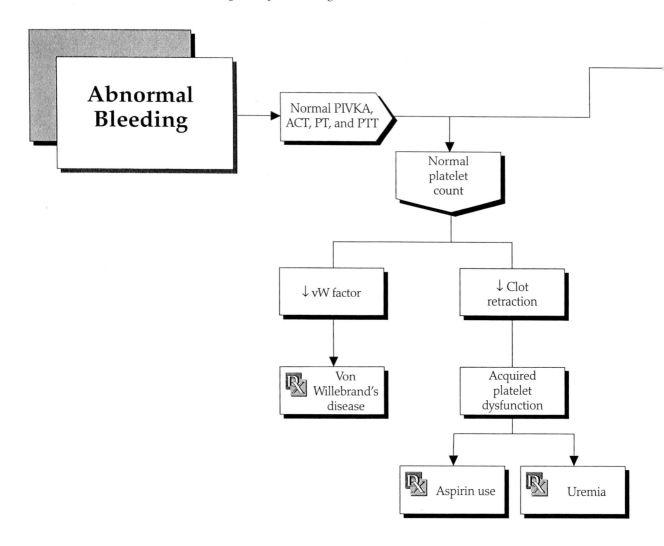

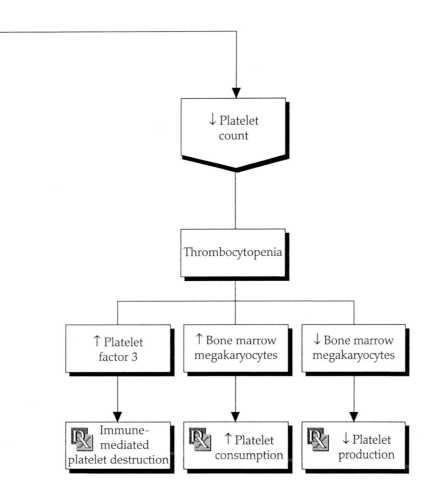

Hematuria

Hematuria can be caused by a coagulation defect or diseases of the genitourinary tract. The site of bleeding can be localized to the kidneys, urerthra, or bladder by obtaining urine samples by cystocentesis, bladder catheterization, and free-catch of urine. True *hematuria* must be distinguished from *hemoglobinuria* and *myoglobinuria.*

The severity of the problem can be judged from its effects on the hemogram. Chronic blood loss can produce anemia with signs of bone marrow response, whereas acute blood loss may show no response for 3 days.

Urinalysis can disclose concurrent infection, tumor cells, and casts. Cytologic examination of urine may show cells suggesting the site of origin, such as the bladder or prostate gland.

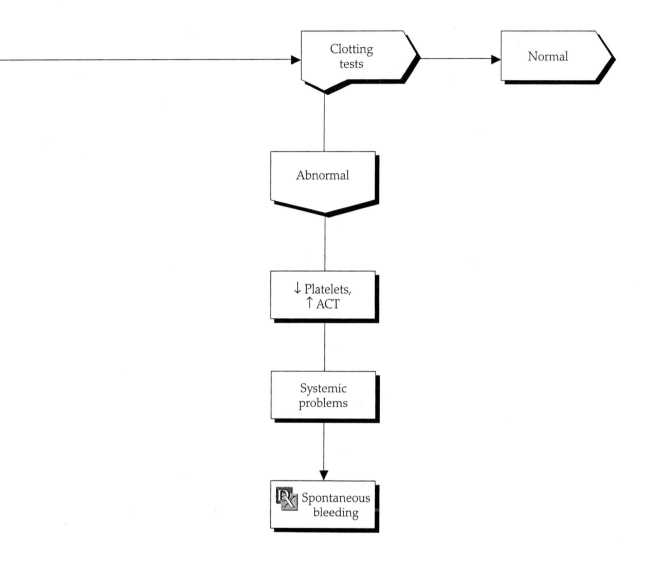

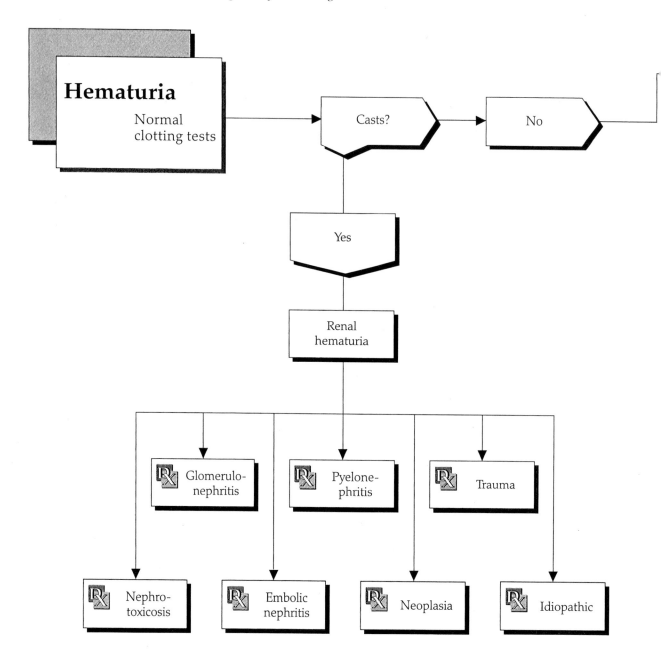

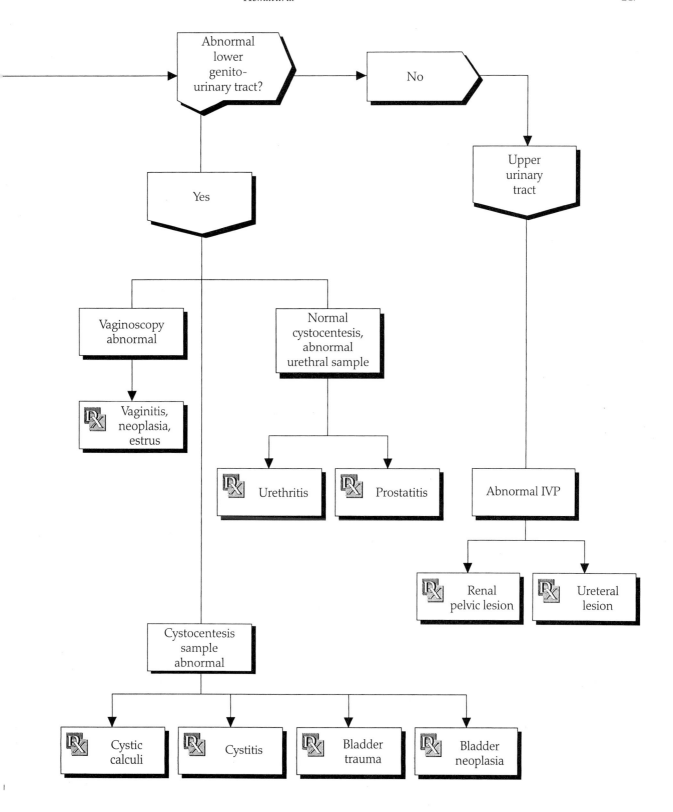

Lipemia

Lipemia is a form of hyperlipidemia characterized by increased serum triglyceride levels. Lipemic blood is pale, resembling tomato soup.

Chylomicrons are the circulating form of dietary triglycerides that can persist in the serum for 14 hours after a meal *(postprandial lipemia). Very-low-density lipoproteins (VLDLs)* are the circulating form of triglycerides synthesized in the liver. They cause the lipemia of fasted animals. Insufficient lipoprotein lipase causes persistence of VLDLs *(pathologic lipemia).*

The *chylomicron test* detects postprandial lipemia. The *heparin test* screens for deficiency of lipoprotein lipase. The *blood panel* may disclose diabetes mellitus, acute pancreatitis, hypothyroidism, or cortisol excess, with accompanying hyperlipidemia of disease.

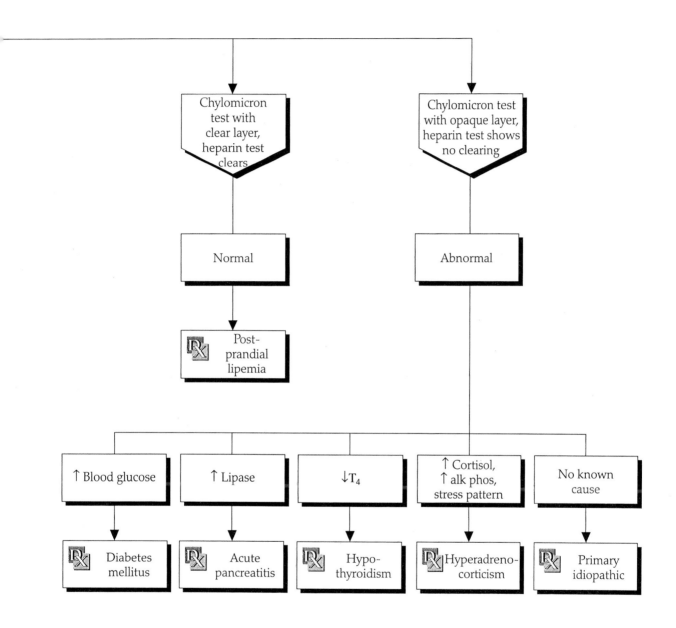

Splenomegaly

Lymphoreticular hyperplasia, hemorrhage, congestion, infection, or neoplastic infiltration can cause splenic enlargement *(splenomegaly)*. Splenomegaly can be detected by palpation, radiography, or ultrasonography.

Reticuloendothelial hyperplasia, causing uniform enlargement, is usually secondary to alterations in RBCs that cause their early removal from circulation. RBCs can be prematurely removed from circulation because of toxic changes (Heinz bodies), parasites *(Babesia, Hemobartonella)*, congenital abnormalities (pyruvate kinase deficiency), or clumping of cells from antibody attachment. The blood panel shows regenerative anemia and thrombocytopenia.

Intrasplenic hemorrhage causes an irregular enlargement, with regenerative anemia, reticulocytosis, and nucleated RBCs. Ultrasonography can reveal irregular splenic enlargement with cavitation.

Secondary splenic congestion in shock, heart failure, or portal hypertension produces a regular enlargement, with hemoconcentration rather than anemia.

Splenic infections or *metastatic tumors* can cause leukocytosis. These are best diagnosed with ultrasound-guided biopsy to allow fine-needle aspiration and cytologic examination.

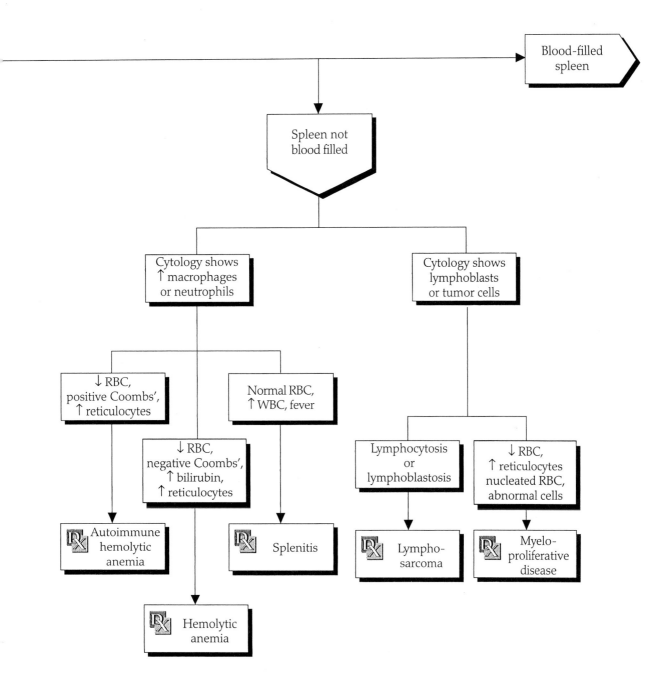

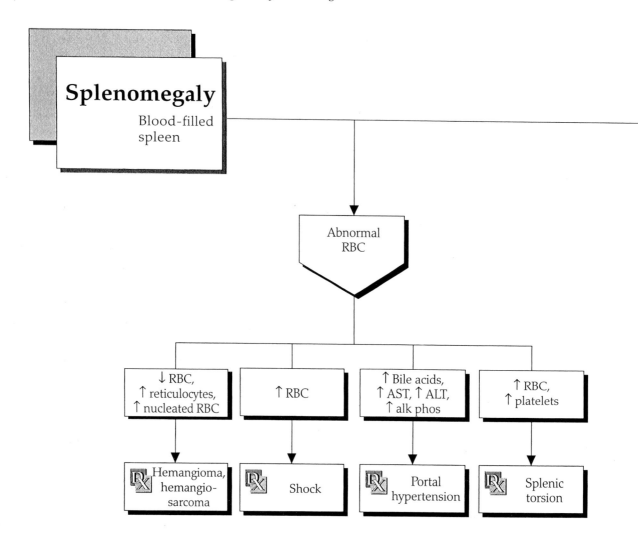

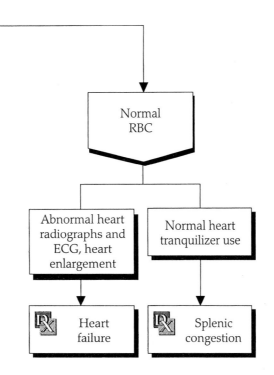

Lymphadenopathy

Normal lymph nodes contain >80% small lymphocytes, with occasional macrophages, large lymphocytes, and plasma cells.

Lymphadenopathy refers to an abnormal size or consistency of a lymph node. A soft, enlarged lymph node suggests abscessation, necrosis, or hemorrhage. A firm, enlarged lymph node suggests hyperplasia or neoplasia. Cytologic examination of the node can determine the cause of lymphadenopathy.

Reactive Conditions

Hyperplasia is a proliferation of normal lymphoid cells from immunologic stimulation, such as vaccinations. Cytologic examination shows a mixture of small lymphocytes, large lymphocytes, and plasma cells.

Lymphadenitis is characterized by infiltration with neutrophils or macrophages. These are drawn to the node by foreign material, bacteria, or fungi. This reaction can be suppurative (neutrophils), granulomatous (macrophages), or pyogranulomatous (mixture of neutrophils and macrophages). Cytologic examination shows increased numbers of neutrophils and macrophages.

Infiltrative Conditions

Nonneoplastic infiltrates from regional skin or mucous membranes can fill the lymph node with red blood cells, mast cells, eosinophils, or pigment-laden macrophages. Cytologic examination shows a mixture of neutrophils, small lymphocytes, and migrating cells.

Neoplastic infiltrates can be caused by lymphosarcoma or metastatic carcinoma, melanomas, or sarcomas. Cytologic examination shows the primary tumor cells. With lymphosarcoma, there is a uniform population of poorly staining lymphoblasts.

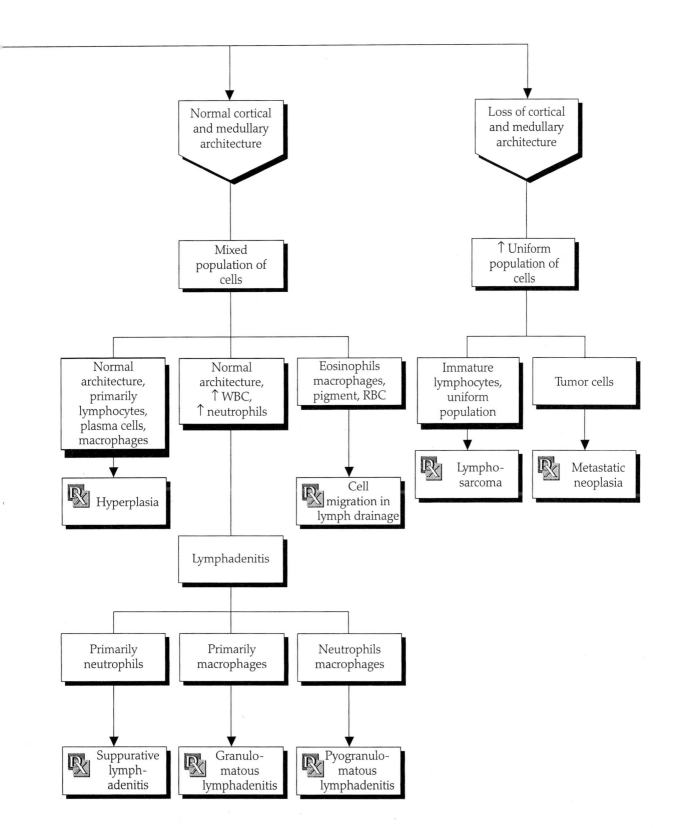

Decreased Bone Density

Such terms as *osteopenia, osteoporosis,* and *osteomalacia* refer to atrophy of bone.

Osteopenia is a radiographic term that includes both *osteoporosis* (atrophy with decreased quantities of normal mineralized bone) and *osteomalacia* (decreased mineralization of bone). Bone density must be reduced by at least 50% before generalized osteopenia can be recognized on radiographs.

Causes of generalized osteopenia include primary hyperparathyroidism, renal secondary hyperparathyroidism, nutritional secondary hyperparathyroidism, hyperadrenocorticism, and disuse atrophy. Tumors, osteitis, and periosteal inflammation cause localized osteopenia.

Disuse causes localized atrophy of several bones in a region. Vascularized lesions cause focal atrophy of bone.

When the serum phosphorus is normal, increased fractional excretion of phosphorus suggests hyperparathyroidism. When the Cl:P ratio is >33, hypercalcemia is more likely due to hyperparathyroidism than by pseudohyperparathyroidism.

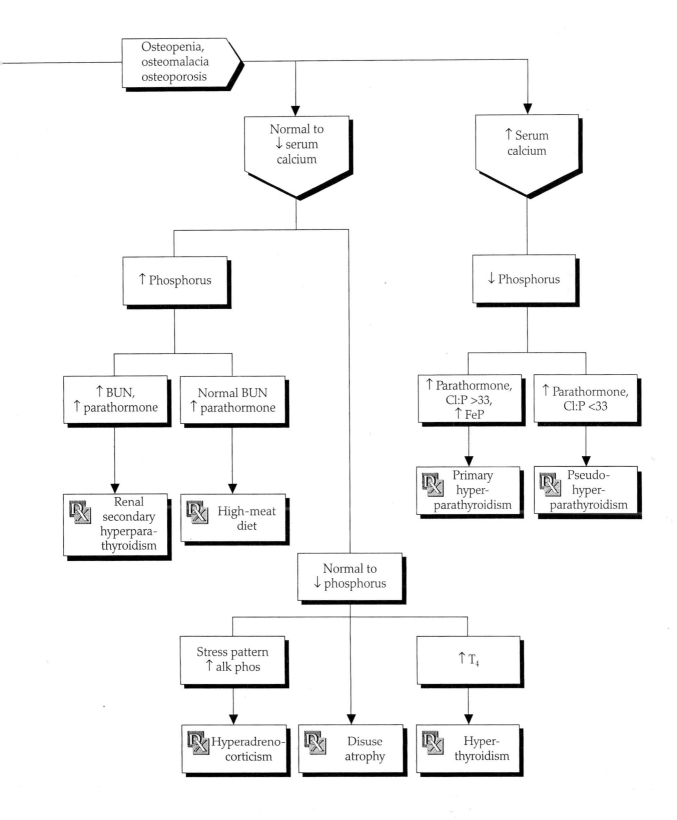

Section 11
Dynamic Testing

Acute Renal Failure

Acute renal failure (ARF) is an abrupt reduction in the glomerular filtration rate manifested by a rise in the plasma creatinine, a rise in the BUN, and a fall in the daily urine volume. It is often caused by an ischemic or toxic insult. Glomerular disease, tubular-interstitial disease, and hypotension are common mechanisms that cause this abrupt reduction in glomerular filtration rate. Clinically, these pathogenic processes are associated with proteinuria, casts, enzymuria, or alterations in the fractional excretion of electrolytes.

Acute renal damage goes through three stages. The induction phase is the time between the renal insult and the development of azotemia. Detection of this stage is important because proper therapy at this time can prevent lethal tubular damage. The maintenance phase occurs when the individual nephrons develop irreversible damage from tubular backleak, vasoconstriction, and decreased glomerular capillary permeability. Therapy at this stage may be lifesaving but does not reverse the renal damage. The recovery phase is associated with some nephron repair, if the basement membrane is intact, and hypertrophy. If 20% of kidney function remains, the animal is able to survive.

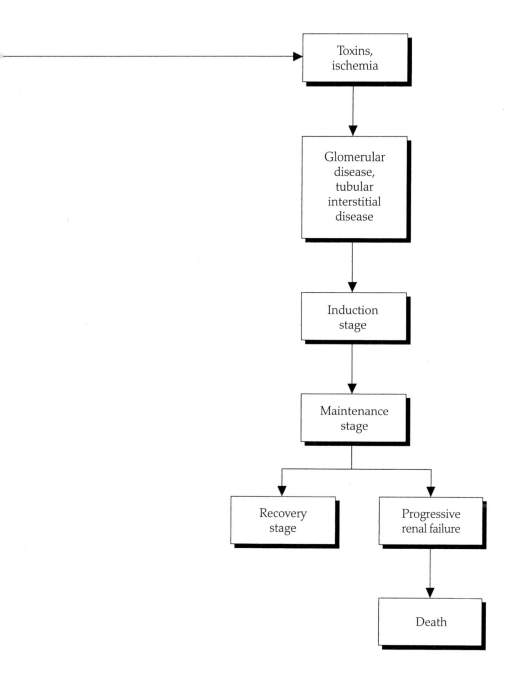

Induction Stage of Acute Renal Failure

The induction stage of acute renal failure is the time from renal insult to development of decreased urine-concentrating capacity and azotemia. Cell damage may be sublethal; however, increasing numbers of tubular epithelial cells sustain lethal injury if intervention is delayed. Early intervention allows the tubular cells to recover and maintain a functional nephron. Clinical detection of the induction phase of ARF is difficult because the clinical signs are vague. Often there is only listlessness with an acute onset of polyuria and polydipsia.

The blood changes are minimal, with only a rise in lipid and cholesterol. The BUN and creatinine are normal. Urine samples taken over a period of time will show a progressive increase in glucosuria, proteinuria, enzymuria, and eventually casts. Key tests for diagnosis are an increased urine GGT:Cr ratio caused by tubular epithelial cell necrosis and an increased fractional excretion of sodium caused by the breakdown of intercellular tight junctions.

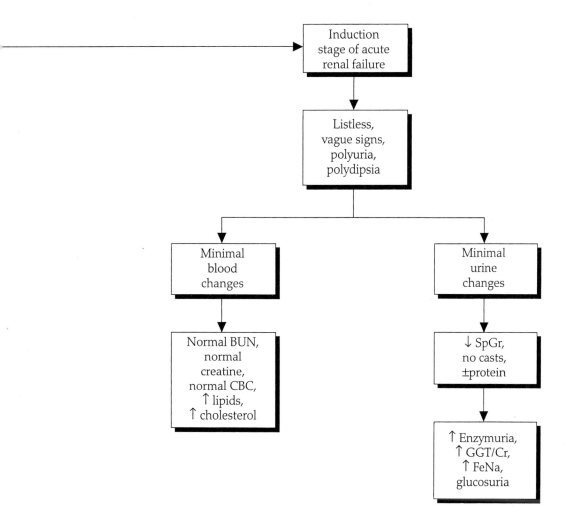

Maintenance Stage of Acute Renal Failure

The maintenance stage of acute renal failure refers to a period of irreversible renal tubular epithelial damage that leads to nephron loss. This stage may be polyuric or oliguric. In the polyuric phase, the patient passes dilute urine and casts and becomes azotemic. At the nephron level, tubular obstruction, tubular backleak, afferent arteriolar vasoconstriction, efferent arteriolar vasodilatation, and decreased glomerular permeability reduce glomerular filtration. This stage may continue if a pathogenic process such as ischemia, urinary toxins, or infection persists.

Laboratory abnormalities start to appear. The urine has a low specific gravity with an active sediment consisting of protein and casts. The glomerular filtration rate decreases, causing a rise in the BUN and creatinine. Often there is dehydration causing a rise in serum sodium, protein, and red blood cells. If the urine is concentrated, this is probably a result of prerenal azotemia and will be corrected by rehydration.

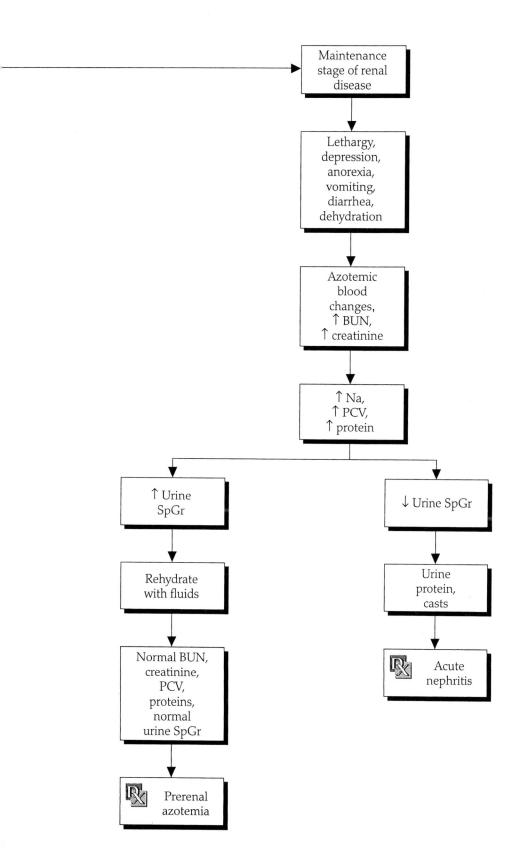

Recovery Stage of Acute Renal Failure

The recovery phase of acute renal failure occurs when the damaging pathologic insult stops and the tubules repair themselves by epithelial proliferation. Nephrons can regenerate if the tubular basement membrane is intact. Usually nephrons do not regenerate if the pathology is severe. Extensive tubular necrosis, interstitial mineralization, disrupted tubular basement membranes, and fibrosis permanently decrease functional nephrons. If the insult stops, the patient no longer passes enzymes, casts, or protein but the urine concentration may be low and the serum BUN and creatinine high because the number of functional nephrons is reduced. If 20% of kidney function remains, the animal is able to survive. The ability to concentrate urine decreases if more than 75% of the functional nephrons are lost.

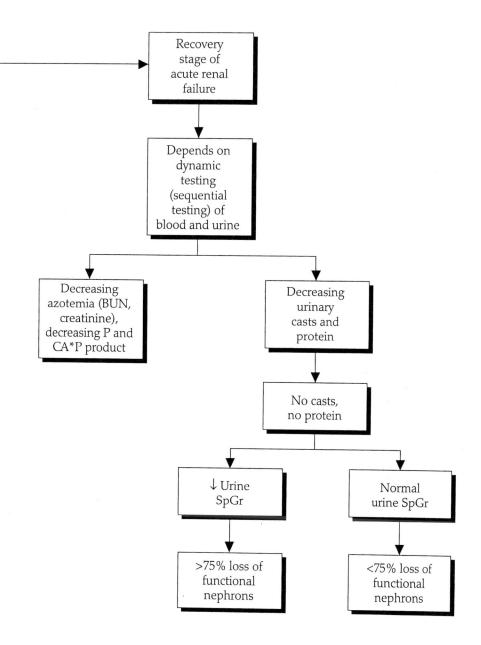

Chronic Renal Failure

Chronic renal failure is a state of progressive and irreversible deterioration of renal function from continued exposure to agents that cause acute renal failure. In addition, hereditary disease, hypertension, hyperparathyroidism, and neoplasia progressively decrease kidney function.

Kidney failure not only causes a rise in urea waste products (BUN and creatinine) but also affects calcium metabolism, acid-base balance, red blood cell production, water balance, electrolyte balance, and neurologic function. Monitoring the presence of an active urine sediment (proteinuria, casts, enzymuria), alterations in the fractional excretion of electrolytes, the results of a renal biopsy for infiltrative disease (tumor or amyloid), the exogenous creatinine clearance, or plotting the serum creatinine (1/Cr) estimates active kidney deterioration. Increased fraction excretion of phosphorus suggests increased parathormone and can be confirmed with a PTH assay. Sequential assays for creatinine, phosphorus, potassium, red blood cells, and bicarbonate give estimates of effective therapy.

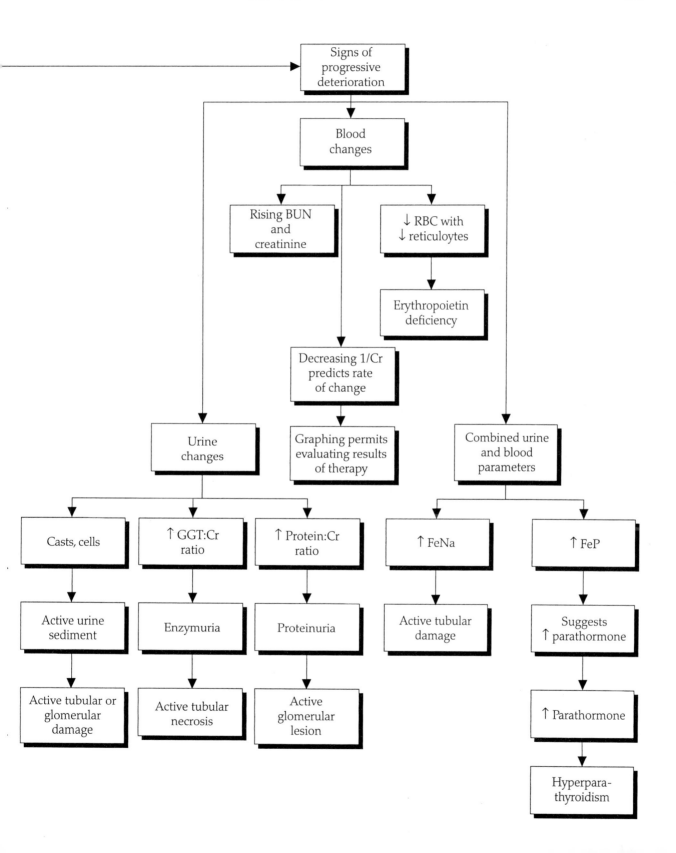

Dynamic Kidney Testing

Kidney function should be evaluated in two ways: (1) deviations from established normal values and (2) deviations from an individual's previous values. The following questions should be answered: Is the patient in renal failure? Is there active kidney disease that can be corrected? What is the cause of the kidney failure? Is the current therapy modifying the progression of the kidney failure?

Common screening tests are the BUN, creatinine, and urine specific gravity. A rising creatinine graphed against time with the formula 1/Cr indicates progressive loss of nephrons. Even a small change suggests early renal disease that necessitates further workup with a urinalysis. A persistent low specific gravity suggests a variety of diseases of kidney or other organ dysfunction. Monitoring common tests and following up with more specific tests such as fractional excretion of sodium, potassium, or phosphorus, protein:creatinine ratios, and urine GGT:creatinine ratios allow early diagnosis of progressive diseases.

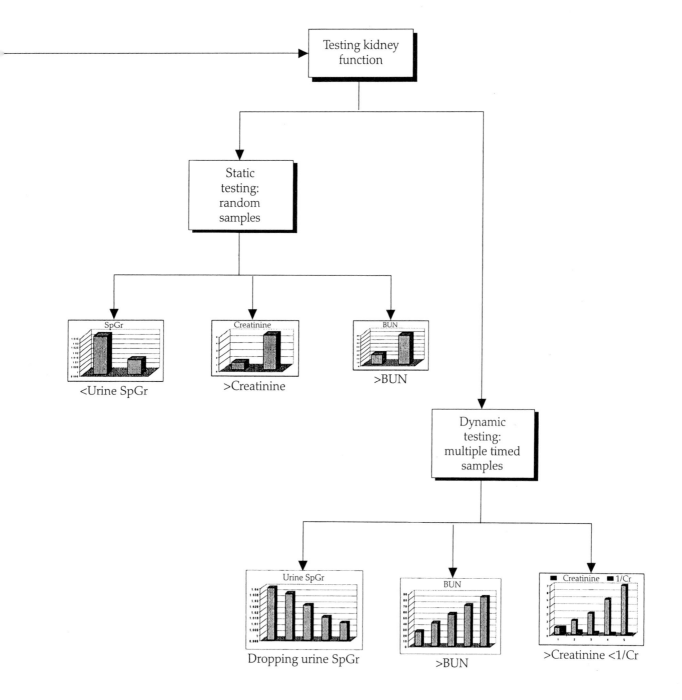

Testing Hepatic Function

The liver is responsible for hundreds of anabolic, catabolic, and storage processes. Clinically we use only a few tests to evaluate liver function. Increased ALT and AST indicate parenchymal damage. Increased SAP and GGT indicate bile stasis or drug reactions (cortisol). Hypoalbuminemia when associated with increased blood ammonia, a low serum BUN concentration, or a low BUN:creatinine ratio indicates functional changes.

Hyperbilirubinemia in nonanemic animals suggests cholestatic liver disease. Increased bile acids indicate vascular shunting. This occurs in acute injury from temporary increased resistance to portal blood flow. Decreasing levels suggest healing, while persistent levels suggest the formation of shunts secondary to hepatic fibrosis. Alpha-fetoprotein is raised in a high percent of dogs with primary or metastatic liver tumors. Rarely, liver disease is severe enough to increase the prothrombin time (PT).

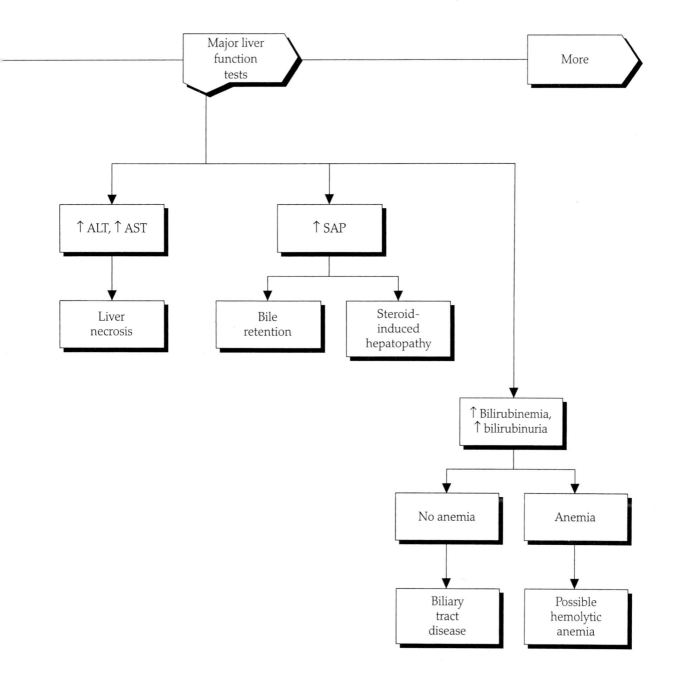

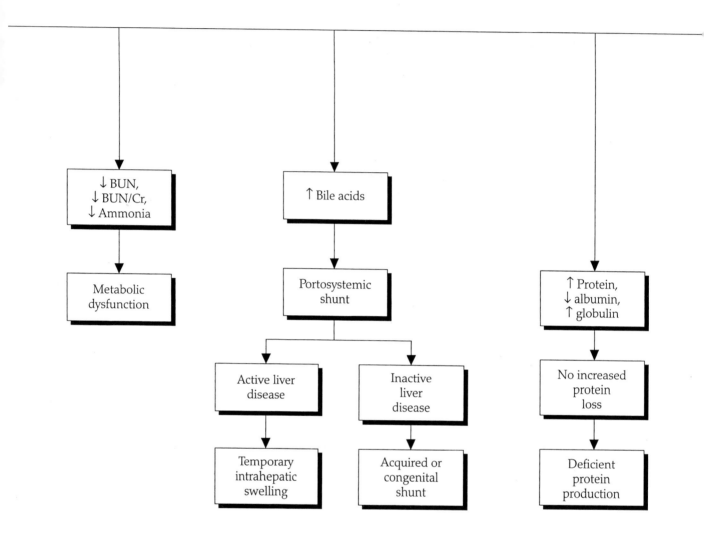

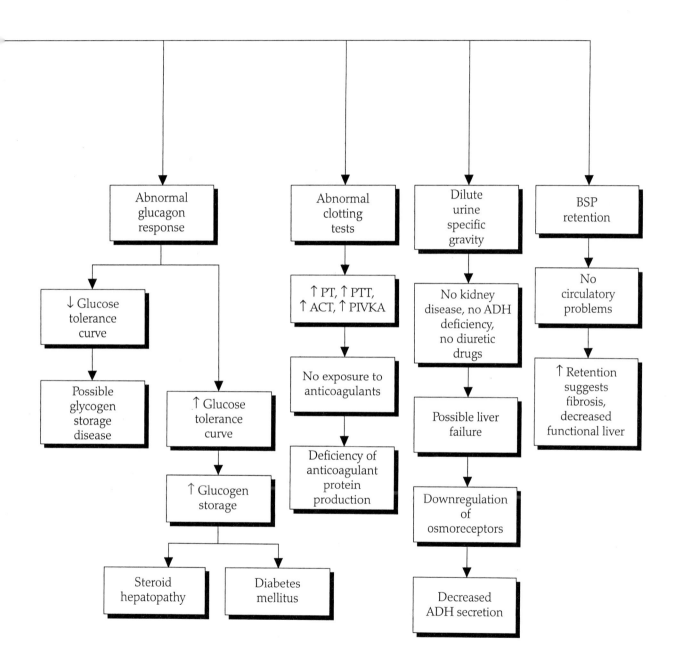

Hepatic Neoplasms

Hepatic neoplasms often impinge on liver sarenchymal cells, causing a rise in ALT and AST, and induce cholestasis. Cholestasis causes a rise in bilirubin, alkaline phosphatase, and GGT. Circulation through the tumor traumatizes the RBCs, causing fragmentation and leptocyte formation.

These are nonspecific signs of liver disease. A markedly elevated alpha-fetoprotein level confirms a liver tumor, but a low level does not rule out a malignancy. If an ultrasound examination shows hypoechoic areas, a diagnosis may be confirmed with cytology of a needle aspirate.

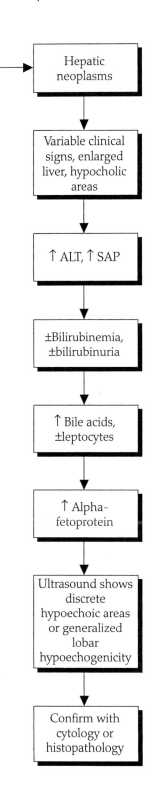

Hepatic
neoplasms

↓

Variable clinical
signs, enlarged
liver, hypocholic
areas

↓

↑ ALT, ↑ SAP

↓

±Bilirubinemia,
±bilirubinuria

↓

↑ Bile acids,
±leptocytes

↓

↑ Alpha-
fetoprotein

↓

Ultrasound shows
discrete
hypoechoic areas
or generalized
lobar
hypoechogenicity

↓

Confirm with
cytology or
histopathology

Hepatic Fibrosis

Massive liver necrosis causes collapse of liver lobules and replacement with fibrous tissue. This is often associated with a cholangiohepatitis as demonstrated by a rise in both the parenchymal enzymes (ALT and AST) and the cholestatic-induced enzymes SAP and GGT. Bile acids are increased because of acquired vascular shunts, but high bilirubin levels mask this rise. Increased BSP levels are a good indicator of decreased liver capacity but are rarely done. Ultrasound examination will show a hyperechoic liver. Fibrosis is confirmed with a liver biopsy. Increased copper levels in this biopsy may differentiate copper toxicosis from other causes of fibrosis.

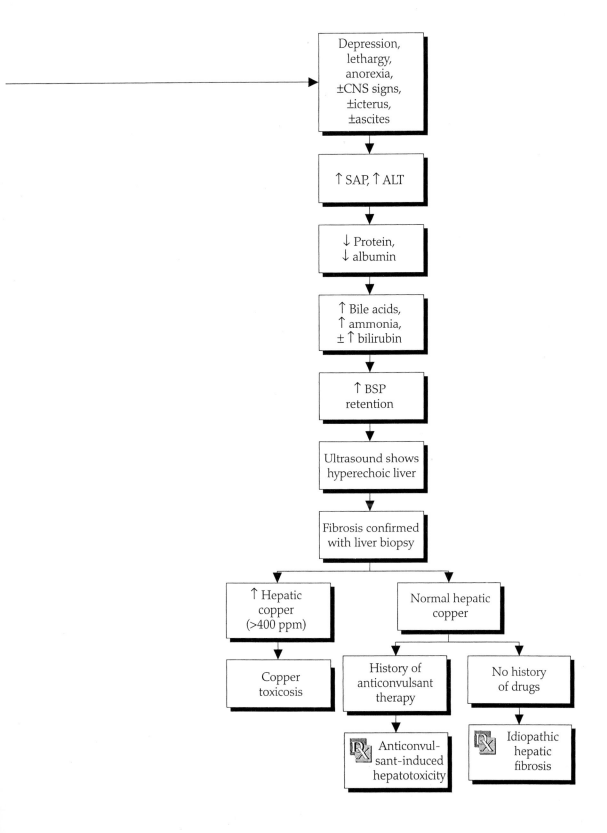

Feline Hepatic Lipidosis

Anorectic cats are at risk for hepatic lipidosis from increased triglyceride deposits. Usually the patient presents with a history of recent weight loss or stress. Increased mobilization of peripheral fat stores during starvation is the probable source of the increased hepatic fat. In severe cases, more than 50% of the liver cells are filled with triglycerides that enlarge the liver and cause jaundice. Usually the alkaline phosphatase is more elevated than GGT and ALT. Since bilirubinuria is always abnormal in the cat, this is an early indicator of a significant liver problem. Bile acids are also a good indicator of early liver disease and may be elevated before there are significant elevations of bilirubin or liver enzymes. The disease may be confirmed by cytologic demonstration of large numbers of fat-filled hepatocytes in a fine needle aspirate.

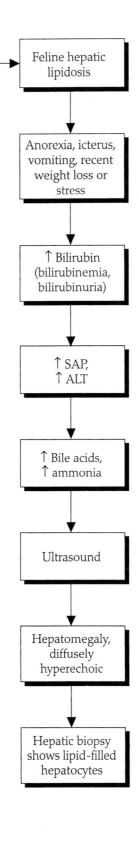

Glucocorticoid-Induced Hepatopathy

The dog liver is sensitive to glucocorticoids. High doses cause increased alkaline phosphatase activity and hepatomegaly within a few weeks. Initial alkaline phosphatase response is due to a liver isoenzyme, but later both biliary alkaline phosphatase and GGT may rise. Early hepatocyte changes are due to distention with glycogen. This marked cell distention can cause membrane devitalization and leakage of ALT. Bile acid levels should be determined if high levels of alkaline phosphatase are found on screening profiles with no other biochemical liver abnormalities. Serum bile acids are often normal but may be slightly elevated. Steroid hepatopathy usually does not cause marked increases. A normal bile acid would suggest steroid induction, while a very high bile acid would suggest other liver pathology. Blood ammonia and ammonia tolerance are usually normal.

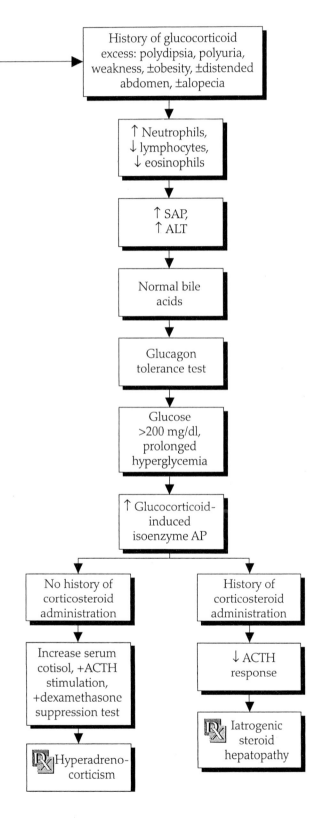

Chronic Hepatitis

A variety of agents (viruses, bacteria, chemicals, and immune reactions) cause the release of liver antigen that activates the immune system. The immune response is mounted against liver membrane antigens to perpetuate nonsuppurative chronic hepatitis. Usually the inflammation starts in the portal areas with inflammation and necrosis. The liver responds with regenerative nodules surrounded by fibrosis and bile duct hyperplasia that together distort the liver architecture.

In dogs, ALT, AST, and SAP are usually increased. In cats the SAP may not increase. If the primary lesion is in the portal area, icterus may occur early. Bile acids are usually increased, and BSP retention is usually markedly elevated.

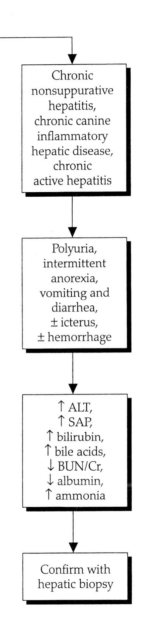

Bile Duct Obstruction

Common causes of bile duct obstruction are neoplasms and inflammation secondary to acute pancreatitis or cholangitis. Obstructed bile flow damages hepatocytes and releases mediators of inflammation. Chronic obstruction causes necrosis and periportal fibrosis. Obstruction for longer than 10 days causes fat malabsorption. This results in a vitamin K deficient coagulopathy.

Marked increases in ALT and AST indicate liver necrosis. Increases in bilirubin, ALP, and GGT indicate bile stasis. Increased bleeding time can be detected by PIVKA, PT, and ACT assays. The dilated bile duct can be confirmed by ultrasound examination. Increased bile acids are masked by the bilirubinemia.

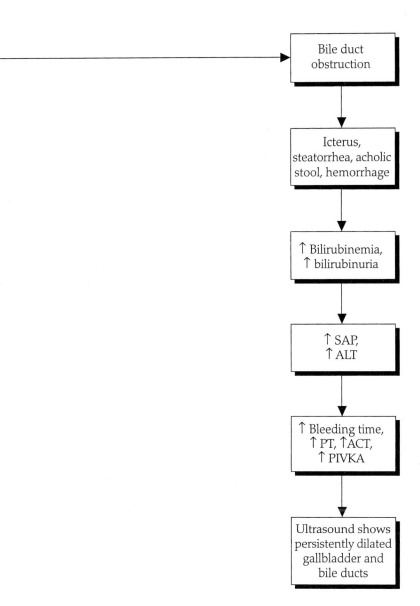

Feline Cholangitis/ Cholangiohepatitis

The cholangitis/cholangiohepatitis syndrome of cats is histologically characterized as nonsuppurative when the cellular infiltrate is lymphocytic or plasmacytic and suppurative when this infiltrate is neutrophilic. Cats with suppurative and plasmacytic cholangitis/cholangiohepatitis have a moderate increase in ALT, AST, and GGT and a slight increase in SAP, whereas cats with lymphocytic cholangitis/cholangiohepatitis have milder increases. The suppurative form usually has a high WBC, whereas the nonsuppurative types have higher serum globulins. Hyperbilirubinuria and hyperbilirubinemia may be detected before the cat is clinically icteric.

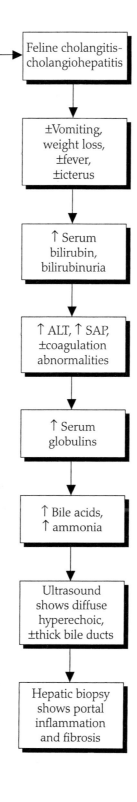

Feline cholangitis-cholangiohepatitis

↓

±Vomiting, weight loss, ±fever, ±icterus

↓

↑ Serum bilirubin, bilirubinuria

↓

↑ ALT, ↑ SAP, ±coagulation abnormalities

↓

↑ Serum globulins

↓

↑ Bile acids, ↑ ammonia

↓

Ultrasound shows diffuse hyperechoic, ±thick bile ducts

↓

Hepatic biopsy shows portal inflammation and fibrosis

Congenital Portosystemic Shunts

Portosystemic shunting occurs from either congenital portal venous malformation or acquired portal hypertension. Both alter hepatic function and cause signs of hepatic encephalopathy. These shunts decrease the portal blood supply to the liver, causing liver atrophy. With congenital shunts, liver enzymes and bilirubin levels are usually normal. Albumin may be slightly low, but globulins are normal. About 30% show hypoglycemia and most have very low serum cholesterol. Many animals develop a microcytic nonregenerative anemia. Urinary abnormalities consist of a low specific gravity that improves with water deprivation and the formation of ammonium urate crystals. Bile acids are consistently elevated. Sometimes these shunts are classified as macroscopic or microvascular. Some macroscopic shunts can be repaired by surgery.

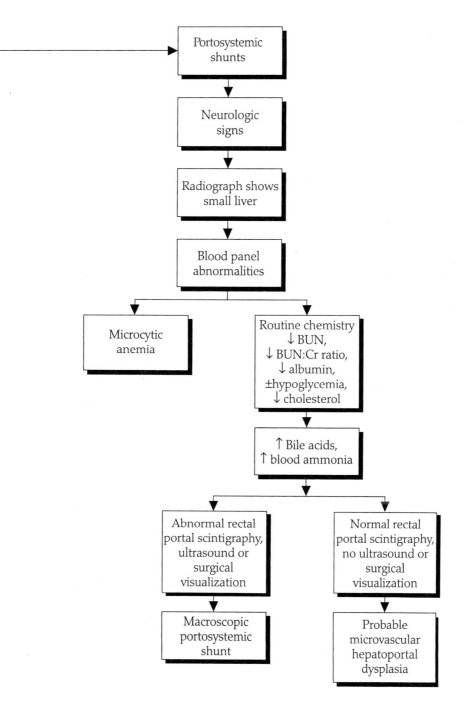

Dynamic Hepatic Function Testing

When we look at liver function dynamically over a period of time we get a sense of progressive liver disease or improved liver function. Persistently elevated or rising ALT levels suggest ongoing liver trauma from disease. Occasionally this enzyme remains elevated after liver disease is resolved when an animal forms macroenzymes. Rising conjugated bilirubin levels with high urine bilirubin are usually associated with continued cholestatic disease. Again there is an exception; *biliprotein* may cause persistently high serum bilirubin levels despite resolution of clinical icterus and bilirubinuria. In these cases functional tests may give a better estimation of liver problems.

Persistently dropping serum albumin levels may indicate chronic liver dysfunction if no source of protein loss is detected. If this is associated with low BUN levels, liver failure is clearly indicated. These levels are best tracked by calculating a BUN:Cr ratio. A persistently low ratio suggests chronic liver failure.

Bile acids are sensitive indicators of improving liver function. Focal injury of the liver causes localized swelling and shunting of the bile acids into the blood. High persistent serum levels suggest the breakdown of liver structure, but dropping levels of bile acids suggest healing of the liver parenchyma.

Vitamin K deficiency may be caused by liver disease or warfarin-type poisoning. They cause clotting disorders secondary to inhibition of liver clotting factors. Improvement of coagulation tests such as ACT, PTT, and PIVKA suggest adequate treatment.

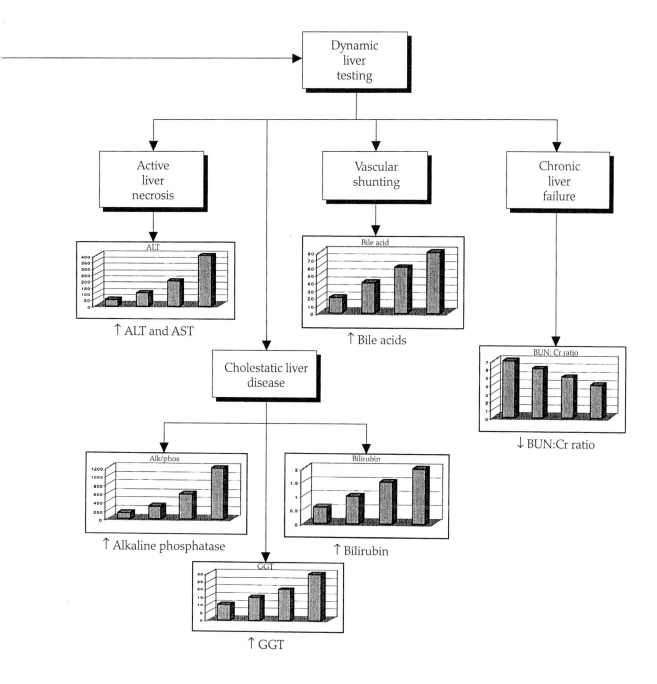

Dynamic Drug Toxicity Testing

Occasionally, adverse reactions follow the administration of therapeutic agents. Acute toxicity is often due to an allergy or idiosyncratic reaction of the patient. More often, reactions to a drug occur after long-term administration because of immunologic reactions or the formation of toxic by-products.

To avoid potential problems, determine a baseline of test values and then periodically test the patient with a battery of organ-specific laboratory tests. This is the safest way of detecting reactions before the drugs cause irreparable damage. The most sensitive indicators of adverse reactions are the following:

- RBCs: may be affected by Heinz bodies, immune anemia, or bone marrow suppression.
- WBCs and platelets: affected by bone marrow suppression or immune reactions to the surface attachment of a drug.
- Blood glucose: may increase with agents such as steroids, which affect glucose metabolism.
- Liver function tests (ALT, SAP, GGT, bilirubin): indicate liver damage or enzyme induction from drugs such as steroids, antiseizure medications, and antiarthritic drugs.
- Renal function tests (BUN, creatinine, urine SpGr): indicate kidney dysfunction from agents such as antibiotics and antiprostaglandins.

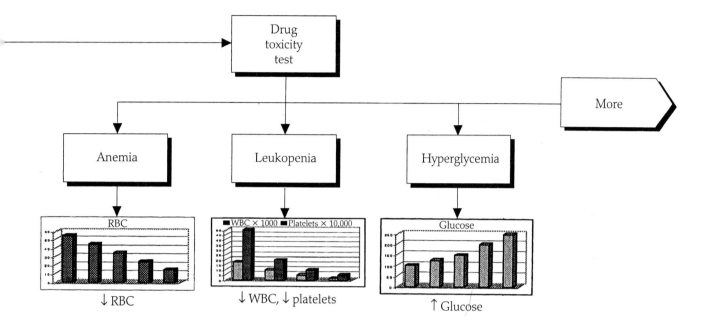

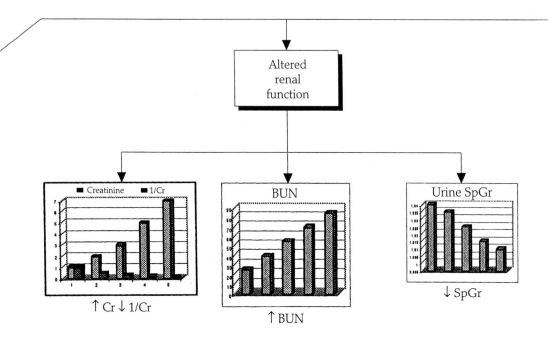

Altered
renal
function

↑ Cr ↓ 1/Cr

↑ BUN

↓ SpGr

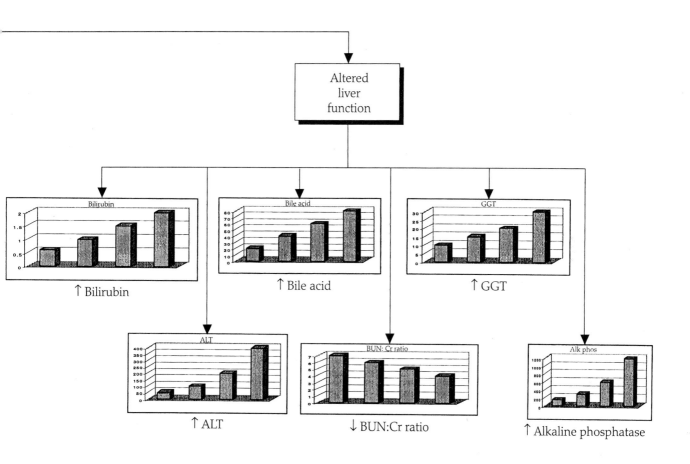

Geriatric Testing

Veterinarians are taught to diagnose, treat, and prevent disease, not monitor and modify the aging process. Most textbooks are disease oriented and discuss testing for organ dysfunction based on large numbers of normal values. Few of these books stress evaluation based on dynamic interpretation of an individual animal's changing test values. Dynamic testing provides a way of disclosing decreasing function before it reaches a disease state.

Although some tests are based on an all or nothing interpretation (FeLV, bacterial cultures, heartworm), many tests are based on average normal values. It is the tests based on averages that have masked early changes that could allow us to deal with aging.

Dynamic changes are best detected if an animal establishes its own normal values for kidney function, liver function, inflammatory disease, red cell production, and liver function. A blood panel run at periodic intervals, ranging from daily samples in sick animals to yearly samples in apparently healthy animals provides an early warning system of pending problems.

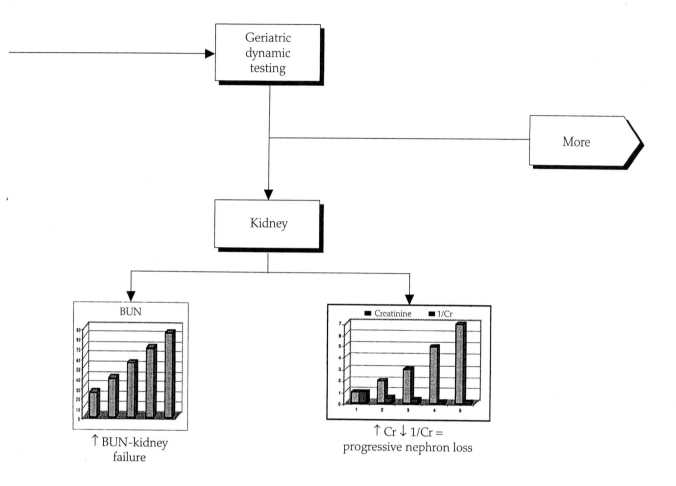

↑ BUN-kidney
failure

↑ Cr ↓ 1/Cr =
progressive nephron loss

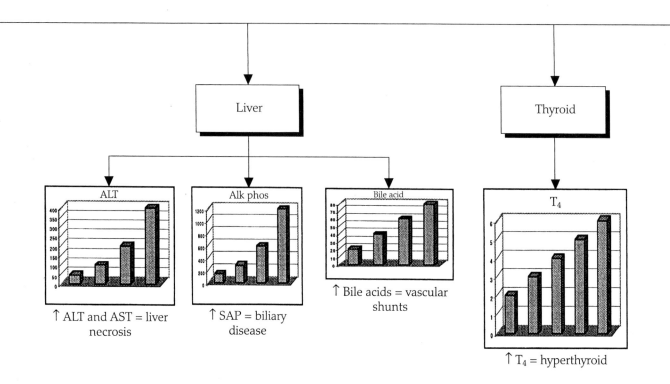

↑ ALT and AST = liver
necrosis

↑ SAP = biliary
disease

↑ Bile acids = vascular
shunts

↑ T₄ = hyperthyroid

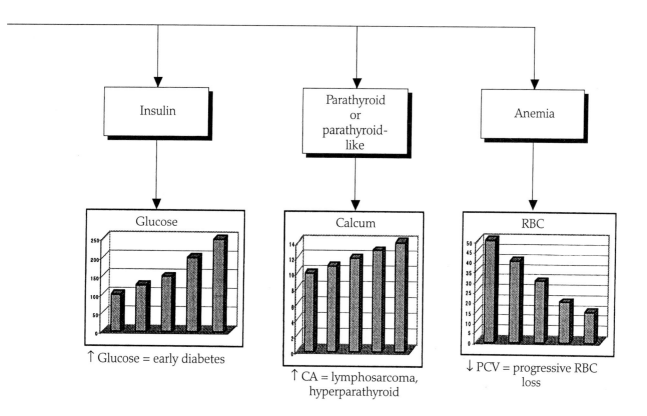

↑ Glucose = early diabetes

↑ CA = lymphosarcoma, hyperparathyroid

↓ PCV = progressive RBC loss

Immune-Mediated Disease

Four types of immune reactions can damage tissues.

Type I: Anaphylactic or immediate hypersensitivity (IgE, IgG) reactions are caused by release of histamine, leukotrienes, prostaglandins, and other agents from mast cells. Examples include anaphylaxis, atopy, and asthma.

Type II: Cytotoxic hypersensitivity reactions (IgG, IgM) caused by binding of antibody to cell-bound antigen, causing lysis of cells. Examples include immune-mediated hemolytic anemia, thrombocytopenia, and pemphigus.

Type III: Immune-complex disease (IgG, IgM) occurs with antibody or antigen excess, leading to formation of circulating immune complexes. These complexes are deposited on vascular endothelium and incite inflammation through activation of complement. Examples include lupus erythematosus, vasculitis, glomerulonephritis, polyarthritis, heartworm disease, feline infectious peritonitis, and feline leukemia virus infection.

Type IV: Cell-mediated or delayed hypersensitivity reactions occur when sensitized T-lymphocytes release lymphokines to cause tissue damage. Examples include contact dermatitis and graft rejection.

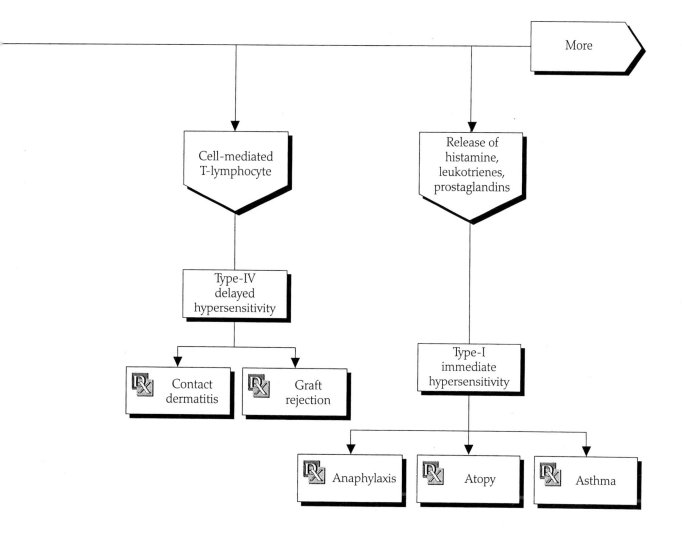

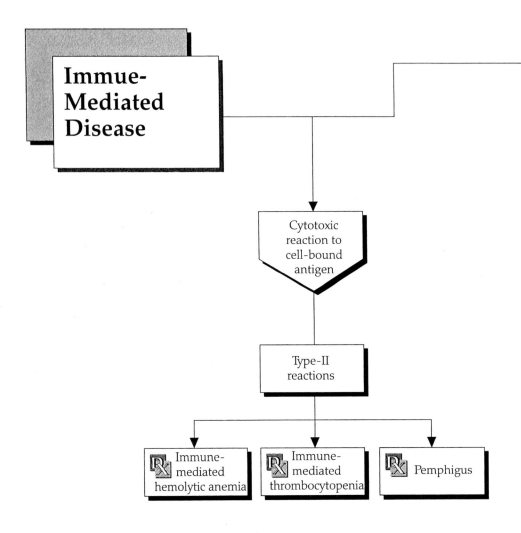

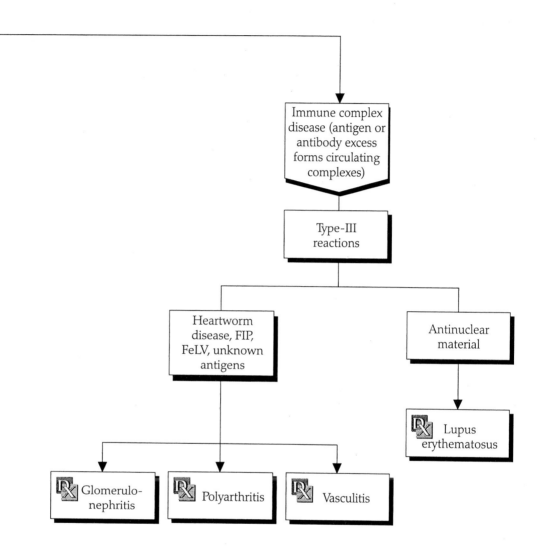

FeLV Infection

FeLV infection is the most common cause of severe illness and death in domestic cats. The virus is usually directly transmitted through the saliva. Following replication in the lymphoid tissue of the pharynx, the virus is either eliminated or the animal becomes viremic and FeLV replicates in the marrow and lymphoid cells. If the immune response is ineffective, the animal becomes a carrier.

The carrier state can be classified according to FeLV antigen test results.

A *latent infection* is present when the virus can be cultivated from the bone marrow but blood tests are negative for FeLV. A *healthy carrier state* exists if ELISA is positive but results of the IFA test on blood marrow cells are negative. A *viremic state* exists if ELISA and IFA tests are both positive.

A positive ELISA or IFA test in a cat showing signs of illness is highly suggestive of FeLV infection, but a positive FeLV test in a healthy cat with a low probability of previous contact with the virus could actually be negative. These cats should be checked again with both ELISA and IFA tests.

The prognosis depends on test results. Cats with persistent viremia, as determined by two consecutive positive IFA tests 4 weeks apart, have an 80% chance of dying from FeLV-related disease within 3 years. Cats with persistently discordant ELISA and IFA test results have approximately a 50% chance of death from FeLV infection within 3 years.

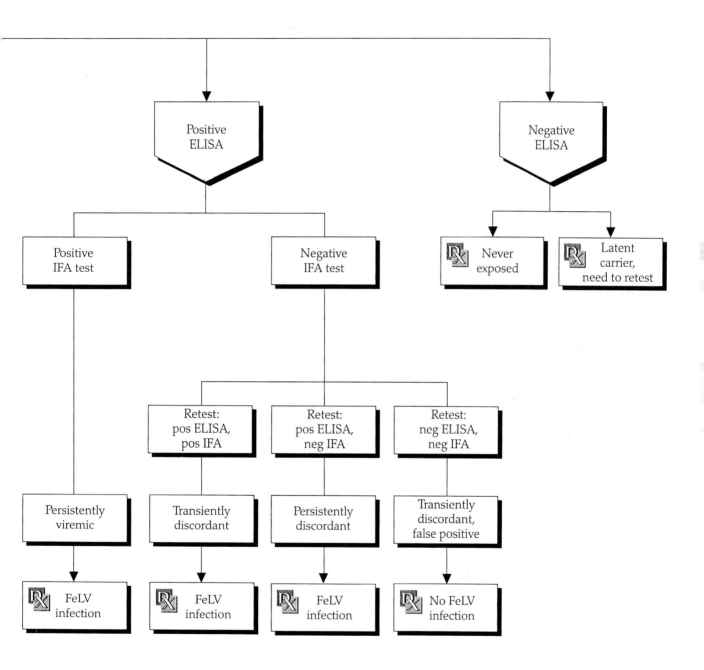

FIP Infection

Feline infectious peritonitis is a complex immunologic disease induced by a mutant feline Corona virus. Many cats carry a nonpathogenic Corona virus that replicates in the intestinal epithelium and is passed in the feces. In immune compromised animals this virus may mutate to produce a viral growth factor (7B protein) that allows the virus to proliferate in macrophages. The modified virus (FIP virus) is passed in the feces and can directly infect normal animals.

Clinical disease is due to type 3 (immune complex) and type 4 (delayed type hypersensitivity) reactions. Type 3 reactions cause vasculitis that results in effusions. Type 4 reactions cause granulomatous lesions typical of the noneffusive FIP. Neither of these immune reactions controls the viral proliferation.

A definitive diagnosis of FIP is difficult. FIP antigen is hard to detect in a clinical case because it is bound to antibody or located in macrophages. Antibody tests tell only that there has been exposure to the Corona or FIP virus. When an FIP-specific antibody is found in a typical FIP case, the probability of a FIP diagnosis is high, but a negative test does not eliminate the diagnosis. Thus the diagnosis of an end stage FIP case may be frustrated by the inability to detect the viral antigen by fecal PCR tests for either Corona virus or FIP virus. An FIP virus shedder is infective to all cats. A Corona virus shedder is potentially dangerous to immune compromised cats such as those with FeLV, kittens, or cats with major diseases.

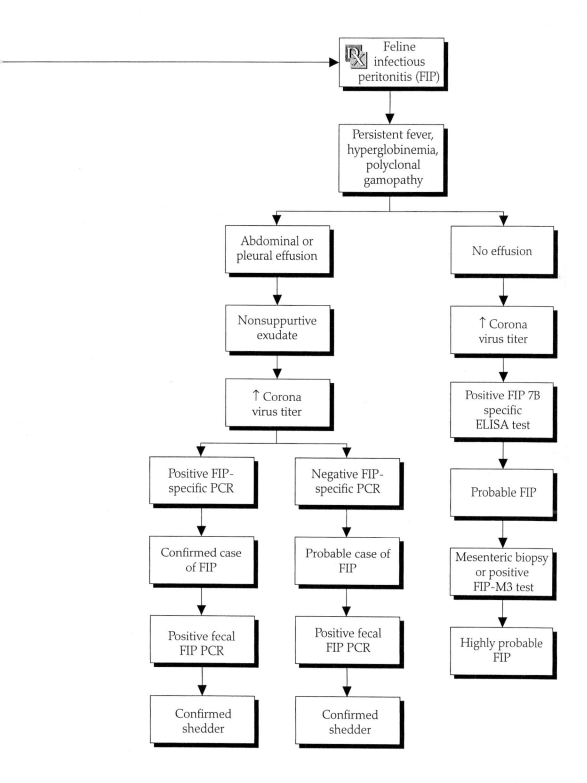

FIP Carrier State

Not all cats that are infected with Corona virus or even the pathogenic FIP virus show signs of disease. These animals may live years without major problems, but they are a threat to other cats.

Detection of the Corona virus carrier or the FIP virus carrier is easy and useful in preventing exposure of uninfected cats. Since the major source of feline coronaviruses is the feces, a carrier cat may be diagnosed by fecal PCR tests for either Corona virus or FIP virus. An FIP virus shedder is infective to all cats. A Corona virus shedder is potentially dangerous to immune compromised cats such as those with FeLV, kittens, or cats with major diseases.

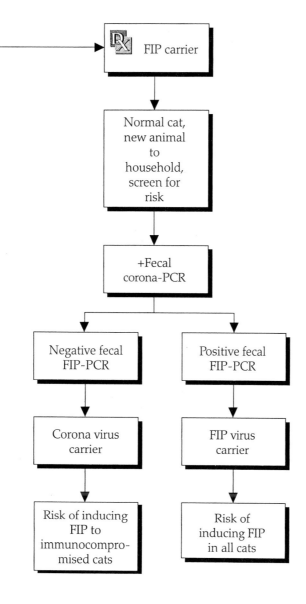

Decreased Adrenal Function (Hypoadrenocorticism)

Weakness, decreased urine production, hemoconcentration, and azotemia can be caused by a number of diseases. Animals with these signs can be quickly screened for adrenal insufficiency using the serum Na:K ratio and the hemogram. If the Na:K ratio is <23 and the eosinophil and lymphocyte counts are high, hypoadrenocorticism (Addison's disease) should be suspected. If the eosinophil and lymphocyte counts are high but the Na:K ratio is >27, partial adrenal insufficiency is possible. The diagnosis can be confirmed by an ACTH stimulation test, which yields low serum cortisol levels in animals with hypoadrenocorticism.

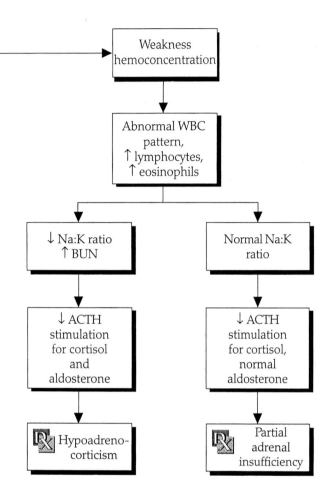

Increased Adrenal Glucocorticoids (Hyperadrenocorticism)

Chronic exposure to excessive amounts of endogenous cortisol and to synthetic corticosteroids has similar effects on the body. Polydipsia, polyuria, weakness, alopecia, muscle wasting, and a stress leukogram are classic signs of corticoid excess.

Excessive adrenal corticoids cause diseases of the liver, pancreas, and kidneys. If no corticosteroids have been administered, the cortisol excess is due to an adrenal or pituitary tumor. These can be distinguished by the ACTH stimulation test or the dexamethasone suppression test. If the excess is due to drugs, the pituitary is suppressed and the animal may actually be deficient in endogenous cortisol and aldosterone.

Excessive cortisol causes diabetes mellitus, nephrogenic diabetes insipidus, corticosteroid-induced hepatopathy, and acute pancreatitis. Sometimes, the underlying cause is first suspected by a stress leukogram and high alkaline phosphatase activity.

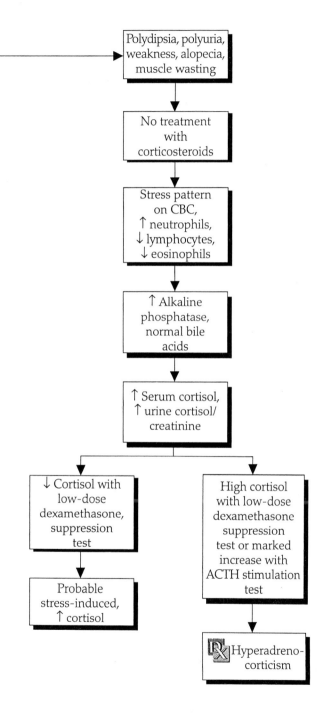

Iatrogenic Hyperadrenocorticism

Iatrogenic hyperadrenocorticism is caused by prolonged use of oral, injectable, or topical corticosteroids. These drugs cause atrophy of the adrenal cortex while producing signs of cortisol excess.

Exogenous corticosteroids inhibit ACTH release and decrease production of endogenous glucocorticoids but not aldosterone. Affected animals show signs of adrenocortical excess, while the adrenal glands are hypofunctional.

The leukogram shows a stress pattern with neutrophilia, lymphopenia, and eosinopenia. The chemistry tests may show a mild hyperglycemia and moderate to marked increase in alkaline phosphatase. Serum cortisol levels are decreased, so dexamethasone suppression tests are not useful. Decreased adrenal function may be confirmed by a decreased response to the ACTH stimulation test.

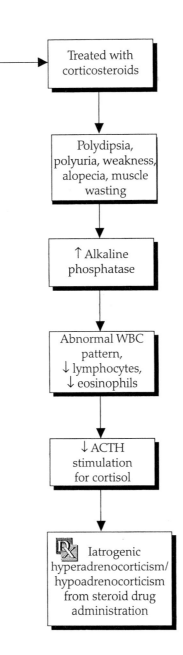

Increased Parathyroid Function (Hyperparathyroidism)

Parathyroid hormone (PTH), calcitriol, and calcitonin act on calcium levels in extracellular fluid and bone reservoirs. High serum calcium levels suppress PTH hormone synthesis and release, whereas low levels increase PTH. An elevated level of serum phosphorus, by lowering serum calcium, secondarily stimulates PTH release. Another calcium regulatory hormone parathyroid-related protein (PTHrP) is the cause of humoral hypercalcemia of malignancy.

Hypercalcemia caused by hyperparathyroid is usually accompanied by a mild hyperchloremic acidosis, that produces a chloride phosphorus ratio greater than 33. Nonhyperparathyroid hypercalcemia is often associated with an elevated serum bicarbonate, producing a chloride phosphorus ratio less than 33. The fractional excretion of phosphorus increases with excess PTH. This test gives a rapid estimation of increased PTH. Measurement of PTH, however, is the most accurate approach to confirm hyperparathyroidism.

In chronic renal failure, low calcium levels secondary to high serum phosphorus can sometimes be controlled with oral phosphate binders. If phosphorus levels are normal, careful use of small doses of vitamin D can control PTH secretion.

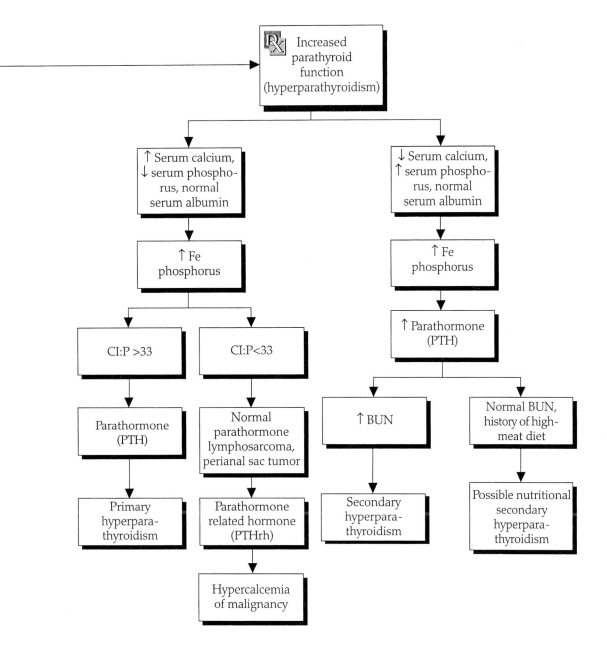

Decreased Thyroid Function (Hypothyroidism)

In most cases the diagnosis of hypothyroidism can be made with three tests (T_4, fT_4d, and cTSH). If the T_4 is normal, hypothyroidism can usually be ruled out. If it is high and there is a high suspicion of hypothyroidism, then thyroid autoantibody tests are run.

If the T_4 is low, this is not sufficient reason to diagnose hypothyroidism. A follow-up test for free T_4 by dialysis (fT_4d) must be run. If this is low, then a diagnosis of hypothyroidism is confirmed. One further test (cTSH) determines if this is primary hypothyroidism (disease of the thyroid) or secondary hypothyroidism (disease of the pituitary).

The TSH stimulation test is no longer available and has been replaced by the TRH stimulation test. This test is rarely done because it is quite expensive and only rules out nonthyroidal disease suppression. This can be inferred by diagnosing concurrent disease by a physical examination with major abnormalities on the blood panel.

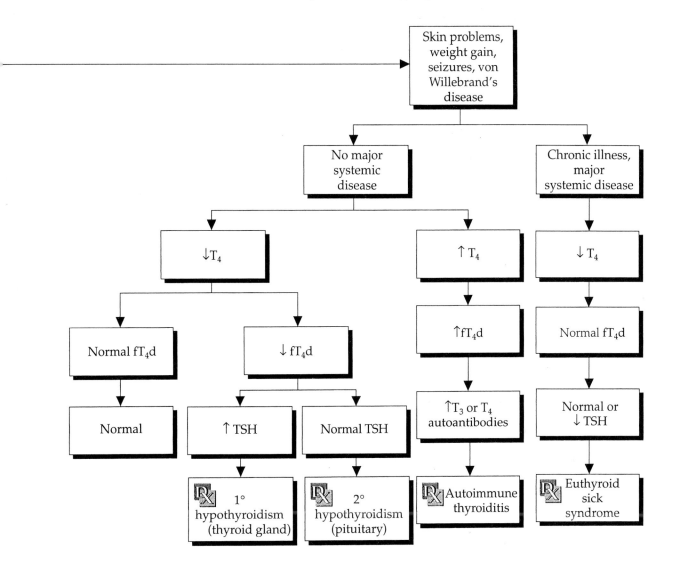

Increased Thyroid Function (Hyperthyroidism)

Hyperthyroidism is common in cats and rare in dogs. In cats, the condition is due to hyperplasia of both glands and occasionally the accessory thyroid tissue. In dogs, it is caused by a malignant thyroid tumor.

Because no feline TSH assays are available, it is not possible to determine if hyperthyroidism is of pituitary origin or a result of a TSH-like substance. The assays for TSH compounds are species specific, so human assays are not diagnostic in dogs and cats.

Markedly elevated T_4 or high fT_4d levels are diagnostic for hyperthyroidism in the cat, but borderline increases may be difficult to separate from high normal values. Because thyroxin levels fluctuate during the day, slight increases can be difficult to distinguish from high normal values. The T_3 suppression test inhibits T_4 levels in normal animals but not in hyperthyroid animals.

A diagnosis of hyperthyroidism may be confirmed with radioisotope thyroid scan.

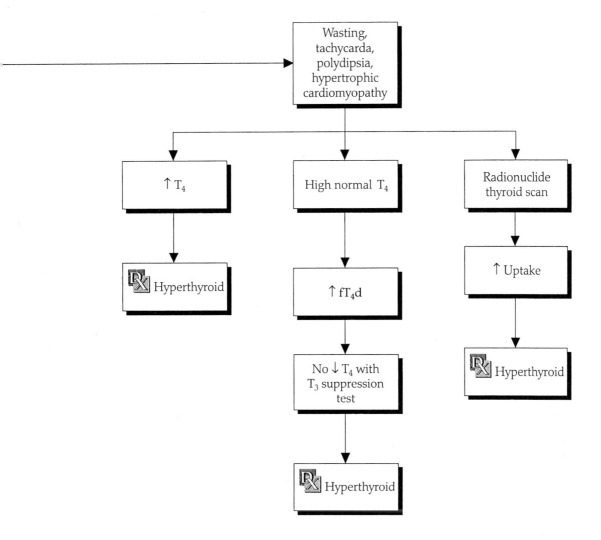

Thyroid Replacement Monitoring

The dog should be monitored for adequate thyroid replacement therapy by testing T_4 and cTSH. The T_4 levels is checked 4 hours after the medicine is administered while the TSH level (cTSH) can be checked at any time. A T_4 in the normal range and a low TSH indicate adequate doses of replacement thyroxin. High levels of T_4 with low TSH levels may indicate overmedication.

High levels of cTSH indicate the dose of replacement hormone is too low.

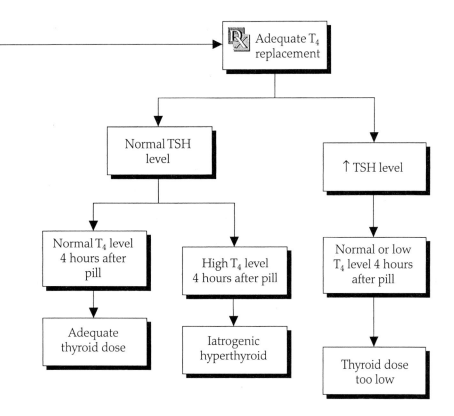

Estrus and Ovulation Prediction

Serum progesterone assay can be combined with vaginal cytology to accurately predict the fertile period in bitches. Serum progesterone levels are below 2 ng/ml, until the LH surge.

Ovulation occurs 2 days after the LH surge and is indicated by a rise in progesterone levels (4-10 ng/ml). To anticipate estrus, begin testing every other day after proestrus is indicated by vaginal cytology or a serosanguineous vulvar discharge, then measure progesterone levels.

Interpretation of Progesterone Levels

Levels <2 ng/ml indicate that the LH peak has not yet occurred.

Levels >2 ng/ml indicate that the luteal surge has occurred and ovulation will occur within 2 days.

Levels 6 to 10 ng/ml indicate that ovulation has already occurred and the fertile period is nearly over.

Levels >15 ng/ml occur after the fertile period.

The week before expected parturition: whelping should occur within 24 hours after the progesterone level falls below 2 ng/ml.

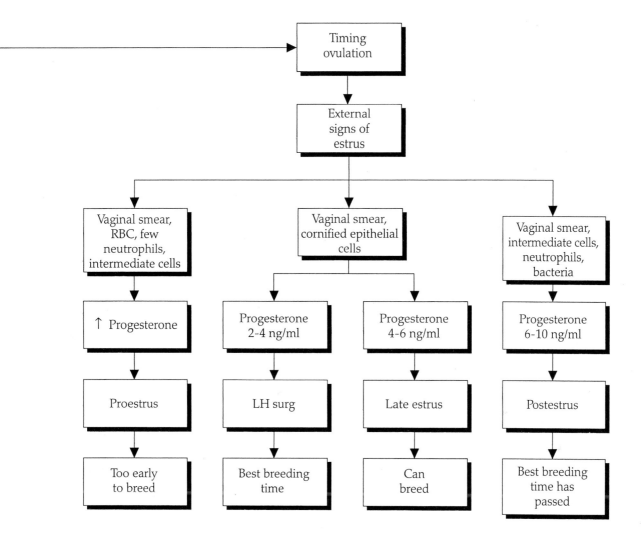

Whelping Prediction

Ultrasound (20 days) and serum relaxin (40 days) can confirm pregnancy in the dog. Serum progesterone levels cannot be used to detect pregnancy because the levels remain elevated following ovulation even if there is no pregnancy. *Assay for acute-phase proteins* can detect pregnancy at 28 to 34 days, but values also increase if there is inflammation from pyometra.

The serum progesterone level is >10 ng/ml during pregnancy and drops below this level just before parturition. To predict whelping, begin daily testing the week before expected parturition. Whelping should occur within 24 hours after the progesterone level falls below 2 ng/ml.

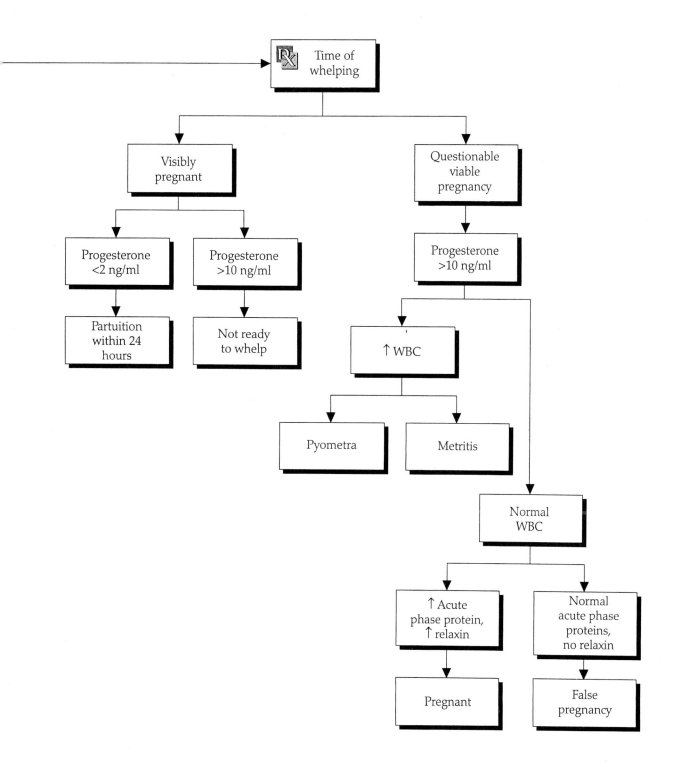

Thrombocytopenia

Insufficiency of platelets (*thrombocytopenia*) commonly causes bleeding. The most common reasons for thrombocytopenia are decreased platelet production, increased platelet destruction by the reticuloendothelial system, disorders of distribution, and increased platelet consumption.

The first step in evaluating a low platelet count is to rule out errors in blood sample collection or in platelet counting. The reference ranges for platelet counts vary with the laboratory, but counts lower than 100,000/µl or falling counts, even in the normal range, can indicate a problem. Increased MPV (mean platelet volume) suggests active bone marrow production without the necessity of a bone marrow aspirate. Platelet bound immunoglobulins are the most accurate method of diagnosing immune thrombocytopenia. Megakaryocyte fluorescence confirms immune destruction of megakaryocytes.

Bleeding can occur at platelet counts from >50,000/µl to 100,000/µl, depending on platelet size, platelet function, concurrent bleeding tendencies, and severity of the challenge.

Concurrent changes in the CBC may suggest blood loss, bone marrow inactivity, and coagulation abnormalities.

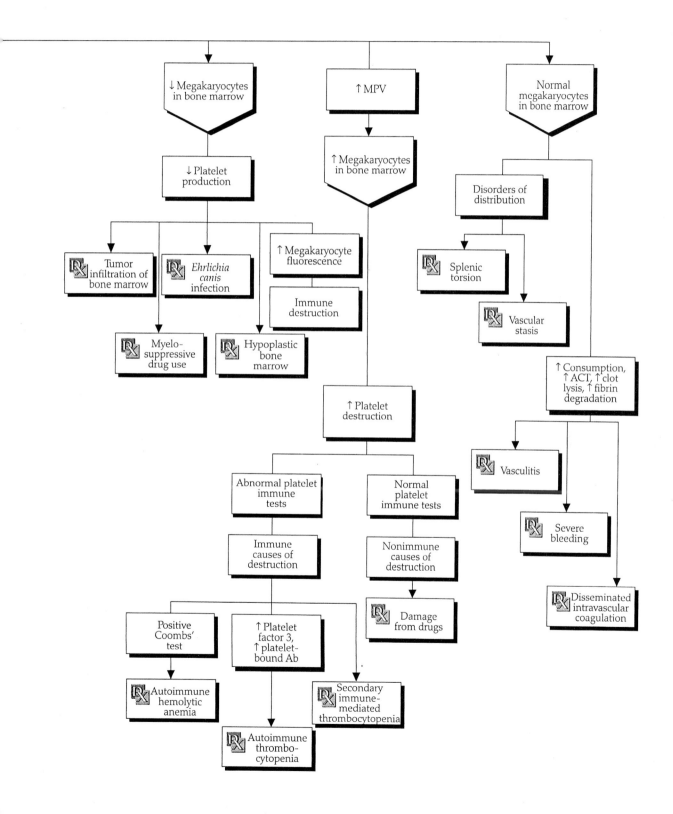

Responsive Anemia

Anemia is a decrease in red cell mass, resulting in insufficient oxygenation of tissues. It is usually secondary to an underlying primary disease. Anemia can be classified by response, by red cell morphology, or by cause.

Regenerative anemia is characterized by large numbers of reticulocytes on blood smears and increased erythrocytic precursors in the bone marrow. If these are not present, the anemia is termed *nonregenerative.* The cause of nonregenerative anemia can be inferred from changes in the blood panel or by bone marrow examination.

A morphologic classification by size and hemoglobin content sometimes suggests specific diseases. *Mean corpuscular volume (MCV)* is used to classify red blood cells by size, such as macrocytic, normocytic, or microcytic. *Mean corpuscular hemoglobin concentration (MCHC)* is used to classify red blood cells as normochromic or hypochromic. The red cell distribution width (RDW) is a sensitive indicator of variable red cells size.

Blood loss, hemolysis, and bone marrow hypoplasia can cause anemia. Occasionally, specific causes can be determined from intracellular parasites, toxic changes, or abnormal RBC shapes.

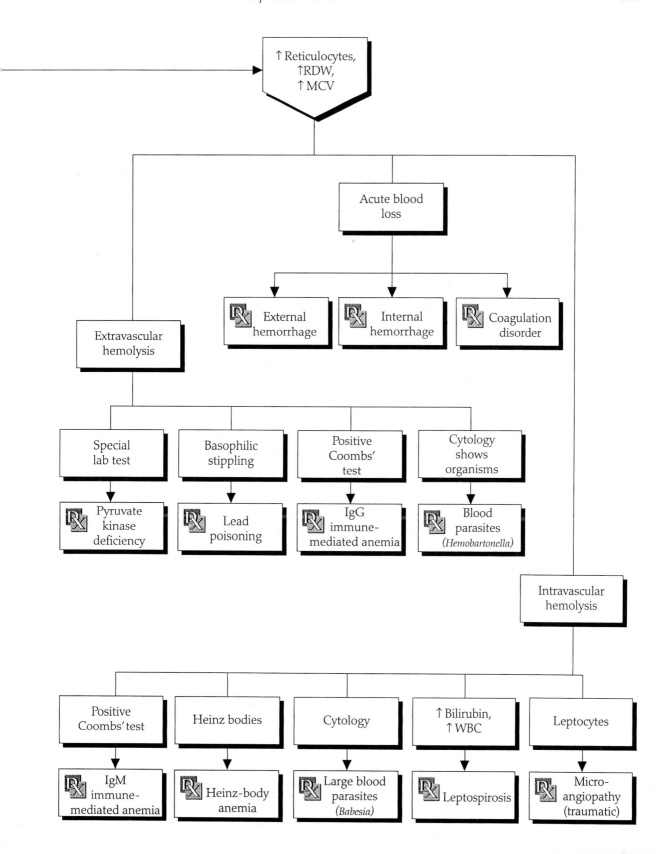

Nonresponsive Anemia

Erythropoiesis can be decreased because of deficient stem cells, erythropoietin, or iron. Severe impairment of erythropoiesis can directly cause nonregenerative anemia, and mild impairment can contribute to anemia caused by hemolysis or bleeding.

The clue to a production defect is a low reticulocyte count, a normal MCV, or a low, or normal RDW. When the response is inadequate, anemia is called *nonresponsive* or *nonregenerative*. These nonregenerative anemias may be associated with at least three vastly different bone marrow states:

- A normal ratio of myeloid cells to erythroid cells (M:E ratio), normal overall cellularity, and a normal pattern of erythroid maturation.
- Virtual absence of normal bone marrow elements caused by aplasia (absence of marrow cells), or by replacement of normal marrow elements by fibrosis, solid tumors, granulomas, or leukemia.
- Erythroid hyperplasia with increased cellularity. Because of defects of erythroid maturation, precursors die in the marrow, and too few cells reach the periphery.

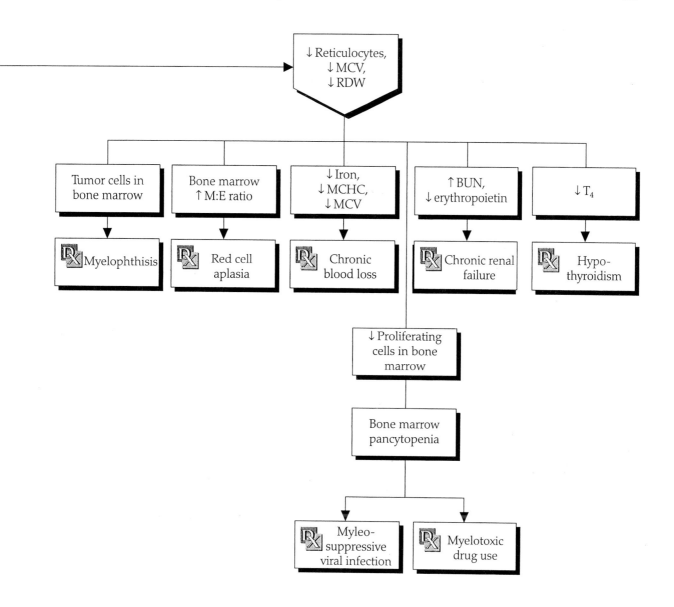

↓ Reticulocytes,
↓ MCV,
↓ RDW

Tumor cells in
bone marrow

Bone marrow
↑ M:E ratio

↓ Iron,
↓ MCHC,
↓ MCV

↑ BUN,
↓ erythropoietin

↓ T$_4$

℞ Myelophthisis

℞ Red cell
aplasia

℞ Chronic
blood loss

℞ Chronic renal
failure

Hypo-
thyroidism

↓ Proliferating
cells in bone
marrow

Bone marrow
pancytopenia

℞ Myleo-
suppressive
viral infection

℞ Myelotoxic
drug use

Polycythemia

Polycythemia is an increase in the number of circulating red blood cells.

Absolute polycythemia is characterized by increased red blood cell numbers with normal plasma fluid levels.

Relative polycythemia occurs with decreased plasma volume from fluid loss or fluid shifts to extravascular areas. This occurs with dehydration secondary to vomiting, diarrhea, hyperventilation, or diminished fluid intake. It also occurs with fluid shifts to interstitial spaces or body cavities secondary to ascites, hypoadrenocorticism, shock, and hemorrhagic gastroenteritis.

Absolute polycythemia occurs when the plasma volume is normal but the red blood cell numbers are elevated. This may occur with normal erythropoietin level in polycythemia vera, or with elevated erythropoietin levels in chronic pulmonary disease, chronic heart failure, and high altitude exposure.

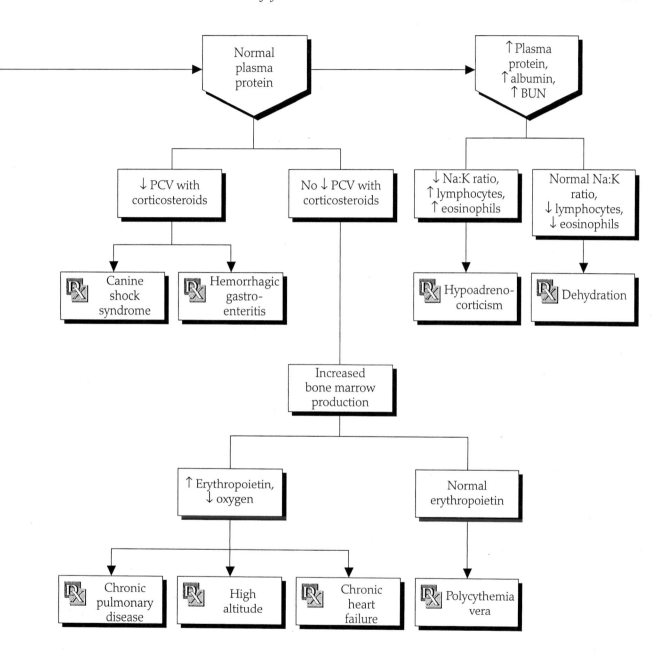

Dynamic RBC Testing

Normal red cell counts vary with age, breed, health, environment, and oxygen content of the air. To base a diagnosis of diseases such as anemia or hemoconcentration on a single static sample may be misleading. A more accurate method is to evaluate the red cell parameters as deviations from known normal values and as deviations from an individual patient's baseline value, which is determined during a period of relative health.

Both marked deviations from established normal values and sudden changes in an individual's values suggest disease. For example, hematocrit values below established normal values indicated anemia, and steps are taken to find the cause. In addition, sudden decreases in hematocrit values even if they are in the normal range for the species, indicate blood loss from hemorrhage or hemolysis that may eventually cause anemia.

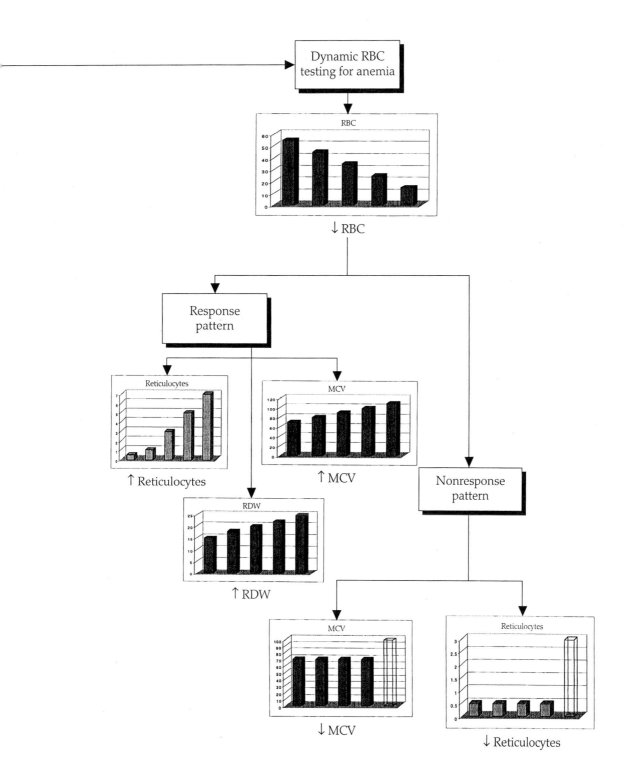

Leukocytosis

Leukocytosis is usually caused by neutrophilia but is occasionally due to lymphocytic or myelogenous leukemia. Three mechanisms are responsible for most neutrophilic reactions: mobilization from the storage or marginal pool, increased neutrophil survival, and increased production of neutrophils.

Acute neutrophilia (physiologic neutrophilia) develops within a few minutes. It is due to mobilization from the marginal or marrow pools, and is caused by excitement, pain, or exercise. Subacute neutrophilia that develops over several hours is due to glucocorticoids and chemotactic factors. These neutrophils are released from marrow stores into the circulating pool.

Continued neutrophil demand causes stem-cell activation and increased neutrophil production. Bacterial infection and diseases that damage tissue are common causes of this chronic neutrophilia.

If the storage pools cannot provide enough neutrophils, immature cells can be released. The presence of immature neutrophils (bands, metamyelocytes, and earlier forms) without an increase in total neutrophil numbers is termed a *degenerative left shift* and suggests an overwhelming septicemia or toxemia.

Neutrophilia with less than 10% band cells is called a *regenerative left shift* and is usually a good prognostic sign.

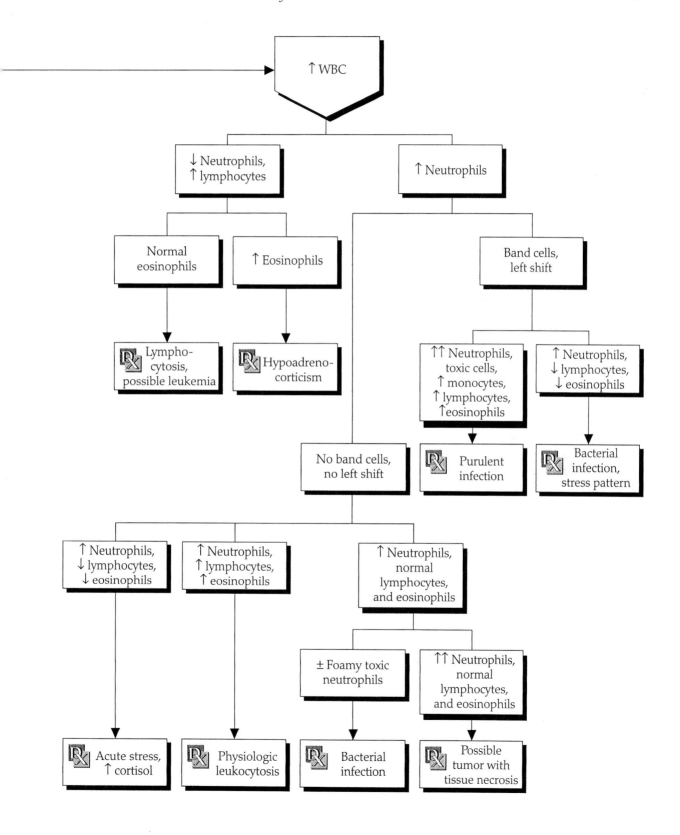

Leukopenia

Leukopenia is almost always due to neutropenia. In some diseases, concurrent lymphopenia and eosinopenia are present. To evaluate abnormalities in the hemogram, both the absolute numbers of each cell type and their percentages should be calculated.

Neutropenia is characterized by an absolute neutrophil count that is consistently below 3000/μl in the dog or 2500/μl in the cat. The pathophysiologic mechanisms of neutropenia can be grouped into three broad categories: defective neutrophil production, accelerated neutrophil removal, and neutrophil redistribution. When the need for neutrophils exceeds the ability of the bone marrow to produce mature cells, young cells (bands, metamyelocytes, myelocytes) appear. This is called *left shift.*

Common infectious causes of neutropenia are feline panleukopenia, feline immunodeficiency virus infection, ehrlichiosis, or canine parvovirus infection. These diseases often depress neutrophil production.

Physical agents, such as radiation, estrogen, fungal toxins, anticonvulsants, and cytotoxic drugs, both decrease neutrophil production and increase neutrophil consumption.

Peracute overwhelming infections, cellulitis, aspiration pneumonia, endotoxemia, peritonitis, acute viral infection, and immune-mediated neutrophil destruction increase consumption by accelerating neutrophil removal.

Neutrophils are redistributed into vascular beds in shock, endotoxemia, and splenomegaly.

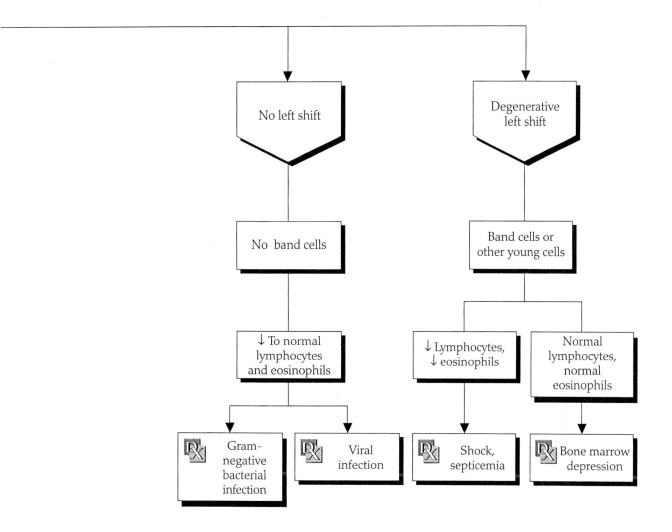

Bone Marrow in Nonresponsive Anemia

The bone marrow can be examined to determine the cause of nonresponsive anemia. For a meaningful interpretation, the marrow must always be evaluated in relation to the expected red blood cell response and the hemogram. The normal response to anemia is hyperplasia of the red cell precursors. This produces a low M:E ratio, with marked cellularity of the marrow.

A practical method of bone marrow examination does not have to be time consuming.

1. Take a core sample to detect fibrosis or tumor infiltration.
2. Squash a fleck of marrow and check the cellularity by comparing the number of fat cells to blood cells. Only in old animals should the fat cells outnumber the blood cells.
3. Count 500 cells and divide them into myeloid or erythroid elements to get the M:E ratio. This will show if there is a shift of the stem cells to granulocytic production. The M:E ratio may be normal if both lines are depressed (pancytopenia).
4. Calculate the EMI (erythroid maturation index) in anemic animals that seem to have large numbers of red blood cell precursors in the marrow. This will indicate a maturation defect.

Depression anemia may be manifested as decreased red blood cell precursor or a maturation defect in which the precursor do not proceed to the mature stage.

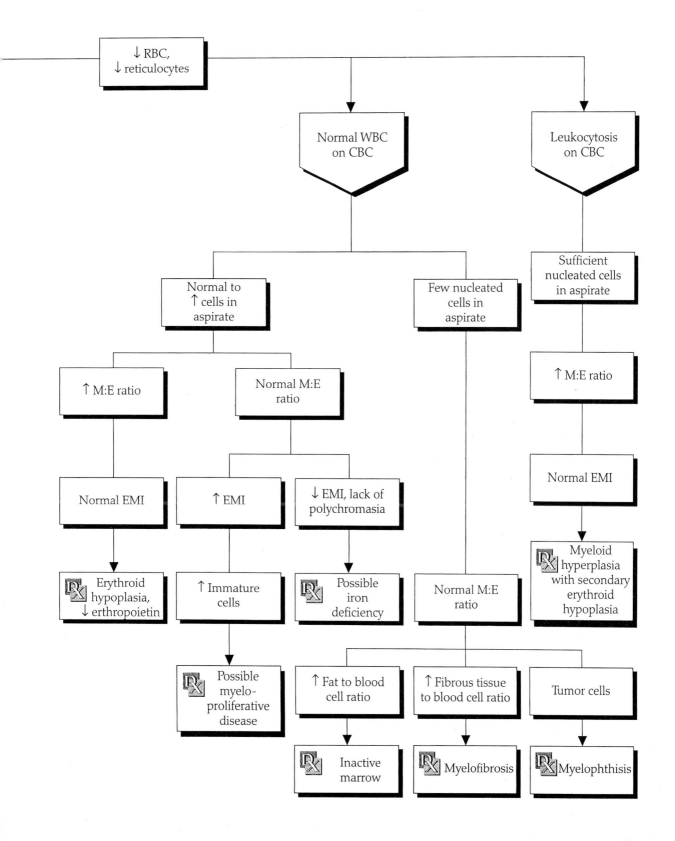

Bone Marrow in Leukopenia and Thrombocytopenia

The marrow is examined to determine the cause of unexpected leukopenia or thrombocytopenia. In cases of neutrophilia, the marrow is not usually examined unless there is a leukemoid reaction.

Several bone marrow patterns may be present in a leukopenic animal.

- Total decrease in bone marrow cells resulting from fibrosis, tumor replacement, or toxicity. This is best seen on histopathologic core samples.
- Highly cellular marrow with few normally maturing white blood cells and many red blood cell precursors. This is seen with an erythrocytic hyperplasia response to anemia.
- Highly cellular marrow with many young proliferating white cells (progranulocytes, granulocytes, and myelocytes) but little progression to metamyelocytes and band cells. This is reflected by a high MMI and indicates increased demand from overwhelming inflammation that is consuming neutrophils.
- Poorly cellular marrow with few proliferating or maturing granulocytes. This indicates stem-cell depression from a virus, antibodies, or toxins.

With thrombocytopenia, megakaryocyte numbers should be elevated. If many are seen, consumptive thrombocytopenia is probable. If few are seen, insufficient production is probable.

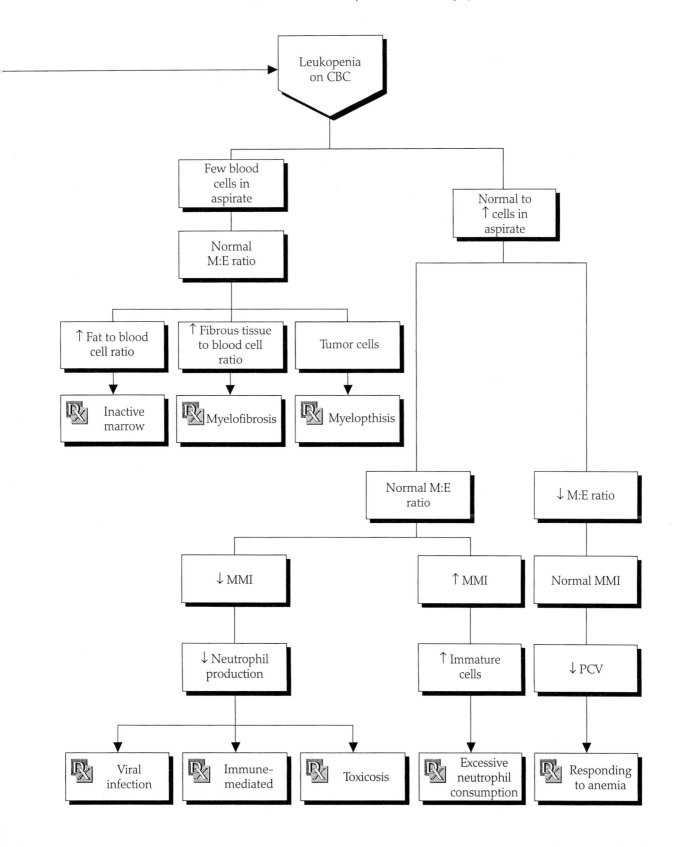

References

Herrewegh AA, et al: Detection of feline coronavirus RNA in feces, tissues, and body fluids of naturally infected cats by reverse transcriptase PCR, *J Clin Microbiol* 33(3):684-689, 1995.

Nishiyama T, et al: Determination of optimal time for mating by artificial insemination, *J Am Vet Med Assoc* 35(4):348-352, 1999.

Paltrinieri S, et al: Type IV hypersensitivity in the pathogenesis of FIPV-induced lesions, *Zentralbl Veterinarmed* [B] 45(3):151-159, 1998.

Vennema H, et al: Feline infectious peritonitis viruses arise by mutation from endemic feline enteric coronaviruses, *Virology* 243(1):150-157, 1998.

Section 12
Laboratory Profiles of Diseases

Liver   526

Urinary System   540

Immune/Infectious Diseases   554

Toxins   560

Adrenal (Primary) Hyperadrenocorticism

adrenal tumors secrete cortisol without stimulation from ACTH

Less than 15% of dogs with spontaneous hyperadrenocorticism have tumors of the adrenal cortex. These tumors secrete cortisol independent of stimulation by ACTH from the pituitary. The tumors are usually unilateral, and 50% are malignant.

Interpretation

The stress pattern on CBC suggests oversecretion of glucocorticoids. In dogs, corticosteroids induce high serum alkaline phosphatase and GGT activities; special tests may reveal a specific corticosteroid-induced isoenzyme of alkaline phosphatase.

Corticosteroids cause hyperlipidemia and can predispose to hepatic lipidosis, pancreatitis, and diabetes mellitus. Low resting serum T_4 levels suggest hypothyroidism, but fT_4d levels are normal.

Resting serum cortisol and urine cortisol levels are high. The response to ACTH stimulation is high in half of affected animals. Lack of high-dosage dexamethasone suppression distinguishes an adrenal tumor from a pituitary tumor. Resting serum ACTH levels are below normal.

Differential Diagnoses
- Pituitary-dependent hyperadrenocorticism: large doses of dexamethasone suppress serum cortisol levels
- Acute renal disease: active kidney lesions, azotemia
- Corticosteroid-induced hepatopathy: high ALT and alkaline phosphatase activities, increased blood glucose level with glucagon stimulation
- Diabetes insipidus: no stress pattern on CBC, no decrease in eosinophil and lymphocyte numbers
- Hypothyroidism: normal fT_4d levels indicate normal thyroid function

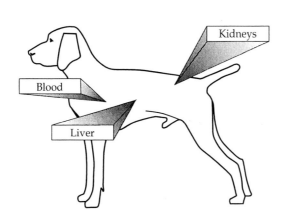

Signs
- Polydipsia
- Polyuria
- Pendulous abdomen
- Bilateral alopecia
- Lethargy
- Weakness
- Thin mineralized skin
- Hyperpigmentation

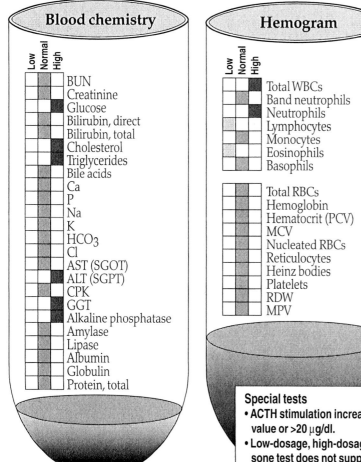

Blood chemistry

	Low	Normal	High	
BUN				
Creatinine				
Glucose				
Bilirubin, direct				
Bilirubin, total				
Cholesterol				
Triglycerides				
Bile acids				
Ca				
P				
Na				
K				
HCO3				
Cl				
AST (SGOT)				
ALT (SGPT)				
CPK				
GGT				
Alkaline phosphatase				
Amylase				
Lipase				
Albumin				
Globulin				
Protein, total				

Hemogram

	Low	Normal	High	
Total WBCs				
Band neutrophils				
Neutrophils				
Lymphocytes				
Monocytes				
Eosinophils				
Basophils				
Total RBCs				
Hemoglobin				
Hematocrit (PCV)				
MCV				
Nucleated RBCs				
Reticulocytes				
Heinz bodies				
Platelets				
RDW				
MPV				

Urinalysis

	Low	Normal / none	High	
pH				
Specific gravity				
Albumin				
Glucose				
Ketones				
Occult blood				
Bilirubin				
WBCs				
RBCs				
Epithelial cells				
Casts				
Crystals				
Bacteria				

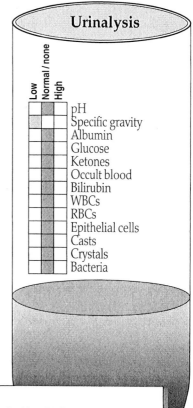

Special tests
- ACTH stimulation increases cortisol level 5 times the baseline value or >20 µg/dl.
- Low-dosage, high-dosage, or very-high-dosage dexamethasone test does not suppress cortisol completely.
- Increased urine cortisol:creatinine ratio.
- Glucose and glucagon tolerance tests show prolonged hyperglycemia.
- Decreased serum T_4, normal fT_4d.

Iatrogenic Hyperadrenocorticism

exogenous corticosteroids depress ACTH release while producing signs of Cushing's disease

Iatrogenic hyperadrenocorticism is caused by prolonged use of oral, injectable, or topical corticosteroids. These drugs cause atrophy of the adrenal cortex while producing signs of cortisol excess.

Exogenous corticosteroids inhibit ACTH release and decrease production of endogenous glucocorticoids but not aldosterone. Affected animals show signs of adrenocortical excess, while the adrenal glands are hypofunctional.

Interpretation
The stress pattern on the CBC suggests glucocorticoid excess. In dogs, corticosteroids induce high serum alkaline phosphatase and GGT activities. Increased lipolysis and decreased lipoprotein lipase activity cause hyperlipidemia.

Low resting serum T_4 levels suggest hypothyroidism, but fT_4d is normal. Resting serum cortisol and urine cortisol levels are low. The low urine specific gravity results from a concentrating defect caused by renal medullary washout of sodium and dysfunction of ADH receptors.

Differential Diagnoses
- Diabetes insipidus: vasopressin administration increases urine specific gravity
- Secondary hypoadrenocorticism: a concurrent problem

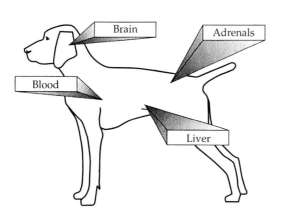

Signs
- Polydipsia
- Polyuria
- Pendulous abdomen
- Bilateral alopecia
- Lethargy
- Weakness
- Thin mineralized skin
- Hyperpigmentation

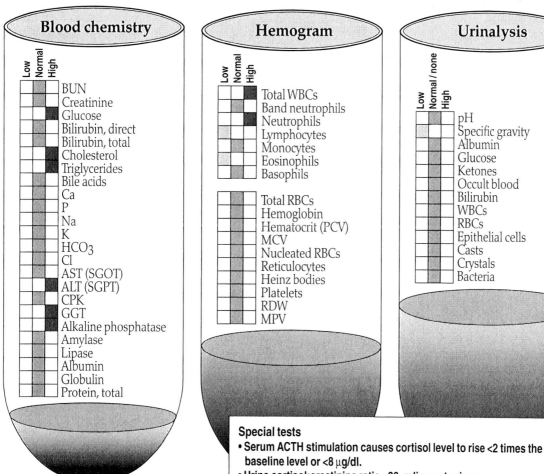

Blood chemistry

	Low	Normal	High	
		■		BUN
		■		Creatinine
			■	Glucose
		■		Bilirubin, direct
		■		Bilirubin, total
			■	Cholesterol
			■	Triglycerides
		■		Bile acids
		■		Ca
		■		P
		■		Na
		■		K
		■		HCO3
		■		Cl
		■		AST (SGOT)
			■	ALT (SGPT)
		■		CPK
			■	GGT
			■	Alkaline phosphatase
		■		Amylase
		■		Lipase
		■		Albumin
		■		Globulin
		■		Protein, total

Hemogram

	Low	Normal	High	
			■	Total WBCs
		■		Band neutrophils
			■	Neutrophils
	■			Lymphocytes
			■	Monocytes
	■			Eosinophils
		■		Basophils

	Low	Normal	High	
		■		Total RBCs
		■		Hemoglobin
		■		Hematocrit (PCV)
		■		MCV
		■		Nucleated RBCs
		■		Reticulocytes
		■		Heinz bodies
		■		Platelets
		■		RDW
		■		MPV

Urinalysis

	Low	Normal / none	High	
		■		pH
	■			Specific gravity
		■		Albumin
		■		Glucose
		■		Ketones
		■		Occult blood
		■		Bilirubin
		■		WBCs
		■		RBCs
		■		Epithelial cells
		■		Casts
		■		Crystals
		■		Bacteria

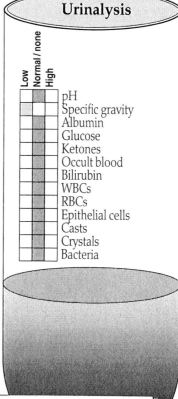

Special tests
- Serum ACTH stimulation causes cortisol level to rise <2 times the baseline level or <8 μg/dl.
- Urine cortisol:creatinine ratio <20, ruling out primary hyperadrenocorticism.
- Serum T_4 level may be low.
- Decreased serum T_4, normal fT_4d.

Pituitary-Dependent Hyperadrenocorticism (Cushing's Disease)

pituitary-
dependent
hyperadreno-
corticism is
diagnosed with
the high-dosage
dexamethasone
suppression test

Bilateral adrenocortical hyperplasia secondary to excessive secretion of ACTH from the pituitary gland is the usual cause of hyperadrenocorticism. ACTH oversecretion can be caused by a pituitary tumor or a brain lesion that secretes corticotropin-releasing factor.

Interpretation
The stress pattern on the CBC suggests oversecretion of glucocorticoids. In dogs, corticosteroids induce high serum alkaline phosphatase and GGT activities.

Corticosteroids cause hyperlipidemia and predispose to hepatic lipidosis, pancreatitis, and diabetes mellitus. A low serum T_4 level suggests hypothyroidism, but fT_4d is normal, indicating the euthyroid sick animal syndrome.

High resting serum cortisol levels and high ACTH-stimulated cortisol levels indicate adrenal hyperfunction. Lack of low-dosage dexamethasone suppression with a positive response to high-dosage dexamethasone suppression or high endogenous ACTH levels is diagnostic for a pituitary lesion.

Differential Diagnoses
- Type-I diabetes mellitus: hyperglycemia with low serum insulin levels
- Type-II diabetes mellitus: hyperglycemia with normal to high serum insulin levels
- Chronic renal failure: high BUN, low urine specific gravity
- Diabetes insipidus: no stress pattern on CBC, normal serum cortisol levels
- Hypothyroidism: decreased fT_4d

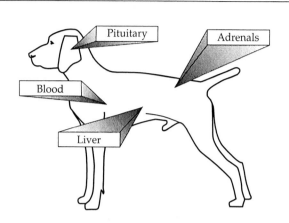

Signs
- Polydipsia
- Polyuria
- Pendulous abdomen
- Bilateral alopecia
- Lethargy
- Weakness
- Thin mineralized skin
- Hyperpigmentation

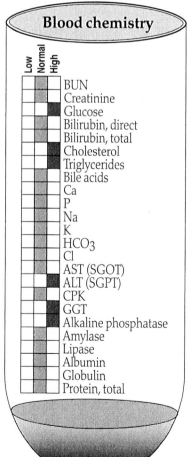

Blood chemistry

	Low	Normal	High	
				BUN
				Creatinine
				Glucose
				Bilirubin, direct
				Bilirubin, total
				Cholesterol
				Triglycerides
				Bile acids
				Ca
				P
				Na
				K
				HCO$_3$
				Cl
				AST (SGOT)
				ALT (SGPT)
				CPK
				GGT
				Alkaline phosphatase
				Amylase
				Lipase
				Albumin
				Globulin
				Protein, total

Hemogram

	Low	Normal	High	
				Total WBCs
				Band neutrophils
				Neutrophils
				Lymphocytes
				Monocytes
				Eosinophils
				Basophils
				Total RBCs
				Hemoglobin
				Hematocrit (PCV)
				MCV
				Nucleated RBCs
				Reticulocytes
				Heinz bodies
				Platelets
				RDW
				MPV

Urinalysis

	Low	Normal / none	High	
				pH
				Specific gravity
				Albumin
				Glucose
				Ketones
				Occult blood
				Bilirubin
				WBCs
				RBCs
				Epithelial cells
				Casts
				Crystals
				Bacteria

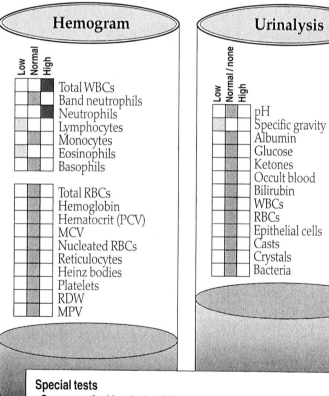

Special tests
- Serum cortisol level >4 µg/dl before and >12 µg/dl after ACTH.
- High urine cortisol:creatinine ratio.
- Low-dosage dexamethasone test does not suppress cortisol level.
- High-dosage dexamethasone test suppresses cortisol level to <50%.
- Serum ACTH level is 40-500 pg/ml.
- Glucose tolerance test shows prolonged hyperglycemia.
- Low serum T$_4$, normal fT$_4$d.

Primary Hypoadrenocorticism (Addison's Disease)

atrophy or destruction of all layers of the adrenal cortex causes deficiency of cortisol and aldosterone; this may occur from immune mechanisms, mitotane therapy, or adrenal disease

Primary hypoadrenocorticism is a failure of the adrenal cortex to secrete glucocorticoids and mineralocorticoids.

Immune-mediated, infectious, vascular, or chemical agents damage the adrenal cortex and cause atrophy or destruction of the cells that produce cortisol or aldosterone.

Interpretation
Eosinophilia, lymphocytosis, and low blood glucose levels suggest corticosteroid deficiency. Aldosterone deficiency causes hyponatremia and hyperkalemia, with low blood pressure causing poor renal perfusion. Poor renal perfusion from decreased vascular volume leads to azotemia. Hypercalcemia is related to an elevated serum albumin level from hemoconcentration.

Cortisol deficiency is confirmed with an ACTH stimulation test. A serum Na:K ratio <23 indicates aldosterone deficiency.

Differential Diagnoses
- Acute renal failure: high BUN, casts in urine, normal Na:K ratio
- Chronic renal failure: high BUN, low urine specific gravity, normal Na:K ratio
- Heart failure: abnormal ECG, pulmonary edema

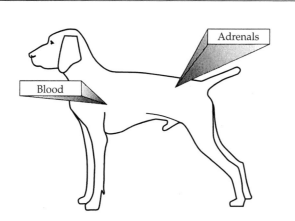

Signs
- Depression
- Weakness
- Lethargy
- Decreased appetite
- Vomiting
- Diarrhea
- Weight loss
- Bradycardia

Adrenals

Blood

Blood chemistry

	Low	Normal	High	
				BUN
				Creatinine
				Glucose
				Bilirubin, direct
				Bilirubin, total
				Cholesterol
				Triglycerides
				Bile acids
				Ca
				P
				Na
				K
				HCO₃
				Cl
				AST (SGOT)
				ALT (SGPT)
				CPK
				GGT
				Alkaline phosphatase
				Amylase
				Lipase
				Albumin
				Globulin
				Protein, total

Hemogram

	Low	Normal	High	
				Total WBCs
				Band neutrophils
				Neutrophils
				Lymphocytes
				Monocytes
				Eosinophils
				Basophils

	Low	Normal	High	
				Total RBCs
				Hemoglobin
				Hematocrit (PCV)
				MCV
				Nucleated RBCs
				Reticulocytes
				Heinz bodies
				Platelets
				RDW
				MPV

Urinalysis

	Low	Normal / none	High	
				pH
				Specific gravity
				Albumin
				Glucose
				Ketones
				Occult blood
				Bilirubin
				WBCs
				RBCs
				Epithelial cells
				Casts
				Crystals
				Bacteria

Special tests
- ACTH stimulation causes cortisol level to rise <2 times the baseline value or <8 µg/dl.
- Na:K ratio <23.

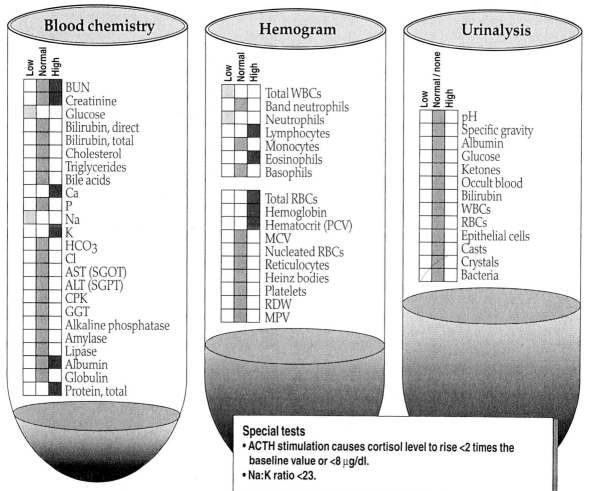

Secondary Hypoadrenocorticism

insufficient ACTH secretion causes glucocorticoid deficiency without mineralocorticoid deficiency; follows abrupt withdrawal of exogenous corticosteroids

Secondary hypoadrenocorticism is characterized by reduced pituitary secretion of ACTH. The most common cause is excessive or prolonged administration of corticosteroids. Occasionally it is caused by lesions in the hypothalamus.

Signs are related to glucocorticoid deficiency, rather than to mineralocorticoid deficiency. Clinical signs occur on withdrawal of exogenous corticosteroids.

Interpretation
Eosinophilia, lymphocytosis, and a low blood glucose level suggest insufficient cortisol production. The insufficiency is confirmed with an ACTH stimulation test. The serum Na:K ratio remains >27 because aldosterone production is normal.

Differential Diagnoses
- Heart failure: abnormal ECG, pulmonary edema
- Renal ischemia: high BUN level that does not respond to fluid therapy
- Hyperadrenocorticism: exogenous corticosteroids can mask the signs of decreased adrenocortical function

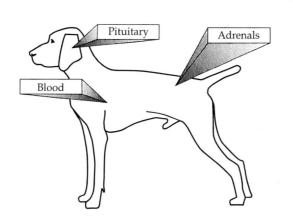

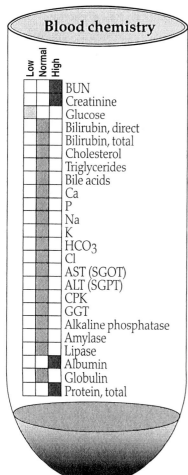

Signs
- Depression
- Weakness
- Lethargy
- Decreased appetite
- Vomiting
- Diarrhea
- Weight loss

Blood chemistry

	Low	Normal	High
BUN			■
Creatinine	■		
Glucose		■	
Bilirubin, direct		■	
Bilirubin, total		■	
Cholesterol		■	
Triglycerides		■	
Bile acids		■	
Ca		■	
P		■	
Na		■	
K		■	
HCO$_3$		■	
Cl		■	
AST (SGOT)		■	
ALT (SGPT)		■	
CPK		■	
GGT		■	
Alkaline phosphatase		■	
Amylase		■	
Lipase		■	
Albumin			■
Globulin		■	
Protein, total			■

Hemogram

	Low	Normal	High
Total WBCs	■		
Band neutrophils		■	
Neutrophils		■	
Lymphocytes			■
Monocytes		■	
Eosinophils			■
Basophils		■	

	Low	Normal	High
Total RBCs			■
Hemoglobin			■
Hematocrit (PCV)			■
MCV		■	
Nucleated RBCs		■	
Reticulocytes		■	
Heinz bodies		■	
Platelets		■	
RDW		■	
MPV		■	

Urinalysis

	Low	Normal / none	High
pH		■	
Specific gravity		■	
Albumin		■	
Glucose		■	
Ketones		■	
Occult blood		■	
Bilirubin		■	
WBCs		■	
RBCs		■	
Epithelial cells		■	
Casts		■	
Crystals		■	
Bacteria		■	

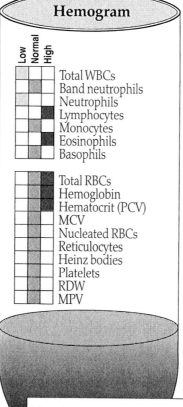

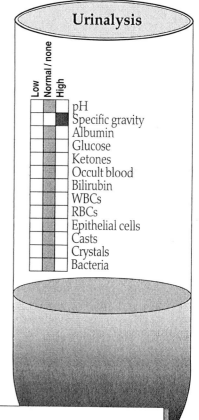

Special tests
- ACTH stimulation causes cortisol level to rise <2 times the baseline value or <8 µg/dl.
- Na:K ratio >27.

Pituitary-Dependent Diabetes Insipidus

insufficient ADH is caused by defective secretion or synthesis

Pituitary-dependent (central) diabetes insipidus, a deficiency of antidiuretic hormone (ADH), causes diuresis and hypotension. ADH is normally released in response to increased serum osmotic pressure, volume depletion, and drugs that increase blood pressure.

A lesion in the hypothalamus or the neurohypophysis of the pituitary causes permanent ADH deficiency. Chemicals (alcohol, xylazine, glucocorticoids) inhibit ADH secretion. Lack of ADH results in very dilute urine.

Interpretation
The blood panel can rule out common causes of polydipsia, such as kidney disease, liver disease, pyometra, and diabetes mellitus. Other causes of dilute urine must be distinguished with special tests.

The exogenous vasopressin test can distinguish between central and nephrogenic diabetes insipidus. To be sure that prolonged polyuria has not washed out the osmotic gradient of the kidneys, a repository vasopressin test should be performed.

Water deprivation can rule out psychogenic water consumption but must not be done in a dehydrated animal. To eliminate problems of urinary washout, the modified water deprivation test is preferred.

Differential Diagnoses
- Diabetes mellitus: hyperglycemia, glycosuria
- Renal failure: anemia, high serum creatinine level, usually a urine specific gravity around 1.010 that does not respond to ADH
- Liver disease: increased serum bile acid levels, no response to ADH
- Hyperadrenocorticism: stress pattern on CBC, high serum cortisol level, high serum alkaline phosphatase activity
- Psychogenic polydipsia: urine specific gravity increases with water deprivation
- Nephrogenic diabetes insipidus: no increase in urine specific gravity after ADH administration
- Renal medullary washout: urine specific gravity returns to normal after injection of repository vasopressin, after the modified water deprivation test, or after IV infusion of concentrated saline (Hickey-Hare test)

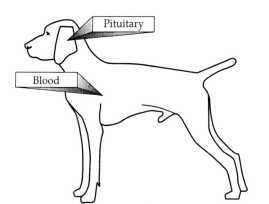

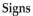

Pituitary

Blood

Signs
- Polyuria
- Polydipsia
- Dehydration

Blood chemistry

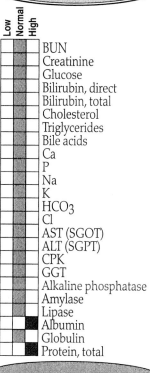

	Low	Normal	High
BUN			
Creatinine			
Glucose			
Bilirubin, direct			
Bilirubin, total			
Cholesterol			
Triglycerides			
Bile acids			
Ca			
P			
Na			
K			
HCO3			
Cl			
AST (SGOT)			
ALT (SGPT)			
CPK			
GGT			
Alkaline phosphatase			
Amylase			
Lipase			
Albumin			
Globulin			
Protein, total			

Hemogram

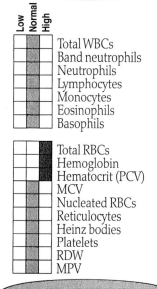

	Low	Normal	High
Total WBCs			
Band neutrophils			
Neutrophils			
Lymphocytes			
Monocytes			
Eosinophils			
Basophils			

	Low	Normal	High
Total RBCs			
Hemoglobin			
Hematocrit (PCV)			
MCV			
Nucleated RBCs			
Reticulocytes			
Heinz bodies			
Platelets			
RDW			
MPV			

Urinalysis

	Low	Normal / none	High
pH			
Specific gravity			
Albumin			
Glucose			
Ketones			
Occult blood			
Bilirubin			
WBCs			
RBCs			
Epithelial cells			
Casts			
Crystals			
Bacteria			

Special tests
- Water deprivation does not increase urine specific gravity.
- Exogenous vasopressin increases urine specific gravity to >1.025.
- Repository vasopressin should be used if the simple vasopressin test is inconclusive.

Primary Hyperparathyroidism

parathyroid-induced hypercalcemia is differentiated from hypercalcemia of malignancy by a Cl:P ratio >33

Elevated serum calcium levels normally inhibit release of parathormone (PTH) from the parathyroid gland. High serum calcium levels do not inhibit PTH secretion by parathyroid tumors or hyperplastic parathyroid tissue.

PTH acts on the bones and kidneys. High serum PTH levels raise blood calcium levels by decalcifying the bones, increasing renal calcium resorption, and increasing renal phosphorus excretion.

Interpretation
Renal failure can cause or result from hypercalcemia. Hypercalcemia and hypophosphatemia are present with both primary hyperparathyroidism and hypercalcemia of malignancy.

A ratio of serum chloride to phosphorus >33 suggests primary hyperparathyroidism because of concurrent hyperchloremic acidosis. A ratio of <33 suggests hypercalcemia induced by malignancy. Definitive diagnosis of a parathyroid tumor requires exploratory surgery of the neck, or high serum PTH levels.

Differential Diagnoses
- Hypercalcemia of malignancy: serum Cl:P ratio <33
- Primary renal failure: hypocalcemia, hyperphosphatemia
- Hypoadrenocorticism: high eosinophil and lymphocyte counts, low serum cortisol level, serum Na:K ratio below 23
- Bone tumors: osteolytic lesion visible on radiographs
- Hemoconcentration: high serum albumin level, high PCV reduced by rehydration

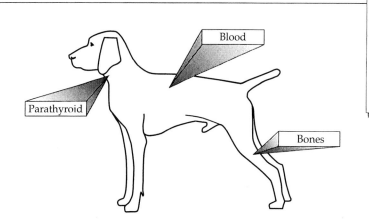

Blood

Parathyroid

Bones

Signs
- Polyuria
- Polydipsia
- Listlessness
- Weakness
- Seizures
- Anorexia

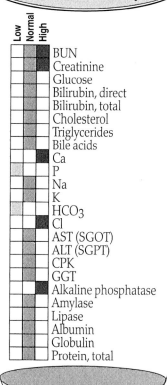

Blood chemistry

	Low	Normal	High	
				BUN
				Creatinine
				Glucose
				Bilirubin, direct
				Bilirubin, total
				Cholesterol
				Triglycerides
				Bile acids
				Ca
				P
				Na
				K
				HCO₃
				Cl
				AST (SGOT)
				ALT (SGPT)
				CPK
				GGT
				Alkaline phosphatase
				Amylase
				Lipase
				Albumin
				Globulin
				Protein, total

Hemogram

	Low	Normal	High	
				Total WBCs
				Band neutrophils
				Neutrophils
				Lymphocytes
				Monocytes
				Eosinophils
				Basophils
				Total RBCs
				Hemoglobin
				Hematocrit (PCV)
				MCV
				Nucleated RBCs
				Reticulocytes
				Heinz bodies
				Platelets
				RDW
				MPV

Urinalysis

	Low	Normal / none	High	
				pH
				Specific gravity
				Albumin
				Glucose
				Ketones
				Occult blood
				Bilirubin
				WBCs
				RBCs
				Epithelial cells
				Casts
				Crystals
				Bacteria

Special tests
- Radiographs may show loss of bone density.
- Adjusted calcium value may be needed if serum albumin levels are abnormally high or low.
- High serum PTH level.
- Serum Cl:P ratio >33.

Renal Secondary Hyperparathyroidism

phosphorus
retention
suppresses
serum calcium
levels, which
stimulates PTH
release

In animals with chronic renal failure, secondary hyperparathyroidism occurs as a result of phosphorus retention and poor calcium absorption. Reaction with phosphorus reduces the serum level of ionized calcium. In addition, reduced activation of vitamin D in the diseased kidneys impairs intestinal absorption of calcium. The low serum calcium level stimulates parathormone release.

Interpretation
Signs of kidney failure predominate, with increased blood urea nitrogen, creatinine, and phosphorus levels. A low serum bicarbonate level and acidic urine indicate acidosis. Nonregenerative anemia is secondary to lack of erythropoietin.

Normal urine sediment and low urine specific gravity suggest chronic renal disease, rather than an acute problem. The danger of soft tissue mineralization is great because the serum calcium $\times$ phosphorus product is >60. Increased fractional excretion of phosphorus and decreased ionized calcium levels suggest increased PTH. This may be confirmed with a direct assay for PTH.

Differential Diagnoses
- Nutritional secondary hyperparathyroidism: hyperphosphatemia, hypocalcemia, no azotemia
- Hypoalbuminemia: normal corrected serum calcium value

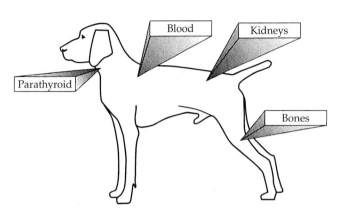

Signs
- Polyuria
- Polydipsia
- Listlessness
- Weakness
- Vomiting
- Anorexia
- Pathologic fractures
- Loose teeth

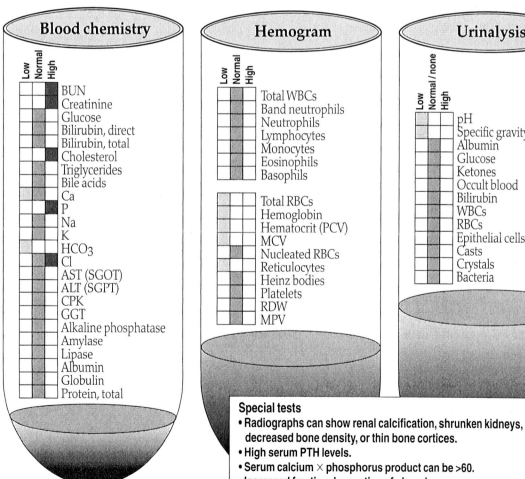

Blood chemistry

	Low	Normal	High
BUN			
Creatinine			
Glucose			
Bilirubin, direct			
Bilirubin, total			
Cholesterol			
Triglycerides			
Bile acids			
Ca			
P			
Na			
K			
HCO$_3$			
Cl			
AST (SGOT)			
ALT (SGPT)			
CPK			
GGT			
Alkaline phosphatase			
Amylase			
Lipase			
Albumin			
Globulin			
Protein, total			

Hemogram

	Low	Normal	High
Total WBCs			
Band neutrophils			
Neutrophils			
Lymphocytes			
Monocytes			
Eosinophils			
Basophils			

	Low	Normal	High
Total RBCs			
Hemoglobin			
Hematocrit (PCV)			
MCV			
Nucleated RBCs			
Reticulocytes			
Heinz bodies			
Platelets			
RDW			
MPV			

Urinalysis

	Low	Normal / none	High
pH			
Specific gravity			
Albumin			
Glucose			
Ketones			
Occult blood			
Bilirubin			
WBCs			
RBCs			
Epithelial cells			
Casts			
Crystals			
Bacteria			

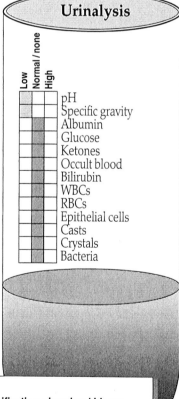

Special tests
- Radiographs can show renal calcification, shrunken kidneys, decreased bone density, or thin bone cortices.
- High serum PTH levels.
- Serum calcium × phosphorus product can be >60.
- Increased fractional excretion of phosphorus.
- Decreased ionized calcium.

Pseudohyper-parathyroidism (Hypercalcemia of Malignancy)

certain malignant tumors cause hypercalcemia, which may be inferred from a Cl:P ratio <33

Pseudohyperparathyroidism occurs when osteolytic substances produced by a nonparathyroid neoplasm elevate serum calcium levels. This hypercalcemia is caused by direct tumor osteolysis, osteolysis by prostaglandins, production of bone resorption substance, or ectopic production of compounds similar to parathyroid hormone.

Interpretation
The primary abnormalities are hypercalcemia and hypophosphatemia, with normal serum alkaline phosphatase activity. Early in the disease, the BUN level is normal, but later dystrophic calcification of the kidneys can elevate BUN and creatinine levels.

A serum chloride/phosphorus ratio below 33 suggests hypercalcemia associated with malignancy. The high serum calcium level causes renal calcification. High PTHrP during episodes of hypercalcemia indicates the hypercalcemia is due to malignancy. Persistently high levels following cancer treatment indicate inadequate control of the tumor. PTH levels are normal.

Differential Diagnoses
- Chronic renal failure: high serum urea nitrogen and phosphorus levels, normal to low serum calcium levels, low urine specific gravity
- Bone tumors: osteolytic lesion visible on radiographs
- Hemoconcentration: high serum calcium level with high serum albumin level
- Hypoadrenocorticism: low serum Na:K ratio (<23)
- Hypervitaminosis D: hypercalcemia, hyperphosphatemia
- Primary hyperparathyroidism: hypercalcemia, hypophosphatemia, Cl:P ratio >33
- Nephrotoxicosis: active urine sediment, renal calcification on radiographs

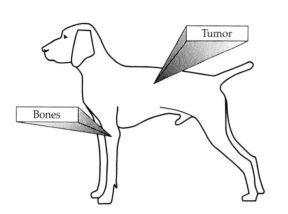

Signs
- Polyuria
- Polydipsia
- Listlessness
- Weakness
- Seizures
- Anorexia
- Weight loss
- Vomiting
- Bradycardia
- Enlarged lymph nodes, spleen, or liver
- Perirectal tumor

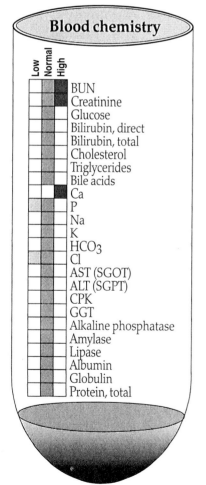

Blood chemistry

	Low	Normal	High
BUN			■
Creatinine			■
Glucose		■	
Bilirubin, direct		■	
Bilirubin, total		■	
Cholesterol		■	
Triglycerides		■	
Bile acids		■	
Ca			■
P	■		
Na		■	
K		■	
HCO3	■		
Cl		■	
AST (SGOT)		■	
ALT (SGPT)		■	
CPK		■	
GGT		■	
Alkaline phosphatase		■	
Amylase		■	
Lipase		■	
Albumin		■	
Globulin		■	
Protein, total		■	

Hemogram

	Low	Normal	High
Total WBCs		■	
Band neutrophils		■	
Neutrophils		■	
Lymphocytes		■	
Monocytes		■	
Eosinophils		■	
Basophils		■	

	Low	Normal	High
Total RBCs		■	
Hemoglobin		■	
Hematocrit (PCV)		■	
MCV		■	
Nucleated RBCs		■	
Reticulocytes		■	
Heinz bodies		■	
Platelets		■	
RDW		■	
MPV		■	

Urinalysis

	Low	Normal / none	High
pH		■	
Specific gravity		■	
Albumin			■
Glucose		■	
Ketones		■	
Occult blood		■	
Bilirubin		■	
WBCs		■	
RBCs		■	
Epithelial cells		■	
Casts			■
Crystals		■	
Bacteria		■	

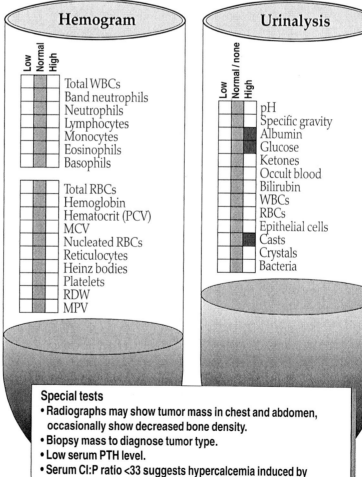

Special tests
- Radiographs may show tumor mass in chest and abdomen, occasionally show decreased bone density.
- Biopsy mass to diagnose tumor type.
- Low serum PTH level.
- Serum Cl:P ratio <33 suggests hypercalcemia induced by malignancy.
- Increased ionized calcium.
- Increased PTH-related protein.

Hypothyroidism of Disease (Euthyroid Sick Syndrome)

severe disease
decreases secre-
tion of TSH and
may give false
indications of
hypothyroidism

Serum T_3 and T_4 levels decrease in many severe or chronic diseases as a compensatory mechanism to conserve essential body tissue in the face of inadequate caloric intake. This condition, called *euthyroid sick syndrome,* is seen with uremia, diabetes mellitus, hyperadrenocorticism, and debilitating diseases.

Interpretation
Thyroid tests show normal to low serum T_3, T_4, and TSH levels. This indicates a normal thyroid gland and a centrally located problem. The fT_4d test is usually normal, indicating normal circulating levels of active hormone.

Differential Diagnoses
- Atrophic hypothyroidism: shows low serum T_4 and fT_4d levels, with normal TSH levels and no antithyroid antibodies
- Immune-mediated hypothyroidism: shows normal to high serum T_4 levels, decreased fT_4d levels, and high serum levels of antithyroid antibodies
- Pituitary-dependent hypothyroidism: shows decreased levels of T_4, fT_4d, and TSH with no antithyroid antibodies
- Severe disease decreases secretion of TSH and release of T_4, giving a false impression of hypothyroidism
- fT_4d is a more accurate test and is usually normal

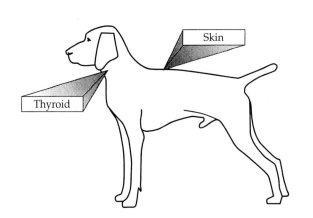

Skin

Thyroid

Signs
• Primarily related to underlying disease

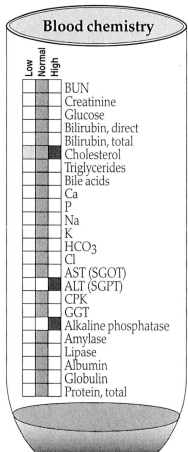

Blood chemistry

	Low	Normal	High	
				BUN
				Creatinine
				Glucose
				Bilirubin, direct
				Bilirubin, total
				Cholesterol
				Triglycerides
				Bile acids
				Ca
				P
				Na
				K
				HCO₃
				Cl
				AST (SGOT)
				ALT (SGPT)
				CPK
				GGT
				Alkaline phosphatase
				Amylase
				Lipase
				Albumin
				Globulin
				Protein, total

Hemogram

	Low	Normal	High	
				Total WBCs
				Band neutrophils
				Neutrophils
				Lymphocytes
				Monocytes
				Eosinophils
				Basophils
				Total RBCs
				Hemoglobin
				Hematocrit (PCV)
				MCV
				Nucleated RBCs
				Reticulocytes
				Heinz bodies
				Platelets
				RDW
				MPV

Urinalysis

	Low	Normal / none	High	
				pH
				Specific gravity
				Albumin
				Glucose
				Ketones
				Occult blood
				Bilirubin
				WBCs
				RBCs
				Epithelial cells
				Casts
				Crystals
				Bacteria

Special tests
• Decreased serum T_3 and T_4 levels.
• Normal levels of fT_4d.
• Decreased serum TSH levels.
• No antithyroid antibody levels.

Pituitary-Dependent Hypothyroidism (Secondary or Central)

drugs, illness, or malnutrition temporarily suppresses TSH secretion by the pituitary; rarely, pituitary disease causes per-manent TSH deficiency

Pituitary-dependent (secondary) hypothyroidism is caused by insufficient secretion of thyroid-stimulating hormone (TSH) by the pituitary gland. This occurs because of dysfunction of the pituitary gland or decreased secretion of thyrotropin-releasing hormone (TRH) from the hypothalamus.

Congenital malformation, tumors, infection, or hemorrhage involving the pituitary can cause permanent deficiencies of TSH. Drugs, illness, or malnutrition can temporarily suppress TSH secretion.

Interpretation
Nonregenerative anemia and high serum cholesterol levels are nonspecific changes present with various metabolic diseases. The slight rise in serum activities of liver-derived enzymes is nonspecific. The blood panel can rule out diseases that cause secondary hypothyroidism (hypothyroidism of disease).

Thyroid tests show a low resting serum T_4 level, low fT_4d, and low TSH. Low circulating serum TSH levels in conjunction with low fT_4d levels indicate abnormal pituitary function.

Differential Diagnoses
- Immune-mediated hypothyroidism: normal or high serum thyroid hormone levels, with high serum levels of antibodies to these hormones
- Atrophic hypothyroidism: low serum thyroid hormone levels, no antithyroglobulin antibodies, thyroid biopsy shows decreased thyroid tissue with increased fat content
- Hypothyroidism of disease: low TSH, low T_4, but normal fT_4d

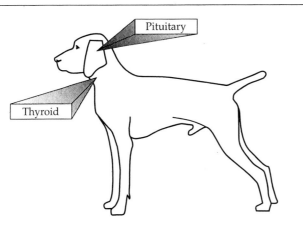

Signs
- Lethargy
- Weight gain
- Alopecia
- Loss of guard hairs
- Dull, dry haircoat
- Slow hair growth
- Hyperkeratosis
- Infertility
- Bradycardia

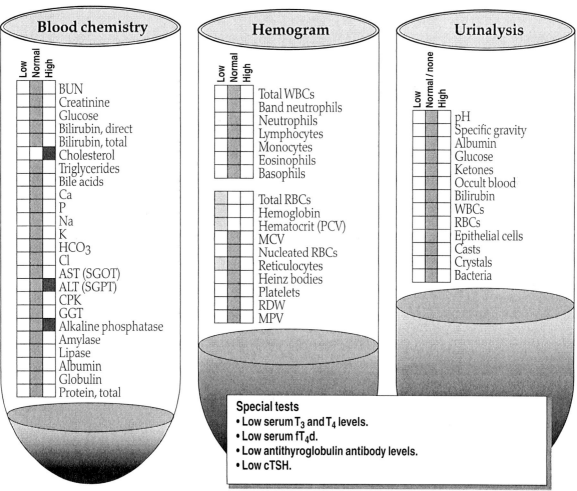

Blood chemistry

	Low	Normal	High	
				BUN
				Creatinine
				Glucose
				Bilirubin, direct
				Bilirubin, total
				Cholesterol
				Triglycerides
				Bile acids
				Ca
				P
				Na
				K
				HCO3
				Cl
				AST (SGOT)
				ALT (SGPT)
				CPK
				GGT
				Alkaline phosphatase
				Amylase
				Lipase
				Albumin
				Globulin
				Protein, total

Hemogram

	Low	Normal	High	
				Total WBCs
				Band neutrophils
				Neutrophils
				Lymphocytes
				Monocytes
				Eosinophils
				Basophils

	Low	Normal	High	
				Total RBCs
				Hemoglobin
				Hematocrit (PCV)
				MCV
				Nucleated RBCs
				Reticulocytes
				Heinz bodies
				Platelets
				RDW
				MPV

Urinalysis

	Low	Normal / none	High	
				pH
				Specific gravity
				Albumin
				Glucose
				Ketones
				Occult blood
				Bilirubin
				WBCs
				RBCs
				Epithelial cells
				Casts
				Crystals
				Bacteria

Special tests
- Low serum T_3 and T_4 levels.
- Low serum fT_4d.
- Low antithyroglobulin antibody levels.
- Low cTSH.

Primary Hypothyroidism

occasionally the thyroid gland atrophies, and glandular tissue is replaced by fat

lymphocytic thyroiditis is an immune-mediated disease in which the thyroid gland is infiltrated by lymphocytes

Thyroid gland atrophy is one cause of primary hypothyroidism. In affected animals, thyroid parenchyma is replaced with adipose tissue. No inflammation or circulating autoantibodies are present. The cause of thyroid atrophy is unknown.

Lymphocytic thyroiditis is another cause of primary hypothyroidism. The thyroid gland is infiltrated by lymphocytes, plasma cells, and macrophages. Circulating antibodies to T_4 can decrease thyroid function despite elevated serum T_4 values.

Interpretation

Nonregenerative anemia, a high serum cholesterol level, and a slight rise in serum activity of liver-derived enzymes are nonspecific findings with other metabolic diseases that cause fatty infiltration of the liver.

Results of basic thyroid tests may be normal because the autoantibodies interfere with the assays. Often the levels of free T_3 and T_4 are higher than normal, but fT_4d is low, and cTSH is increased. The key diagnostic finding for immune thyroiditis is high levels of antithyroid antibodies.

Differential Diagnoses

- Hypothyroidism of disease: normal response to TSH stimulation, no antithyroid antibodies
- Secondary hypothyroidism: normal response to TSH stimulation, no antithyroid antibodies, low TSH levels

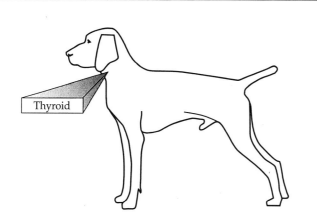

Signs
- Lethargy
- Weight gain
- Alopecia
- Loss of guard hairs
- Dull, dry haircoat
- Slow hair growth
- Hyperkeratosis
- Infertility
- Bradycardia

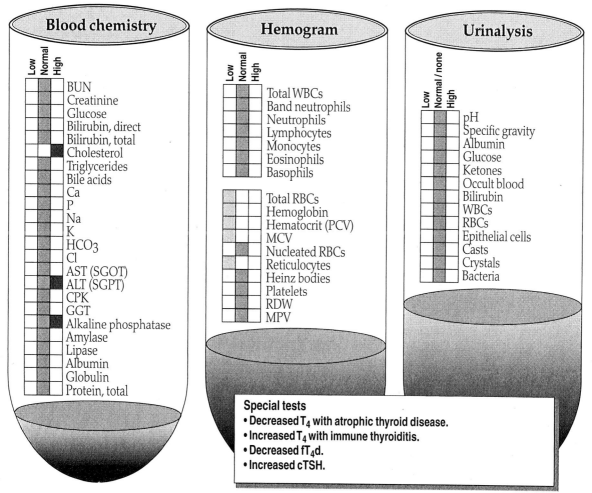

Blood chemistry

	Low	Normal	High	
				BUN
				Creatinine
				Glucose
				Bilirubin, direct
				Bilirubin, total
				Cholesterol
				Triglycerides
				Bile acids
				Ca
				P
				Na
				K
				HCO$_3$
				Cl
				AST (SGOT)
				ALT (SGPT)
				CPK
				GGT
				Alkaline phosphatase
				Amylase
				Lipase
				Albumin
				Globulin
				Protein, total

Hemogram

	Low	Normal	High	
				Total WBCs
				Band neutrophils
				Neutrophils
				Lymphocytes
				Monocytes
				Eosinophils
				Basophils
				Total RBCs
				Hemoglobin
				Hematocrit (PCV)
				MCV
				Nucleated RBCs
				Reticulocytes
				Heinz bodies
				Platelets
				RDW
				MPV

Urinalysis

	Low	Normal / none	High	
				pH
				Specific gravity
				Albumin
				Glucose
				Ketones
				Occult blood
				Bilirubin
				WBCs
				RBCs
				Epithelial cells
				Casts
				Crystals
				Bacteria

Special tests
- Decreased T$_4$ with atrophic thyroid disease.
- Increased T$_4$ with immune thyroiditis.
- Decreased fT$_4$d.
- Increased cTSH.

Diabetic Ketoacidosis

without insulin, metabolism of fat for energy produces ketosis and acidosis

Diabetic ketoacidosis is a metabolic disorder that develops from decompensated diabetes mellitus. Lipolysis increases serum free fatty acids, which are converted by the liver to ketones in the diabetic animal. Release of stress-related hormones, such as glucagon, cortisol, growth hormone, and epinephrine, increases this tendency.

Interpretation
A blood glucose level above 250 mg/dl and a large amount of glucose in the urine indicate diabetes mellitus. Ketones in the blood and urine indicate severe alterations in metabolism. High serum activities of liver-derived enzymes and high serum cholesterol and triglyceride levels reflect concurrent hepatomegaly caused by lipidosis. Dehydration elevates the PCV and total plasma protein level. The modified urine ketone test demonstrated ketonuria in severe cases.

Kidney damage leads to high BUN and creatinine levels. Concurrent infections can cause leukocytosis. Localized infections can occur in the urinary bladder.

Diuresis and shifts from acidosis cause acid-base and serum electrolyte abnormalities. Elevated serum beta-hydroxybutyrate levels are the best indicators of ketoacidosis. The usual qualitative tests for ketones detect only acetoacetate and acetone.

Differential Diagnoses
- Kidney failure: usually no hyperglycemia or ketosis
- Liver failure: low serum albumin and glucose levels

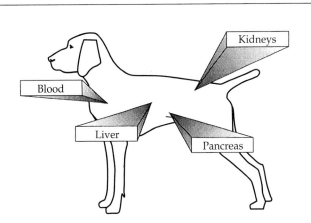

Signs
- Previous polyuria, polydipsia, polyphagia, weight loss
- Anorexia
- Vomiting
- Diarrhea
- Dehydration
- Depression

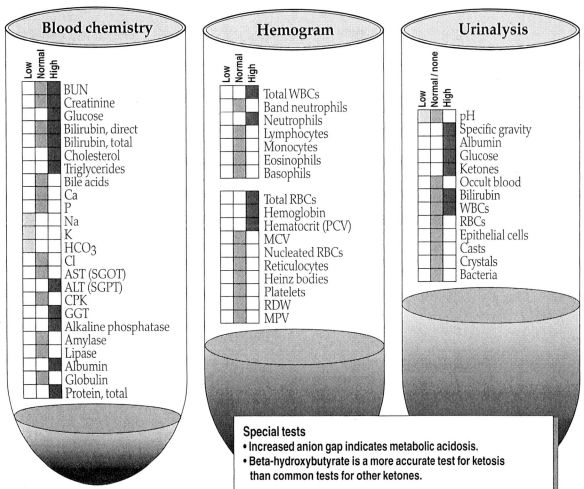

Blood chemistry

	Low	Normal	High
BUN			
Creatinine			
Glucose			
Bilirubin, direct			
Bilirubin, total			
Cholesterol			
Triglycerides			
Bile acids			
Ca			
P			
Na			
K			
HCO_3			
Cl			
AST (SGOT)			
ALT (SGPT)			
CPK			
GGT			
Alkaline phosphatase			
Amylase			
Lipase			
Albumin			
Globulin			
Protein, total			

Hemogram

	Low	Normal	High
Total WBCs			
Band neutrophils			
Neutrophils			
Lymphocytes			
Monocytes			
Eosinophils			
Basophils			
Total RBCs			
Hemoglobin			
Hematocrit (PCV)			
MCV			
Nucleated RBCs			
Reticulocytes			
Heinz bodies			
Platelets			
RDW			
MPV			

Urinalysis

	Low	Normal / none	High
pH			
Specific gravity			
Albumin			
Glucose			
Ketones			
Occult blood			
Bilirubin			
WBCs			
RBCs			
Epithelial cells			
Casts			
Crystals			
Bacteria			

Special tests
- Increased anion gap indicates metabolic acidosis.
- Beta-hydroxybutyrate is a more accurate test for ketosis than common tests for other ketones.

Type I Diabetes Mellitus (Insulin-Dependent)

type I diabetes is characterized by insufficient circulating insulin and requires insulin for control

Type I diabetes mellitus, the most common form of diabetes mellitus in dogs, results from insulin deficiency. It is caused by a genetic predisposition, pancreatitis, viral infection, or immune-mediated destruction of pancreatic beta cells. Type I diabetes mellitus requires administration of insulin for control.

Interpretation

Hyperglycemia and glycosuria are usually diagnostic. High serum lipase and amylase activities suggest concurrent pancreatitis. High serum activities of liver-derived enzymes, high serum cholesterol, and high triglyceride levels reflect concurrent hepatomegaly caused by lipidosis.

Dehydration causes a high PCV and an elevated total plasma protein level. A low serum bicarbonate level with an anion gap indicates metabolic acidosis.

Differential Diagnoses

- Chronic renal failure: no hyperglycemia or glycosuria, low urine specific gravity
- Diabetes insipidus: no hyperglycemia or glycosuria, low urine specific gravity
- Type II or III diabetes mellitus: hyperglycemia with normal to high serum insulin levels

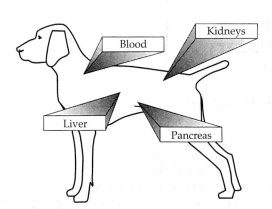

Signs
- Polyuria
- Polydipsia
- Polyphagia
- Weight loss
- ±Cataracts

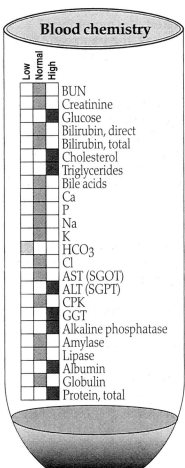

Blood chemistry

	Low	Normal	High	
				BUN
				Creatinine
				Glucose
				Bilirubin, direct
				Bilirubin, total
				Cholesterol
				Triglycerides
				Bile acids
				Ca
				P
				Na
				K
				HCO3
				Cl
				AST (SGOT)
				ALT (SGPT)
				CPK
				GGT
				Alkaline phosphatase
				Amylase
				Lipase
				Albumin
				Globulin
				Protein, total

Hemogram

	Low	Normal	High	
				Total WBCs
				Band neutrophils
				Neutrophils
				Lymphocytes
				Monocytes
				Eosinophils
				Basophils

	Low	Normal	High	
				Total RBCs
				Hemoglobin
				Hematocrit (PCV)
				MCV
				Nucleated RBCs
				Reticulocytes
				Heinz bodies
				Platelets
				RDW
				MPV

Urinalysis

	Low	Normal / none	High	
				pH
				Specific gravity
				Albumin
				Glucose
				Ketones
				Occult blood
				Bilirubin
				WBCs
				RBCs
				Epithelial cells
				Casts
				Crystals
				Bacteria

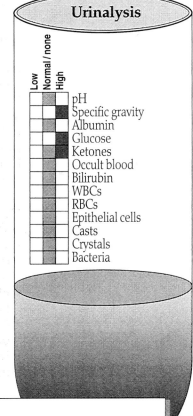

Special tests
- Increased anion gap indicates metabolic acidosis from organic acids.
- Blood insulin levels are usually low but rarely measured.
- Low blood insulin level (<26 μU/ml) with a high blood glucose indicates type I diabetes mellitus.
- Glucose or glucagon tolerance test shows prolonged hyperglycemia in questionable cases.

Type III Diabetes Mellitus (Secondary Diabetes)

type III diabetes is induced by drugs or hormones

Type III (secondary) diabetes mellitus is caused by prolonged gluconeogenesis induced by administration of glucagon, growth hormone, glucocorticoids, or progestins.

Initially, serum insulin levels are elevated. With prolonged exposure to these diabetogenic substances, the pancreatic islet cells become unresponsive, and serum insulin levels decline.

Interpretation
Glucose levels in blood and urine are high, but serum insulin levels are normal or low. This results in a low serum insulin/glucose ratio. Blood glucose levels return to normal following a short term of insulin therapy and withdrawal of the offending drug. Specific tests for adrenal hormones or a history of drug therapy is needed for diagnosis. Usually there is no ketonuria.

Differential Diagnoses
- Type I diabetes mellitus: low serum insulin level
- Type II diabetes mellitus: normal to high serum insulin level, no history of diabetogenic drug use, suspected but unidentified glucogenic substance
- Hyperadrenocorticism: increased serum cortisol levels, history of adrenocorticotropic drug use
- Chronic renal failure: no hyperglycemia or glycosuria, low urine specific gravity
- Diabetes insipidus: no hyperglycemia or glycosuria, low urine specific gravity

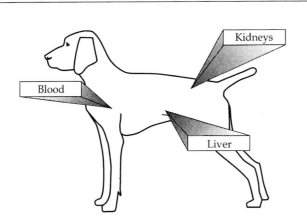

Signs
- Polyuria
- Polydipsia
- Polyphagia
- Weight loss
- History of drug or hormone administration

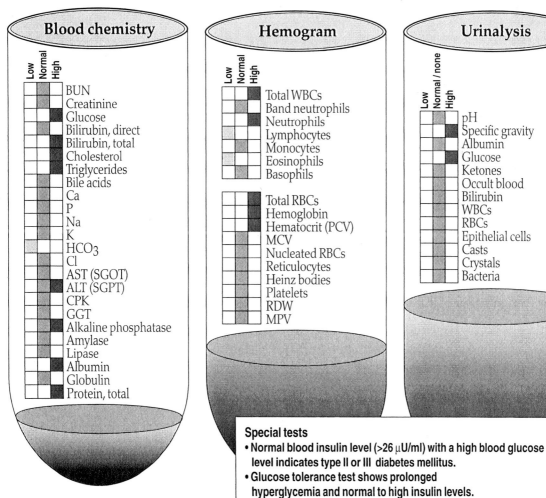

Blood chemistry

	Low	Normal	High	
				BUN
				Creatinine
				Glucose
				Bilirubin, direct
				Bilirubin, total
				Cholesterol
				Triglycerides
				Bile acids
				Ca
				P
				Na
				K
				HCO₃
				Cl
				AST (SGOT)
				ALT (SGPT)
				CPK
				GGT
				Alkaline phosphatase
				Amylase
				Lipase
				Albumin
				Globulin
				Protein, total

Hemogram

Low / Normal / High

- Total WBCs
- Band neutrophils
- Neutrophils
- Lymphocytes
- Monocytes
- Eosinophils
- Basophils

- Total RBCs
- Hemoglobin
- Hematocrit (PCV)
- MCV
- Nucleated RBCs
- Reticulocytes
- Heinz bodies
- Platelets
- RDW
- MPV

Urinalysis

Low / Normal / none / High

- pH
- Specific gravity
- Albumin
- Glucose
- Ketones
- Occult blood
- Bilirubin
- WBCs
- RBCs
- Epithelial cells
- Casts
- Crystals
- Bacteria

Special tests
- Normal blood insulin level (>26 μU/ml) with a high blood glucose level indicates type II or III diabetes mellitus.
- Glucose tolerance test shows prolonged hyperglycemia and normal to high insulin levels.

Kidneys

Blood

Liver

Islet-Cell Tumors

islet-cell tumors are malignant beta cells that secrete insulin without regulation; common metastatic sites are the mesenteric lymphatics, lymph nodes, liver, and serosal surfaces

Pancreatic islet-cell tumors are often malignant. They occur most often in middle-aged dogs. Clinical signs are related to hypoglycemia, which is caused by secretion of excessive insulin. Hyperinsulinemia inhibits glycogenolysis and gluconeogenesis, resulting in hypoglycemia.

Interpretation
The blood panel rules out several other conditions, such as hypoadrenocorticism, hypokalemia, hypocalcemia, and anemia. Normal serum bile acid levels shows there is no evidence of liver vascular shunts. A normal ECG rules out continuous arrhythmias as a cause of seizures. Electrocardiographic monitoring for 24 hours may be needed for complete analysis.

A high serum insulin/glucose ratio during a seizure episode or with a glucose or glucagon tolerance test is diagnostic.

Differential Diagnoses
• Primary brain disorder: no hypoglycemia
• Myasthenia gravis: no hypoglycemia, positive Tensilon (edrophonium) test
• Hypoadrenocorticism: low serum Na:K ratio, high eosinophil and lymphocyte counts
• Arrhythmias: abnormal ECG
• Hypokalemia: low serum potassium level
• Liver failure: low serum albumin level, high serum bile acid levels
• Anemia: low PCV

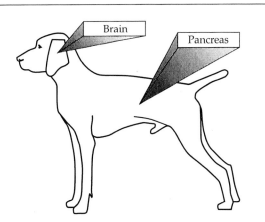

Signs
- Fatigue
- Episodic weakness
- Behavior changes
- Ataxia
- Collapse
- Seizures
- Blindness
- Coma

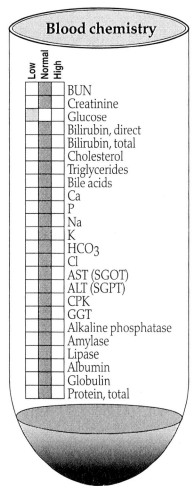

Blood chemistry

	Low	Normal	High	
				BUN
				Creatinine
				Glucose
				Bilirubin, direct
				Bilirubin, total
				Cholesterol
				Triglycerides
				Bile acids
				Ca
				P
				Na
				K
				HCO3
				Cl
				AST (SGOT)
				ALT (SGPT)
				CPK
				GGT
				Alkaline phosphatase
				Amylase
				Lipase
				Albumin
				Globulin
				Protein, total

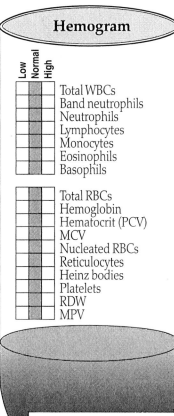

Hemogram

	Low	Normal	High	
				Total WBCs
				Band neutrophils
				Neutrophils
				Lymphocytes
				Monocytes
				Eosinophils
				Basophils
				Total RBCs
				Hemoglobin
				Hematocrit (PCV)
				MCV
				Nucleated RBCs
				Reticulocytes
				Heinz bodies
				Platelets
				RDW
				MPV

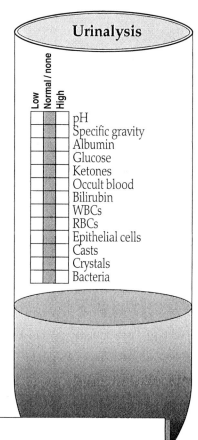

Urinalysis

	Low	Normal / none	High	
				pH
				Specific gravity
				Albumin
				Glucose
				Ketones
				Occult blood
				Bilirubin
				WBCs
				RBCs
				Epithelial cells
				Casts
				Crystals
				Bacteria

Special tests
- Amended insulin:glucose ratio >30 indicates insulin excess.
- Glucose tolerance test shows a rapid drop in the blood glucose level, with high insulin levels.
- Fasting glucose <60 mg/dl with an insulin level >20 μU/ml.

Exocrine Pancreatic Insufficiency

reduced digestive enzymes cause maldigestion, mucosal atrophy, and bacterial overgrowth in the small intestine

Exocrine pancreatic insufficiency occurs in young animals as congenital pancreatic hypoplasia. It is also seen in adults with idiopathic pancreatic acinar atrophy and after recurrent attacks of pancreatitis.

Reduced production of digestive enzymes causes maldigestion, mucosal atrophy, and bacterial overgrowth in the small intestine. This results in diarrhea and weight loss, despite a good appetite.

Interpretation
Most results of the serum chemistry panel are normal. Results of special digestive tests are abnormal. Xylose absorption is normal, indicating maldigestion rather than malabsorption. Intestinal bacterial overgrowth is a concurrent problem causing decreased vitamin B_{12} with increased folic acid.

The definitive test in dogs is low trypsin-like immunoreactivity (TLI). Fecal trypsin and fecal proteolytic activity are rapid screening tests but have questionable accuracy.

Differential Diagnoses
• Malabsorption: detected with xylose absorption, or a fatty meal incubated with pancreatic enzymes, normal TLI

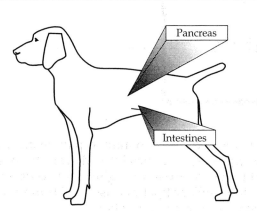

Signs
- Weight loss
- Good appetite
- Diarrhea
- Voluminous stools

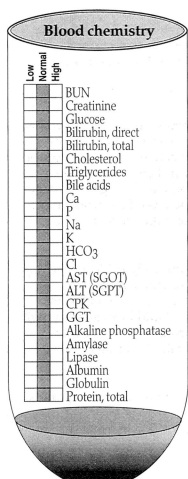

Blood chemistry

Low / Normal / High

BUN
Creatinine
Glucose
Bilirubin, direct
Bilirubin, total
Cholesterol
Triglycerides
Bile acids
Ca
P
Na
K
HCO₃
Cl
AST (SGOT)
ALT (SGPT)
CPK
GGT
Alkaline phosphatase
Amylase
Lipase
Albumin
Globulin
Protein, total

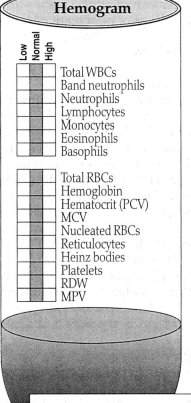

Hemogram

Low / Normal / High

Total WBCs
Band neutrophils
Neutrophils
Lymphocytes
Monocytes
Eosinophils
Basophils

Total RBCs
Hemoglobin
Hematocrit (PCV)
MCV
Nucleated RBCs
Reticulocytes
Heinz bodies
Platelets
RDW
MPV

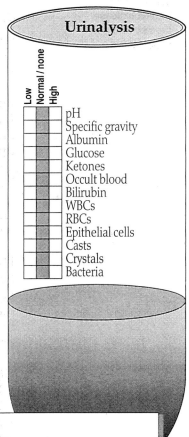

Urinalysis

Low / Normal / none / High

pH
Specific gravity
Albumin
Glucose
Ketones
Occult blood
Bilirubin
WBCs
RBCs
Epithelial cells
Casts
Crystals
Bacteria

Special tests
- Decreased fecal proteolytic activity.
- Decreased trypsin-like immunoreactivity.
- Decreased fat absorption.
- Normal xylose absorption.
- Decreased vitamin A absorption.
- Increased folic acid and decreased vitamin B_{12}.
- Decreased TLI.

Acute Pancreatitis

hyperlipidemia, glucocorticoids, organophosphate insecticides, biliary disease, and trauma increase the risk of acute pancreatitis

Pancreatitis occurs when injured pancreatic acinar cells release digestive enzymes into adjacent tissues. Hyperlipidemia, exogenous glucocorticoids, organophosphate insecticides, biliary tract disease, and trauma increase the risk of pancreatic enzyme activation.

The pattern of attacks varies from single episodes with little destruction of pancreatic glandular tissue, to recurrent episodes with progressive destruction of the pancreatic parenchyma.

Interpretation
High serum amylase and lipase activities suggest pancreatitis but also can be increased in animals with renal disease or upper GI inflammation. High serum activities of liver-derived enzymes indicate hepatic cell injury and cholangitis from ischemia and absorption of toxic products through the portal blood. TLI increased within 24 hours. It tends to peak before and to decrease more rapidly than activities of lipase and amylase.

Hypercholesterolemia and high serum triglyceride levels may be either the cause or the result of enzyme leakage. Hyperglycemia and glucosuria can be a sign of concurrent diabetes mellitus or glucagon release. Fluid loss causes a high PCV and an elevated total plasma protein level. Calcium deposition in saponified fats causes mild hypocalcemia.

Differential Diagnoses
- Intestinal foreign body: normal TLI, abnormal radiographs
- Renal failure: increased BUN
- Acute intestinal viral infections: low WBC, normal serum lipase, and TLI

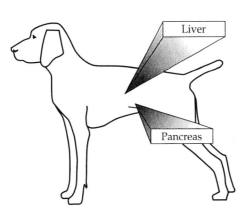

Signs
- Anorexia
- Vomiting
- Depression
- Abdominal pain
- Fever
- Occasionally signs of shock
- Diarrhea
- Polyuria

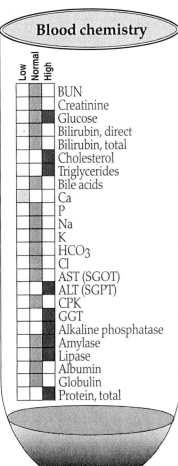

Blood chemistry

	Low	Normal	High	
				BUN
				Creatinine
				Glucose
				Bilirubin, direct
				Bilirubin, total
				Cholesterol
				Triglycerides
				Bile acids
				Ca
				P
				Na
				K
				HCO$_3$
				Cl
				AST (SGOT)
				ALT (SGPT)
				CPK
				GGT
				Alkaline phosphatase
				Amylase
				Lipase
				Albumin
				Globulin
				Protein, total

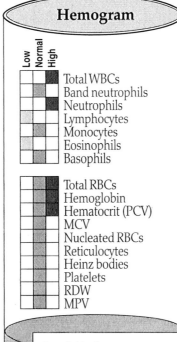

Hemogram

	Low	Normal	High	
				Total WBCs
				Band neutrophils
				Neutrophils
				Lymphocytes
				Monocytes
				Eosinophils
				Basophils
				Total RBCs
				Hemoglobin
				Hematocrit (PCV)
				MCV
				Nucleated RBCs
				Reticulocytes
				Heinz bodies
				Platelets
				RDW
				MPV

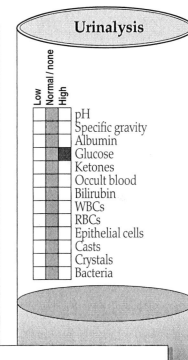

Urinalysis

	Low	Normal / none	High	
				pH
				Specific gravity
				Albumin
				Glucose
				Ketones
				Occult blood
				Bilirubin
				WBCs
				RBCs
				Epithelial cells
				Casts
				Crystals
				Bacteria

Special tests
- Radiographs may show focal peritonitis in the area of the pancreas and rule out other causes of vomiting and acute abdominal pain.
- Cytologic examination of peritoneal fluid shows primarily neutrophils.
- Analysis of peritoneal fluid shows a high protein content (>2.5 g/dl).
- Amylase and lipase activities are high, suggesting pancreatitis.
- Serum is often lipemic.
- Increased TLI.
- Increased urine trypsinogen activation test (TAP).

Chronic Active Hepatitis (Chronic Canine Inflammatory Hepatic Disease)

after initial injury the liver may be continuously damaged by immune mechanism, persistent infectious agents, or persistent toxins

Chronic active hepatitis is a progressive inflammatory disease with several possible causes. Infectious or toxic agents bind to and alter the surface of hepatocytes. Several factors such as abnormal immune responses, retention of toxic substances, or stimulation of fibrogenesis cause continued inflammation. This hepatic inflammation, regeneration, and fibrosis result in portal hypertension and portal systemic shunts, which promote ascites and hepatic encephalopathy.

Interpretation
Serum ALT activity can be up to 10 times normal, indicating large areas of active liver necrosis. Increased serum AST activity confirms disruption of liver cells. High serum direct bilirubin, alkaline phosphatase, and GGT values indicate cholestatic disease. Low serum albumin, glucose, and BUN levels suggest chronic liver disease and liver failure. Increased bile acids are associated with portal shunts.

Differential Diagnoses
- Corticosteroid-induced hepatopathy: polyphagia, weight gain, vacuoles in hepatocytes, exaggerated glucagon tolerance test
- Drug or toxin-induced hepatopathy: normal copper content in liver biopsies, normal CBC
- Cholangiohepatitis: serum activity of ALT not so markedly elevated, moderate rise in alkaline phosphatase activity
- Cirrhosis: liver biopsy shows more fibrosis and less active necrosis; high serum bile acid levels suggest shunting

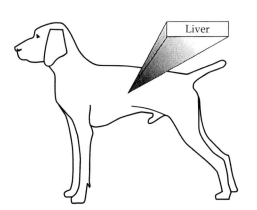

Signs
- Depression
- Anorexia
- Vomiting
- Icterus
- Weight loss
- Polydipsia
- Ascites

Liver

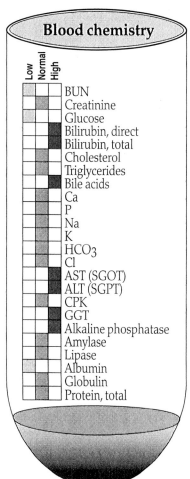

Blood chemistry

	Low	Normal	High	
				BUN
				Creatinine
				Glucose
				Bilirubin, direct
				Bilirubin, total
				Cholesterol
				Triglycerides
				Bile acids
				Ca
				P
				Na
				K
				HCO₃
				Cl
				AST (SGOT)
				ALT (SGPT)
				CPK
				GGT
				Alkaline phosphatase
				Amylase
				Lipase
				Albumin
				Globulin
				Protein, total

Hemogram

	Low	Normal	High	
				Total WBCs
				Band neutrophils
				Neutrophils
				Lymphocytes
				Monocytes
				Eosinophils
				Basophils
				Total RBCs
				Hemoglobin
				Hematocrit (PCV)
				MCV
				Nucleated RBCs
				Reticulocytes
				Heinz bodies
				Platelets
				RDW
				MPV

Urinalysis

	Low	Normal / none	High	
				pH
				Specific gravity
				Albumin
				Glucose
				Ketones
				Occult blood
				Bilirubin
				WBCs
				RBCs
				Epithelial cells
				Casts
				Crystals
				Bacteria

Special tests
- Radiographs show a large liver (acute cases) or a small liver (chronic cases).
- Liver biopsy shows normal copper content of <200 μg/g.
- Histopathologic examination of liver biopsies shows bridging necrosis, piecemeal necrosis with destruction of limiting plates, active cirrhosis, infiltration of lymphocytes, eosinophils in the portal area.
- Increased blood ammonia level.

Corticosteroid-Induced Hepatopathy

in dogs, glucocorticoids cause hepatic glycogen accumulation and increases of induced and intracellular liver enzymes; this hepatopathy is usually reversible

Endogenous glucocorticoids from an adrenal tumor or exogenous glucocorticoids can cause hepatopathy in dogs by inhibiting phosphorylating enzymes. This increases glycogen storage in the liver and decreases glycogen mobilization. The liver enlarges because of increased storage of glycogen.

Interpretation

The blood panel indicates liver disease, with a glucocorticoid-induced stress pattern on the CBC. The stress pattern on the CBC and the high blood glucose level suggest cortisol excess.

High serum activity of AST and ALT indicates hepatic cell injury with enzyme leakage. High serum alkaline phosphatase activity is caused by a corticosteroid-induced enzyme and may be related to glycogen synthesis. Elevated serum GGT activity indicates portal obstruction and physiologic enzyme induction. Increased serum bile acid levels suggest bile stasis from portal constriction.

Cytologic examination of fine-needle liver aspirates shows vacuolated parenchymal cells with a reticular pattern but no lipid vacuoles. Glucagon injection produces an exaggerated glucose tolerance curve.

Differential Diagnoses
- Fatty liver: usually anorexia, liver biopsy shows fat rather than glycogen
- Cholangiohepatitis: usually higher bilirubin level and WBC count
- Toxic liver disease: higher bilirubin level, no vacuolation on liver biopsy

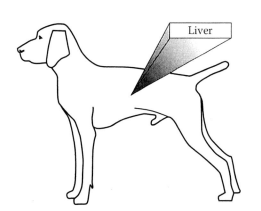

Signs
- Anorexia
- Vomiting
- Polydipsia
- Polyuria
- Obesity
- Abdominal distention
- Weakness

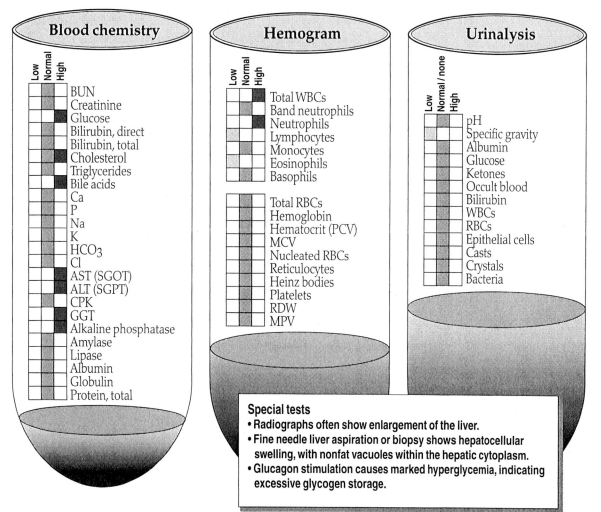

Blood chemistry

	Low	Normal	High	
BUN		■		
Creatinine		■		
Glucose			■	
Bilirubin, direct		■		
Bilirubin, total		■		
Cholesterol			■	
Triglycerides			■	
Bile acids		■		
Ca		■		
P		■		
Na		■		
K		■		
HCO3		■		
Cl		■		
AST (SGOT)			■	
ALT (SGPT)			■	
CPK		■		
GGT			■	
Alkaline phosphatase			■	
Amylase		■		
Lipase		■		
Albumin		■		
Globulin		■		
Protein, total		■		

Hemogram

	Low	Normal	High	
Total WBCs			■	
Band neutrophils		■		
Neutrophils			■	
Lymphocytes	■			
Monocytes		■		
Eosinophils		■		
Basophils		■		
Total RBCs		■		
Hemoglobin		■		
Hematocrit (PCV)		■		
MCV		■		
Nucleated RBCs		■		
Reticulocytes		■		
Heinz bodies		■		
Platelets		■		
RDW		■		
MPV		■		

Urinalysis

	Low	Normal / none	High	
pH		■		
Specific gravity	■			
Albumin		■		
Glucose		■		
Ketones		■		
Occult blood		■		
Bilirubin		■		
WBCs		■		
RBCs		■		
Epithelial cells		■		
Casts		■		
Crystals		■		
Bacteria		■		

Special tests
- Radiographs often show enlargement of the liver.
- Fine needle liver aspiration or biopsy shows hepatocellular swelling, with nonfat vacuoles within the hepatic cytoplasm.
- Glucagon stimulation causes marked hyperglycemia, indicating excessive glycogen storage.

Hepatic Fibrosis (Cirrhosis)

acute and chronic liver necrosis can lead to hepatic fibrosis

Conditions that cause massive liver necrosis destroy normal hepatic architecture, causing lobule collapse and fibrosis. In addition, many chronic liver disorders cause the deposition of fibrous tissue within the hepatic parenchyma. This fibrotic tissue compromises hepatic function and contributes significantly to hepatic failure. Progressive fibrosis leads to death from hepatic failure. Concurrent problems can include kidney failure, increased portal pressure, hypersplenism, portosystemic shunting, and bleeding.

Interpretation
High serum AST and ALT activities indicate hepatic cell necrosis. Portal constriction from fibrosis induces high serum alkaline phosphatase and GGT activities. The high serum bilirubin level indicates loss of bile duct integrity and intrahepatic obstruction.

An abnormal coagulation profile, elevated serum bile acid levels, ammonia retention, and hypoalbuminemia without urinary loss indicate vascular shunts and impairment of multiple liver functions. The anemia is nonresponsive despite active hemorrhage.

Differential Diagnoses
- Cholangiohepatitis: high WBC count, normal serum albumin level, normal coagulation tests
- Copper toxicosis: hemolytic anemia, high tissue copper level
- Anticoagulant poisoning: coagulopathy without signs of liver necrosis

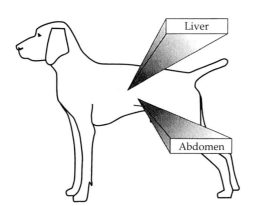

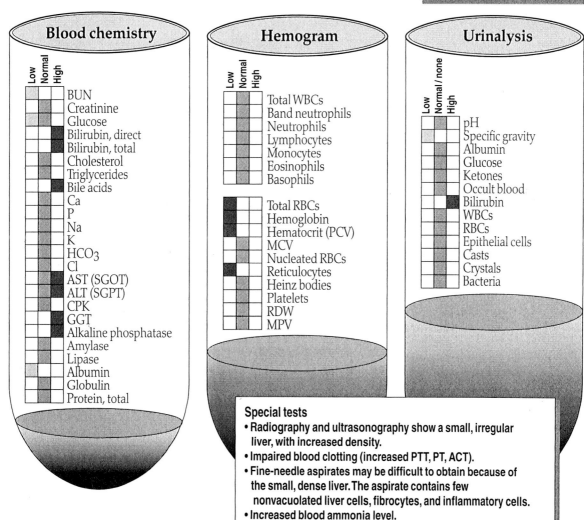

Signs
- Depression
- Anorexia
- Vomiting
- Icterus
- Weight loss
- Hemorrhage (melana, bleeding tendency)
- Abdominal distention from ascites (transudate)
- Intolerance of tranquilizers
- Polyuria
- Polydipsia

Blood chemistry

Low	Normal	High	
			BUN
			Creatinine
			Glucose
			Bilirubin, direct
			Bilirubin, total
			Cholesterol
			Triglycerides
			Bile acids
			Ca
			P
			Na
			K
			HCO₃
			Cl
			AST (SGOT)
			ALT (SGPT)
			CPK
			GGT
			Alkaline phosphatase
			Amylase
			Lipase
			Albumin
			Globulin
			Protein, total

Hemogram

Low	Normal	High	
			Total WBCs
			Band neutrophils
			Neutrophils
			Lymphocytes
			Monocytes
			Eosinophils
			Basophils

Low	Normal	High	
			Total RBCs
			Hemoglobin
			Hematocrit (PCV)
			MCV
			Nucleated RBCs
			Reticulocytes
			Heinz bodies
			Platelets
			RDW
			MPV

Urinalysis

Low	Normal / none	High	
			pH
			Specific gravity
			Albumin
			Glucose
			Ketones
			Occult blood
			Bilirubin
			WBCs
			RBCs
			Epithelial cells
			Casts
			Crystals
			Bacteria

Special tests
- Radiography and ultrasonography show a small, irregular liver, with increased density.
- Impaired blood clotting (increased PTT, PT, ACT).
- Fine-needle aspirates may be difficult to obtain because of the small, dense liver. The aspirate contains few nonvacuolated liver cells, fibrocytes, and inflammatory cells.
- Increased blood ammonia level.

Metastatic Hepatic Tumors

lymphosarcoma, hemangiosar- coma, and pancreatic carcinoma are common metastatic tumors of the liver

Common metastatic tumors of the liver are lymphosarcoma, hemangiosarcoma, and pancreatic carcinoma. These neoplasms induce cholangiohepatitis, cirrhosis, and, occasionally, acute hemorrhage.

Interpretation

High serum AST and ALT activities indicate hepatic cell necrosis. High serum alkaline phosphatase and GGT activities indicate bile stasis and bile duct obstruction. In many cases these elevations are minimal because relatively small amounts of liver tissue are involved. A high serum bilirubin level indicates loss of bile duct integrity.

Hepatic insufficiency is minimal and usually there are no abnormalities in the coagulation profile or ammonia retention. A serum alpha-fetoprotein level of 100 to 200 ng/ml suggests metastatic liver tumors. A nonresponsive anemia can develop.

Differential Diagnoses

- Primary liver tumors: cytologic examination shows tumor cells and very high serum alpha-fetoprotein levels (>250 ng/ml)
- Cholangiohepatitis: normal pattern on ultrasonographic examination
- Bile duct obstruction: pale stools, no increase in serum alpha-protein levels, dilated bile ducts on ultrasonographic examination

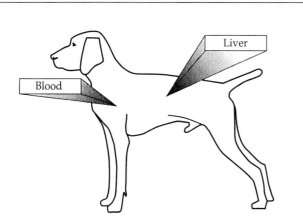

Signs
• Variable

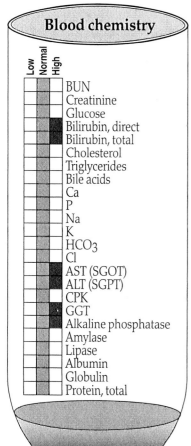

Blood chemistry

	Low	Normal	High	
				BUN
				Creatinine
				Glucose
				Bilirubin, direct
				Bilirubin, total
				Cholesterol
				Triglycerides
				Bile acids
				Ca
				P
				Na
				K
				HCO₃
				Cl
				AST (SGOT)
				ALT (SGPT)
				CPK
				GGT
				Alkaline phosphatase
				Amylase
				Lipase
				Albumin
				Globulin
				Protein, total

Hemogram

	Low	Normal	High	
				Total WBCs
				Band neutrophils
				Neutrophils
				Lymphocytes
				Monocytes
				Eosinophils
				Basophils

	Low	Normal	High	
				Total RBCs
				Hemoglobin
				Hematocrit (PCV)
				MCV
				Nucleated RBCs
				Reticulocytes
				Heinz bodies
				Platelets
				RDW
				MPV

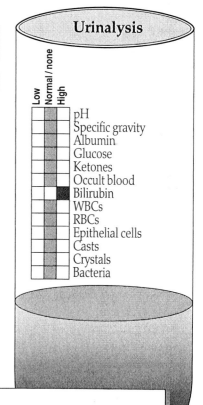

Urinalysis

	Low	Normal / none	High	
				pH
				Specific gravity
				Albumin
				Glucose
				Ketones
				Occult blood
				Bilirubin
				WBCs
				RBCs
				Epithelial cells
				Casts
				Crystals
				Bacteria

Special tests
• Ultrasonography shows hypoechoic areas in the liver.
• Cytologic or histopathologic examination identifies the type of tumor.
• Alpha-fetoprotein 100-200 ng/ml suggests metastatic liver tumors.
• ±Abnormal RBC cytology, shistocytes.
• Abnormal clotting tests.

Portosystemic Shunts

portosystemic shunts can be congenital or acquired through sustained resistance to portal flow from fibrotic liver disease

Portosystemic shunts are vascular connections between the portal veins and the systemic circulation that bypass the liver. These shunts can be congenital or acquired through sustained resistance to portal flow from fibrotic liver disease. Shunted portal blood delivers enteric waste products to the general circulation, resulting in hepatic encephalopathy. If shunting is suspected but a macrovascular anomaly cannot be identified and the liver is of normal size, there may be a disordered microscopic vascular arrangement termed hepatic microvascular dysplasia.

Interpretation
Decreased BUN, albumin, and glucose levels with normal serum AST and ALT activities suggest chronic liver disease. This is a pattern of liver failure without active liver disease.

High serum GGT and alkaline phosphatase activities suggest biliary disease.

High serum bile acid levels are the best indicators of liver shunting in a nonicteric animal. A high blood ammonia level is also characteristic of failure to process digestive products.

Differential Diagnoses
- CNS disease (encephalitis, epilepsy): no increase in serum bile acid levels
- Acute liver disease: high serum ALT and AST activities
- Hepatic lipidosis in cats: lipid-filled hepatocytes in fine-needle aspirates of the liver
- Primary hyperammonemia (enzyme defect): no increase in serum bile acid levels
- Primary hepatic tumors: liver biopsy shows fibrosis and neoplastic cells; ultrasonographic examination shows hypoechoic areas with abnormal architecture

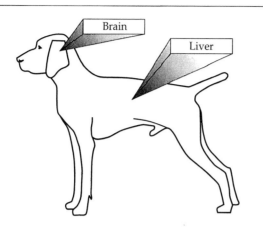

Signs
- Lethargy
- Weakness
- Ataxia
- Seizure
- Blindness
- Vomiting
- Diarrhea
- Polyuria
- Polydipsia

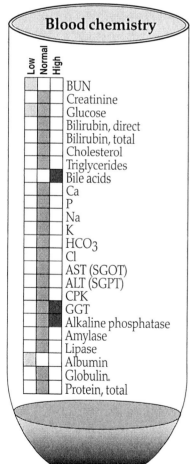

Blood chemistry

	Low	Normal	High	
				BUN
				Creatinine
				Glucose
				Bilirubin, direct
				Bilirubin, total
				Cholesterol
				Triglycerides
				Bile acids
				Ca
				P
				Na
				K
				HCO₃
				Cl
				AST (SGOT)
				ALT (SGPT)
				CPK
				GGT
				Alkaline phosphatase
				Amylase
				Lipase
				Albumin
				Globulin
				Protein, total

Hemogram

	Low	Normal	High	
				Total WBCs
				Band neutrophils
				Neutrophils
				Lymphocytes
				Monocytes
				Eosinophils
				Basophils
				Total RBCs
				Hemoglobin
				Hematocrit (PCV)
				MCV
				Nucleated RBCs
				Reticulocytes
				Heinz bodies
				Platelets
				RDW
				MPV

Urinalysis

	Low	Normal / none	High	
				pH
				Specific gravity
				Albumin
				Glucose
				Ketones
				Occult blood
				Bilirubin
				WBCs
				RBCs
				Epithelial cells
				Casts
				Crystals
				Bacteria

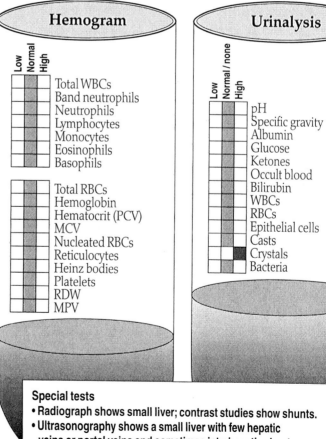

Special tests
- Radiograph shows small liver; contrast studies show shunts.
- Ultrasonography shows a small liver with few hepatic veins or portal veins and sometimes intrahepatic shunts.
- Ammonia tolerance test shows increased blood ammonia level.
- Cold-urine crystal analysis shows ammonium biurate or urate crystals.
- ±Uroliths.
- Confirm with portogram or rectal portal scintigraphy.

Primary Hepatic Tumors

alpha-fetoprotein
value above
250 ng/ml is
diagnostic for
primary liver
tumors

The most common primary liver tumors are hepatocellular adenomas, hepatocellular carcinomas, bile duct carcinomas, and hepatic carcinoids. Nodular hyperplasia is common in older dogs and is difficult to distinguish from adenomas.

Early liver tumors may be masked by secondary liver disease. Hepatic neoplasms can induce cholangiohepatitis, cirrhosis, and occasionally acute hemorrhage.

Interpretation
High serum AST and ALT activities indicate hepatic cell necrosis. In some cases these elevations are minimal because the altered tumor cells do not release enzymes and their growth is slow.

High serum bilirubin, alkaline phosphatase, and GGT values indicate portal compression and cholestasis. A serum alpha-fetoprotein value above 250 ng/ml is diagnostic for primary liver tumors, such as hepatocellular carcinoma and cholangiocarcinoma.

Differential Diagnoses
- Cholangiohepatitis: distinguished by cytologic examination and ultrasonographic pattern
- Metastatic liver tumors: cytologic examination of ultrasound-guided biopsies shows cell type; serum levels of alpha-fetoprotein may be slightly increased

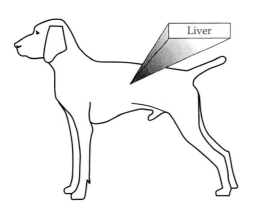

Signs
- Depression
- Anorexia
- Vomiting
- Icterus
- Weight loss
- Polydipsia
- Polyuria
- Abdominal distention
- Hemorrhage
- Intolerance to tranquilizers

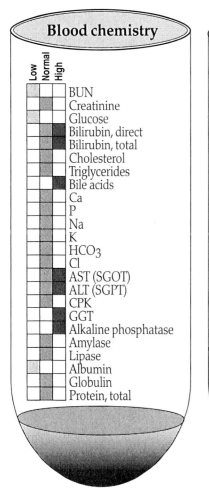

Blood chemistry

	Low	Normal	High	
				BUN
				Creatinine
				Glucose
				Bilirubin, direct
				Bilirubin, total
				Cholesterol
				Triglycerides
				Bile acids
				Ca
				P
				Na
				K
				HCO$_3$
				Cl
				AST (SGOT)
				ALT (SGPT)
				CPK
				GGT
				Alkaline phosphatase
				Amylase
				Lipase
				Albumin
				Globulin
				Protein, total

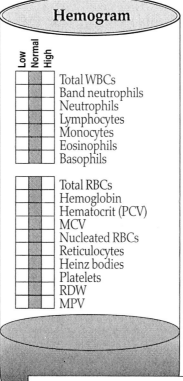

Hemogram

	Low	Normal	High	
				Total WBCs
				Band neutrophils
				Neutrophils
				Lymphocytes
				Monocytes
				Eosinophils
				Basophils
				Total RBCs
				Hemoglobin
				Hematocrit (PCV)
				MCV
				Nucleated RBCs
				Reticulocytes
				Heinz bodies
				Platelets
				RDW
				MPV

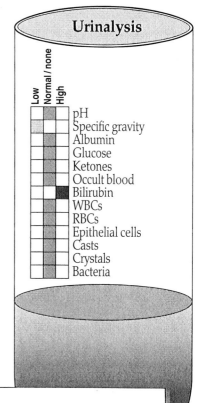

Urinalysis

	Low	Normal / none	High	
				pH
				Specific gravity
				Albumin
				Glucose
				Ketones
				Occult blood
				Bilirubin
				WBCs
				RBCs
				Epithelial cells
				Casts
				Crystals
				Bacteria

Special tests
- Liver biopsy shows fibrosis and neoplastic cells.
- Ultrasonography shows hypoechoic areas with abnormal architecture.
- Cytologic examination of the fine-needle liver aspirate shows tumor cells.
- Alpha-fetoprotein level >250 ng/ml is diagnostic for primary liver tumors.
- Ascitic fluid analysis shows a transudate.

Hepatic Response to Septicemia and Endotoxemia

the RE system responds to toxemia by hyperplasia; septic emboli may bypass the RE system by entering through the hepatic artery and produce liver abscess

Septicemia causes congestion of hepatic sinusoids, dilatation of hepatic veins, necrosis, and fatty vacuolation. Later, neutrophils infiltrate the hepatic parenchyma and portal area, possibly leading to microabscess formation. As the condition persists, the reticuloendothelial cells hypertrophy.

Interpretation
Marked septicemia or endotoxemia can overwhelm the bone marrow, producing a degenerative left shift in the neutrophilic response. The combination of accelerated RBC removal by the hyperactive reticuloendothelial system and bone marrow depression produces nonresponsive anemia.

Liver necrosis causes high serum ALT and AST activities. Biliary inflammation and cholestasis elevate the serum alkaline phosphatase, GGT, and bilirubin values.

Differential Diagnoses
• Primary liver disease: no splenomegaly

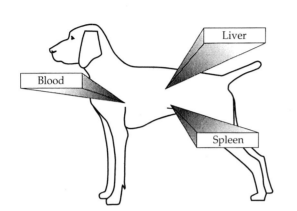

Signs
- Hepatomegaly
- Splenomegaly
- Fever
- Depression
- ±Icterus

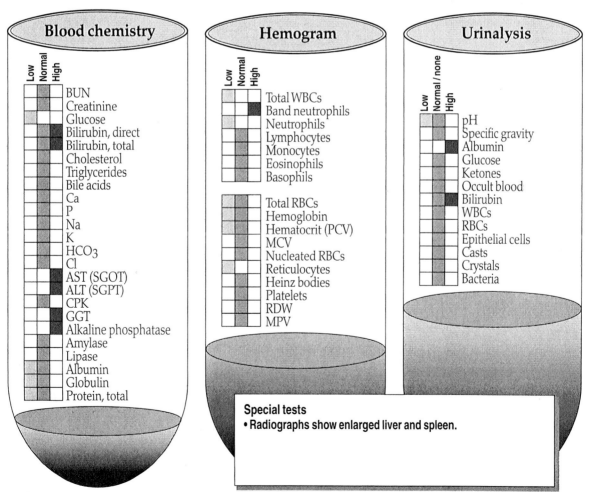

Blood chemistry

	Low	Normal	High	
				BUN
				Creatinine
				Glucose
				Bilirubin, direct
				Bilirubin, total
				Cholesterol
				Triglycerides
				Bile acids
				Ca
				P
				Na
				K
				HCO₃
				Cl
				AST (SGOT)
				ALT (SGPT)
				CPK
				GGT
				Alkaline phosphatase
				Amylase
				Lipase
				Albumin
				Globulin
				Protein, total

Hemogram

	Low	Normal	High	
				Total WBCs
				Band neutrophils
				Neutrophils
				Lymphocytes
				Monocytes
				Eosinophils
				Basophils
				Total RBCs
				Hemoglobin
				Hematocrit (PCV)
				MCV
				Nucleated RBCs
				Reticulocytes
				Heinz bodies
				Platelets
				RDW
				MPV

Urinalysis

	Low	Normal / none	High	
				pH
				Specific gravity
				Albumin
				Glucose
				Ketones
				Occult blood
				Bilirubin
				WBCs
				RBCs
				Epithelial cells
				Casts
				Crystals
				Bacteria

Special tests
- Radiographs show enlarged liver and spleen.

Acute Toxic Hepatopathy

adverse hepatic reactions are usually idio-syncratic; a high degree of suspicion is needed to determine a cause

Reactions to drugs, chemicals, or plant toxins may damage the liver by direct hepatic injury or by disturbances of hepatocellular hemostasis. Risks are increased by poor nutritional status and female gender. Some agents cause rapid hepatic injury while others must accumulate to cause damage. Histopathologic lesions consist of centrilobular necrosis or periportal inflammation. Dynamic testing consisting of comparing values before and after administration of a drug is the earliest way of detecting liver toxicity.

Interpretation
Laboratory results are typical of mild, moderate, or severe liver parenchymal cell damage. This is suggested by high levels of ALT and AST. Increased levels of alkaline phosphatase and GGT suggest biliary involvement, but this is variable. Increased levels of bilirubin are caused by hepatocellular damage rather than by biliary stasis. In nonicteric animals early changes are detected by high bile acid levels.

Differential Diagnoses
- Chronic hepatopathies: increased liver fibrosis, evident on ultrasound, biopsy, or increased BSP retention
- Endotoxic or anaphylactic shock: hemoconcentration, normal serum bilirubin level

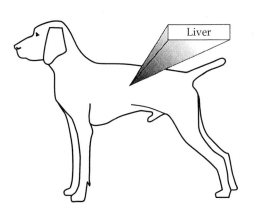

Signs
- Anorexia
- Vomiting
- Icterus
- Depression
- Hemorrhagic diarrhea
- Death

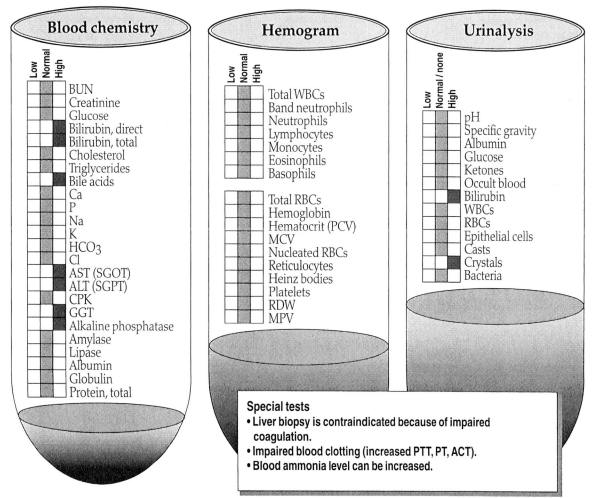

Blood chemistry

	Low	Normal	High	
				BUN
				Creatinine
				Glucose
				Bilirubin, direct
				Bilirubin, total
				Cholesterol
				Triglycerides
				Bile acids
				Ca
				P
				Na
				K
				HCO₃
				Cl
				AST (SGOT)
				ALT (SGPT)
				CPK
				GGT
				Alkaline phosphatase
				Amylase
				Lipase
				Albumin
				Globulin
				Protein, total

Hemogram

	Low	Normal	High	
				Total WBCs
				Band neutrophils
				Neutrophils
				Lymphocytes
				Monocytes
				Eosinophils
				Basophils
				Total RBCs
				Hemoglobin
				Hematocrit (PCV)
				MCV
				Nucleated RBCs
				Reticulocytes
				Heinz bodies
				Platelets
				RDW
				MPV

Urinalysis

	Low	Normal / none	High	
				pH
				Specific gravity
				Albumin
				Glucose
				Ketones
				Occult blood
				Bilirubin
				WBCs
				RBCs
				Epithelial cells
				Casts
				Crystals
				Bacteria

Special tests
- Liver biopsy is contraindicated because of impaired coagulation.
- Impaired blood clotting (increased PTT, PT, ACT).
- Blood ammonia level can be increased.

Chronic Toxic Hepatitis

long-term or heavy exposure to certain drugs can destroy entire liver lobules and collapse the portal areas; this results in fibrosis and loss of liver tissue

The anticonvulsant drugs primidone and phenytoin can be hepatotoxic. They sometimes can cause hypertrophy, internal cell changes, intrahepatic cholestasis, cirrhosis, and liver failure. The toxic effect of these drugs is dose related. Phenobarbital induces increased liver enzyme activity but causes no histologic evidence of hepatic disease.

Interpretation
High serum AST and ALT activities indicate hepatic cell necrosis. High serum bilirubin, alkaline phosphatase, and GGT values indicate portal disease with intrahepatic cholestasis. The severity of hepatic insufficiency is indicated by an abnormal coagulation profile and ammonia retention. Abnormal clotting from liver failure leads to blood-loss anemia.

Differential Diagnoses
- Cholangiohepatitis: no anemia
- Corticosteroid-induced hepatopathy: polyphagia, weight gain, vacuoles in hepatocytes, exaggerated glucagon tolerance test
- Copper toxicosis: high copper content in liver biopsies
- Platelet dysfunction: abnormal platelet function tests

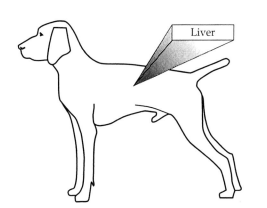

Liver

Signs
- Depression
- Anorexia
- Vomiting
- Icterus
- Weight loss
- Polydipsia
- Polyuria
- Ascites (transudate)
- Hemorrhage (melena, bleeding tendency)

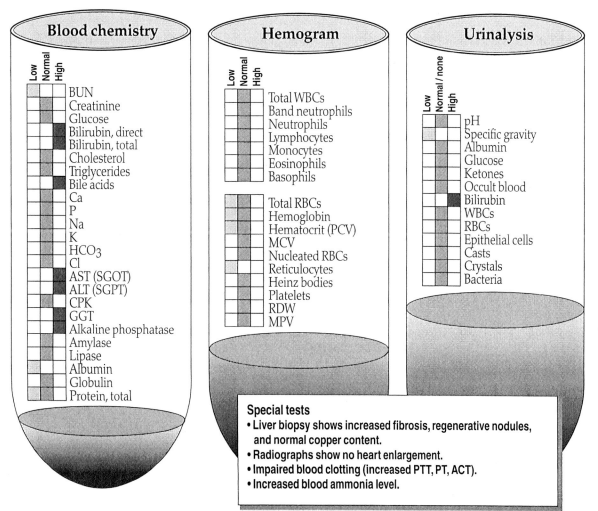

Blood chemistry

	Low	Normal	High	
				BUN
				Creatinine
				Glucose
				Bilirubin, direct
				Bilirubin, total
				Cholesterol
				Triglycerides
				Bile acids
				Ca
				P
				Na
				K
				HCO3
				Cl
				AST (SGOT)
				ALT (SGPT)
				CPK
				GGT
				Alkaline phosphatase
				Amylase
				Lipase
				Albumin
				Globulin
				Protein, total

Hemogram

	Low	Normal	High	
				Total WBCs
				Band neutrophils
				Neutrophils
				Lymphocytes
				Monocytes
				Eosinophils
				Basophils
				Total RBCs
				Hemoglobin
				Hematocrit (PCV)
				MCV
				Nucleated RBCs
				Reticulocytes
				Heinz bodies
				Platelets
				RDW
				MPV

Urinalysis

	Low	Normal / none	High	
				pH
				Specific gravity
				Albumin
				Glucose
				Ketones
				Occult blood
				Bilirubin
				WBCs
				RBCs
				Epithelial cells
				Casts
				Crystals
				Bacteria

Special tests
- Liver biopsy shows increased fibrosis, regenerative nodules, and normal copper content.
- Radiographs show no heart enlargement.
- Impaired blood clotting (increased PTT, PT, ACT).
- Increased blood ammonia level.

Hepatitis from Copper Toxicosis

hepatic copper accumulation causes acute hepatitis that progresses to chronic hepatitis and cirrhosis

Genetic and chronic cholestatic disorders cause the liver to retain dietary copper. Copper accumulations eventually become toxic, producing focal areas of necrosis and mild inflammation. The necrotic areas enlarge and then fibrose. Progressive fibrosis eventually causes liver failure.

Genetic predispositions have been reported in Bedlington Terriers, Doberman Pinschers, and West Highland Terriers.

Interpretation
High serum ALT and AST activities indicate acute liver necrosis. High serum direct bilirubin, alkaline phosphatase, and GGT indicate cholestatic disease. Bilirubinuria indicates that the bilirubin is of hepatic origin.

When hemolytic anemia occurs, both the direct and indirect bilirubin levels can be high. Decreasing serum albumin, glucose, and urea nitrogen values with high ammonia and bile acid levels indicate hepatic failure, fibrosis, and shunting of blood. Nonresponsive anemia develops.

Differential Diagnoses
- Corticosteroid-induced hepatopathy: polyphagia, weight gain, vacuoles in hepatocytes, exaggerated glucagon tolerance test
- Drug-induced or toxin-induced hepatopathy: normal copper content in liver biopsies
- Chronic active hepatitis: bridging necrosis, with infiltration of lymphocytes and eosinophils in portal area, normal copper content in liver biopsies
- Cholangiohepatitis: no hemolytic anemia
- Cirrhosis: normal copper content in liver biopsies
- Autoimmune hemolytic anemia: positive Coombs' test

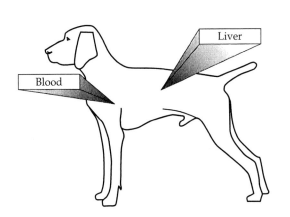

Signs
- Depression
- Anorexia
- Vomiting
- Icterus
- Weight loss
- Polydipsia
- Ascites
- Pale mucous membranes

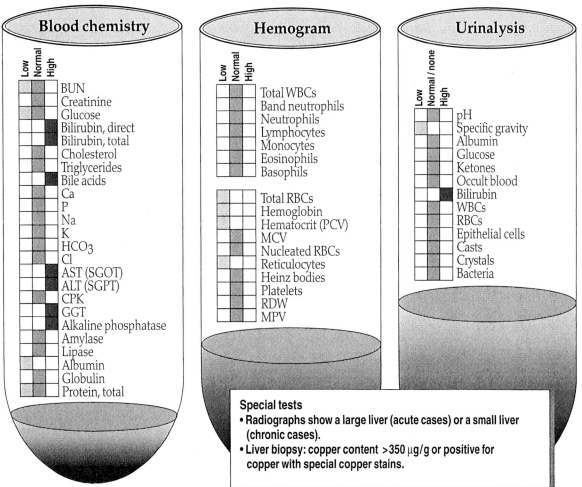

Blood chemistry

	Low	Normal	High	
				BUN
				Creatinine
				Glucose
				Bilirubin, direct
				Bilirubin, total
				Cholesterol
				Triglycerides
				Bile acids
				Ca
				P
				Na
				K
				HCO3
				Cl
				AST (SGOT)
				ALT (SGPT)
				CPK
				GGT
				Alkaline phosphatase
				Amylase
				Lipase
				Albumin
				Globulin
				Protein, total

Hemogram

	Low	Normal	High	
				Total WBCs
				Band neutrophils
				Neutrophils
				Lymphocytes
				Monocytes
				Eosinophils
				Basophils

	Low	Normal	High	
				Total RBCs
				Hemoglobin
				Hematocrit (PCV)
				MCV
				Nucleated RBCs
				Reticulocytes
				Heinz bodies
				Platelets
				RDW
				MPV

Urinalysis

	Low	Normal / none	High	
				pH
				Specific gravity
				Albumin
				Glucose
				Ketones
				Occult blood
				Bilirubin
				WBCs
				RBCs
				Epithelial cells
				Casts
				Crystals
				Bacteria

Special tests
- Radiographs show a large liver (acute cases) or a small liver (chronic cases).
- Liver biopsy: copper content >350 µg/g or positive for copper with special copper stains.

Hypergastrinemia

hypergastrinemia is caused by excessive dietary calcium, renal failure, and, rarely, a gastrinoma

G-cells in the gastric pit produce the hormone gastrin, which stimulates release of gastric hydrochloric acid. G-cell hypertrophy causes gastric ulceration, mucosal hypertrophy, and delayed gastric emptying.

Interpretation
Blood tests are used to rule out abdominal organ dysfunction, such as chronic liver disease, kidney disease, and pancreatitis. Responsive anemia occurs with chronic gastric ulceration.

Differential Diagnoses
- Gastritis: no increase in serum gastrin levels following calcium injection
- Azotemia: high serum urea nitrogen and creatinine levels
- Intestinal obstruction: radiographs reveal intestinal abnormalities

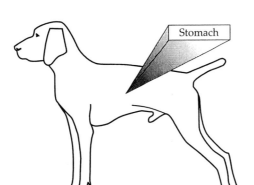

Signs
- Vomiting
- Melena
- Diarrhea
- Steatorrhea

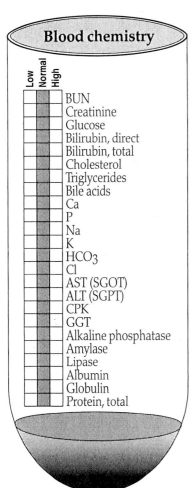

Blood chemistry

	Low	Normal	High	
				BUN
				Creatinine
				Glucose
				Bilirubin, direct
				Bilirubin, total
				Cholesterol
				Triglycerides
				Bile acids
				Ca
				P
				Na
				K
				HCO$_3$
				Cl
				AST (SGOT)
				ALT (SGPT)
				CPK
				GGT
				Alkaline phosphatase
				Amylase
				Lipase
				Albumin
				Globulin
				Protein, total

Hemogram

	Low	Normal	High	
				Total WBCs
				Band neutrophils
				Neutrophils
				Lymphocytes
				Monocytes
				Eosinophils
				Basophils

				Total RBCs
				Hemoglobin
				Hematocrit (PCV)
				MCV
				Nucleated RBCs
				Reticulocytes
				Heinz bodies
				Platelets
				RDW
				MPV

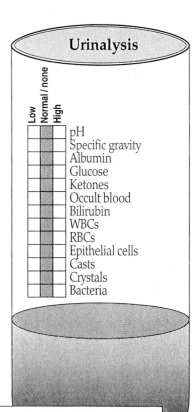

Urinalysis

	Low	Normal / none	High	
				pH
				Specific gravity
				Albumin
				Glucose
				Ketones
				Occult blood
				Bilirubin
				WBCs
				RBCs
				Epithelial cells
				Casts
				Crystals
				Bacteria

Special tests
- Endoscopy may show distal esophagitis, mucosal thickening, edema, hyperemia, ulceration, or hemorrhage.
- Contrast radiographs may show decreased rugal folds, large rugal folds, nodular areas, ulcers, and decreased emptying time.
- IV calcium gluconate (1 mg/lb) increases serum gastrin level by >2 baseline values with gastrinoma.
- Fasting or stimulated gastrin levels >500 pg/ml.

Primary Hyperlipidemia

primary hyper-
chylomicronemia
increases the
risk of acute
pancreatitis

Primary hyperlipidemia is an inherited disease in which lipid levels in a fasting blood sample are increased without underlying endocrine or metabolic disease.

Hypertriglyceridemia with hyperchylomicronemia causes serious clinical disease. Primary hypercholesterolemia does not cause clinical illness.

Interpretation
The blood panel can rule out some common causes of secondary hyperlipidemia. Serum triglyceride levels could indicate hyperlipidemia if there is no visible lipemia. Lipemic blood samples that fail to clear following heparin injection indicate a lipoprotein lipase deficiency.

Differential Diagnoses
- Postprandial hyperlipidemia: ruled out by withholding food for at least 24 hours
- Acute pancreatitis: high serum lipase and amylase activities
- Diabetes mellitus: hyperglycemia, glycosuria
- Hyperadrenocorticism: stress pattern on CBC, cortisol excess can induce a lipoprotein lipase deficiency

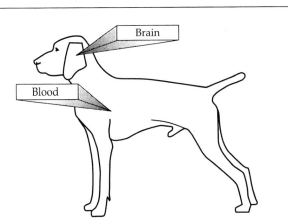

Signs
- Seizures
- Paralysis
- Predisposition to pancreatitis
- Subcutaneous nodules
- Diarrhea
- Abdominal pain

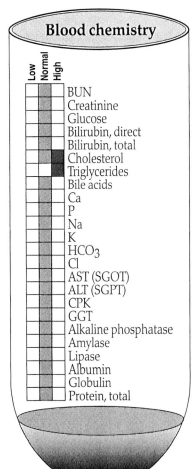

Blood chemistry

	Low	Normal	High	
				BUN
				Creatinine
				Glucose
				Bilirubin, direct
				Bilirubin, total
				Cholesterol
				Triglycerides
				Bile acids
				Ca
				P
				Na
				K
				HCO3
				Cl
				AST (SGOT)
				ALT (SGPT)
				CPK
				GGT
				Alkaline phosphatase
				Amylase
				Lipase
				Albumin
				Globulin
				Protein, total

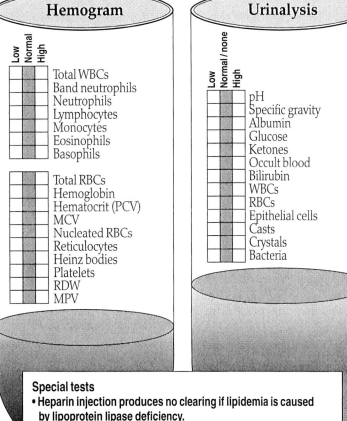

Hemogram

	Low	Normal	High	
				Total WBCs
				Band neutrophils
				Neutrophils
				Lymphocytes
				Monocytes
				Eosinophils
				Basophils

	Low	Normal	High	
				Total RBCs
				Hemoglobin
				Hematocrit (PCV)
				MCV
				Nucleated RBCs
				Reticulocytes
				Heinz bodies
				Platelets
				RDW
				MPV

Urinalysis

	Low	Normal / none	High	
				pH
				Specific gravity
				Albumin
				Glucose
				Ketones
				Occult blood
				Bilirubin
				WBCs
				RBCs
				Epithelial cells
				Casts
				Crystals
				Bacteria

Special tests
- Heparin injection produces no clearing if lipidemia is caused by lipoprotein lipase deficiency.
- Chylomicron test can show both a cream layer and lactescence in fasting blood sample.
- Normal amylase and lipase activities.
- Normal T_4 and fT_4d.

Secondary Hyperlipidemia

fasting
hyperlipidemia
indicates
abnormal lipid
metabolism

Fasting hyperlipidemia indicates abnormal lipid metabolism. This is usually secondary to metabolic disease, such as diabetes mellitus, acute pancreatitis, hypothyroidism, hyperadrenocorticism, liver disease, or nephrotic syndrome.

Interpretation
Not all possible serum chemistry abnormalities are present in every affected animal. The blood panel can detect primary disease that is causing the hyperlipidemia.

High serum triglyceride levels could indicate hyperlipidemia if there is no visible lipemia. With lipemia, the chylomicron test confirms chylomicronemia. Lipemic blood samples that fail to clear following heparin injection indicate a lipoprotein lipase deficiency.

Differential Diagnoses
- Primary hyperlipidemia: high blood lipids with no other metabolic disease
- Diabetes mellitus: hyperglycemia, glycosuria
- Acute pancreatitis: usually high serum lipase, amylase, and TLI
- Cholestatic liver disease: abnormal serum activity of liver-derived enzymes, high serum bilirubin levels
- Nephrotic syndrome: low serum albumin level, proteinuria
- Postprandial hyperlipidemia: ruled out by withholding food for at least 12 hours

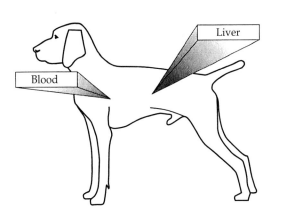

Signs
- Obvious lipemia
- Abdominal pain
- Seizures
- Vomiting
- Diarrhea
- Hepatomegaly
- Lipid-laden aqueous humor
- Corneal dystrophy
- Lethargy
- Anorexia

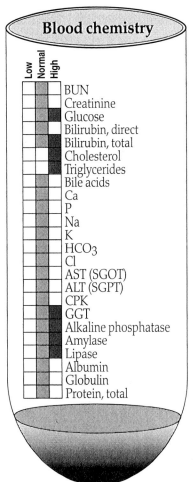

Blood chemistry

	Low	Normal	High	
				BUN
				Creatinine
				Glucose
				Bilirubin, direct
				Bilirubin, total
				Cholesterol
				Triglycerides
				Bile acids
				Ca
				P
				Na
				K
				HCO3
				Cl
				AST (SGOT)
				ALT (SGPT)
				CPK
				GGT
				Alkaline phosphatase
				Amylase
				Lipase
				Albumin
				Globulin
				Protein, total

Hemogram

	Low	Normal	High	
				Total WBCs
				Band neutrophils
				Neutrophils
				Lymphocytes
				Monocytes
				Eosinophils
				Basophils

	Low	Normal	High	
				Total RBCs
				Hemoglobin
				Hematocrit (PCV)
				MCV
				Nucleated RBCs
				Reticulocytes
				Heinz bodies
				Platelets
				RDW
				MPV

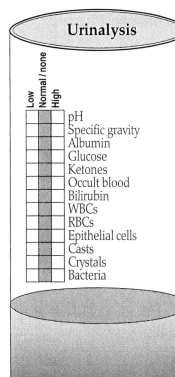

Urinalysis

	Low	Normal / none	High	
				pH
				Specific gravity
				Albumin
				Glucose
				Ketones
				Occult blood
				Bilirubin
				WBCs
				RBCs
				Epithelial cells
				Casts
				Crystals
				Bacteria

Special tests
- **Heparin injection does not clear the serum, indicating a primary or secondary problem.**
- **Chylomicron test shows a cream layer and lactescence in fasting blood sample, suggesting abnormal fat metabolism or lipolysis.**
- **Amylase and lipase assays to screen for acute pancreatitis.**
- **Low serum T_4, low fT_4d, and poor response to ACTH stimulation with hypothyroidism.**

Intestinal Histoplasmosis

histoplasma causes malabsorption because of thickened intestinal walls and lymphatic obstruction

Histoplasmosis is a systemic fungal disease. Microconidia are inhaled or ingested, develop into yeast form within macrophages, and then disseminate throughout the body.

The disease is usually self-limiting unless the animal has a defective immune response. Gastrointestinal dysfunction is the most common sign in dogs, while pulmonary involvement is more common in cats. Final diagnosis depends on observation of the fungus on cytologic smears.

Interpretation
High serum bilirubin, GGT, and alkaline phosphatase values indicate cholestatic liver disease. Leukocytosis with monocytosis indicates a chronic infection. Cytologic examination of rectal smears or lymph node aspirates is required for diagnosis.

Differential Diagnoses
- Colitis from whipworm infection: whipworm ova in feces, positive response to whipworm treatment
- Colitis from protozoal infection: protozoa in feces, positive response to antiprotozoal treatment
- Exocrine pancreatic insufficiency: abnormal digestion tests
- Intestinal malabsorption from lymphangiectasia or lymphosarcoma: intestinal biopsy

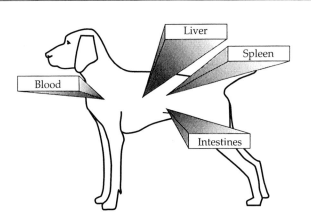

Signs
- Chronic diarrhea
- Emaciation
- Cough
- Dyspnea

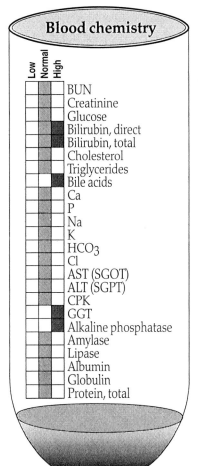

Blood chemistry

	Low	Normal	High	
		■		BUN
		■		Creatinine
		■		Glucose
			■	Bilirubin, direct
		■		Bilirubin, total
		■		Cholesterol
		■		Triglycerides
	■		■	Bile acids
		■		Ca
		■		P
		■		Na
		■		K
		■		HCO3
		■		Cl
		■		AST (SGOT)
		■		ALT (SGPT)
		■		CPK
	■		■	GGT
			■	Alkaline phosphatase
		■		Amylase
		■		Lipase
		■		Albumin
		■		Globulin
		■		Protein, total

Hemogram

	Low	Normal	High	
		■		Total WBCs
		■		Band neutrophils
			■	Neutrophils
	■			Lymphocytes
			■	Monocytes
	■			Eosinophils
		■		Basophils

	Low	Normal	High	
		■		Total RBCs
		■		Hemoglobin
		■		Hematocrit (PCV)
		■		MCV
		■		Nucleated RBCs
		■		Reticulocytes
		■		Heinz bodies
		■		Platelets
		■		RDW
		■		MPV

Urinalysis

	Low	Normal / none	High	
		■		pH
		■		Specific gravity
		■		Albumin
		■		Glucose
		■		Ketones
		■		Occult blood
			■	Bilirubin
		■		WBCs
		■		RBCs
		■		Epithelial cells
		■		Casts
		■		Crystals
		■		Bacteria

Special tests
- Radiographs may show mesenteric lymphadenopathy, splenomegaly, hepatomegaly, ascites, interstitial pulmonary densities, and hilar lymphadenopathy; also occasional lytic bone lesions.
- Cytologic examination of rectal scrapings, buffy coat smears or aspirates of liver, lung, spleen and bone marrow show fungal organisms.
- Abnormal fat absorption.
- Serologic diagnosis is unreliable because of cross-reaction with other fungi; need rising titers.

Viral Enteritis in Dogs

parvovirus, coronavirus, and distemper virus cause significant intestinal lesions in dogs

Three viral agents cause significant intestinal lesions in dogs. Parvovirus destroys proliferating cells in the crypts of the intestinal villi, causing severe damage to the absorptive surface of the small intestine. Coronavirus damages the tips of villi, resulting in villus blunting and loss of absorptive surface. Distemper virus invades the nonvillus epithelial cells but does not blunt the villi. All lead to diarrhea, decreased absorption, and exudation.

Interpretation
A low WBC count suggests viral infection. The animal may be dehydrated, but severe vomiting and diarrhea can reduce the total plasma protein level and mask hemoconcentration. The total plasma protein level is low, but the relative serum levels of sodium, potassium, and chloride are normal.

Parvovirus infection and distemper are diagnosed with specific antigen or antibody tests.

Differential Diagnoses
- Hemorrhagic gastroenteritis: hemoconcentration with normal total plasma protein levels
- Salmonellosis: cytologic examination of feces shows many neutrophils, positive fecal culture
- Intestinal obstruction: antigen/antibody tests are negative for parvovirus or distemper virus, obstruction visible on radiographs

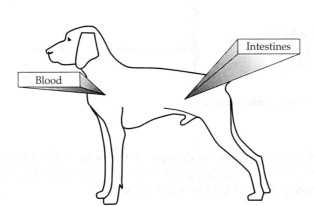

Signs
- Fever
- Depression
- Anorexia
- Vomiting
- Diarrhea
- Dehydration

Blood chemistry

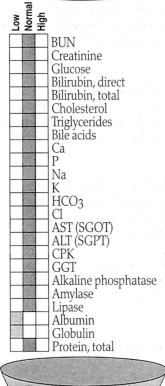

Low / Normal / High

BUN
Creatinine
Glucose
Bilirubin, direct
Bilirubin, total
Cholesterol
Triglycerides
Bile acids
Ca
P
Na
K
HCO₃
Cl
AST (SGOT)
ALT (SGPT)
CPK
GGT
Alkaline phosphatase
Amylase
Lipase
Albumin
Globulin
Protein, total

Hemogram

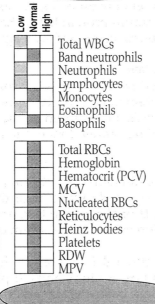

Low / Normal / High

Total WBCs
Band neutrophils
Neutrophils
Lymphocytes
Monocytes
Eosinophils
Basophils

Total RBCs
Hemoglobin
Hematocrit (PCV)
MCV
Nucleated RBCs
Reticulocytes
Heinz bodies
Platelets
RDW
MPV

Urinalysis

Low / Normal / none / High

pH
Specific gravity
Albumin
Glucose
Ketones
Occult blood
Bilirubin
WBCs
RBCs
Epithelial cells
Casts
Crystals
Bacteria

Special tests
- Confirm parvovirus infection with a fecal antigen test, a stool hemagglutination test >1:64, or a serum IgM titer.
- Confirm canine distemper with IgM titer or fluorescent antibody test for distemper virus on cells of the conjunctiva, tonsils, or buffy coat during the first 3 weeks of illness.
- There is no specific test for acute coronavirus infection, but it may be diagnosed by a rising coronavirus titer.

Protein-Losing Enteropathy

the key to early diagnosis of intestinal protein loss is the alpha-1 protease inhibitor test

Inflammatory bowel disease, neoplastic infiltration of the bowel, increased lymphatic pressure, and lymphosarcoma can cause protein loss from the bowel.

Normally, proteins lost in the small intestine are digested and absorbed farther distally in the tract to make new protein. If normal protein loss is increased by mucosal diseases or obstruction of lymphatics, loss of albumin and globulin reduces serum protein levels. Early detection of enteric protein loss requires testing for fecal alpha-1 protease inhibitor.

Interpretation
The blood panel can rule out common causes of hypoproteinemia. Liver tests show no sign of active necrosis, biliary stasis, or retention of bile pigments. A normal BUN level and no protein loss in the urine indicate normal kidney function.

Fecal examination can rule out parasites as a cause of the bowel disease. Results of digestive enzyme tests are normal, but results of absorption tests are abnormal. Decreased fat absorption causes a low serum cholesterol level.

A low serum calcium level is related to low serum albumin levels. A positive fecal alpha-1 protease inhibitor test confirms protein loss before serum albumin is affected.

Differential Diagnoses
- Chronic liver disease: usually high serum globulin and bile acid levels
- Glomerulonephritis: protein in the urine
- Intestinal parasitism: ova or parasites on fecal examination
- Bleeding problems: anemia, melena
- Inflammatory bowel disease: bowel biopsy usually shows inflammatory-cell infiltration and causative organism

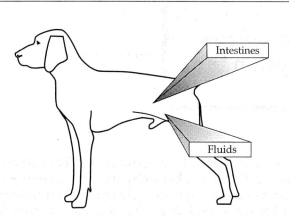

Signs
- Chronic diarrhea
- ±Hemorrhage
- ±Vomiting
- Weight loss
- Edema
- Ascites
- Hydrothorax

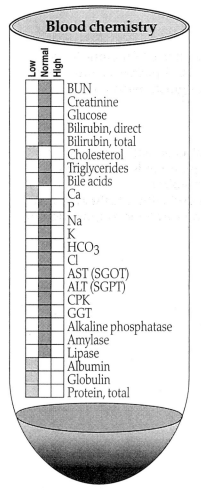

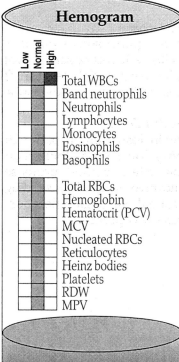

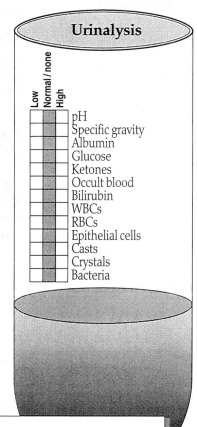

Blood chemistry

Low / Normal / High

- BUN
- Creatinine
- Glucose
- Bilirubin, direct
- Bilirubin, total
- Cholesterol
- Triglycerides
- Bile acids
- Ca
- P
- Na
- K
- HCO₃
- Cl
- AST (SGOT)
- ALT (SGPT)
- CPK
- GGT
- Alkaline phosphatase
- Amylase
- Lipase
- Albumin
- Globulin
- Protein, total

Hemogram

Low / Normal / High

- Total WBCs
- Band neutrophils
- Neutrophils
- Lymphocytes
- Monocytes
- Eosinophils
- Basophils

- Total RBCs
- Hemoglobin
- Hematocrit (PCV)
- MCV
- Nucleated RBCs
- Reticulocytes
- Heinz bodies
- Platelets
- RDW
- MPV

Urinalysis

Low / Normal / none / High

- pH
- Specific gravity
- Albumin
- Glucose
- Ketones
- Occult blood
- Bilirubin
- WBCs
- RBCs
- Epithelial cells
- Casts
- Crystals
- Bacteria

Special tests
- Fecal examination for common worms to determine if parasitic cause.
- Fecal cytologic examination for such organisms as *Giardia* or *Histoplasma*.
- Intestinal biopsy to distinguish inflammatory from neoplastic infiltrate.
- Fecal alpha-1 protease inhibitor >0 indicates intestinal protein loss.

Maldigestion versus Malabsorption

special tests can distinguish between malabsorption and maldigestion

Exocrine pancreatic insufficiency, biliary obstruction, gastric hyperacidity, and bacterial overgrowth of the small intestine can cause maldigestion. Chronic inflammatory bowel disease, infiltrative bowel diseases, infections, and endoparasitism cause malabsorption.

Interpretation
The blood panel shows mainly the effects of malnutrition, with altered levels of serum proteins, cholesterol, and triglycerides. Special tests can distinguish between malabsorption and maldigestion.

Differential Diagnoses
- Protein-losing enteropathy: diagnosed with intestinal biopsy, low serum albumin and globulin levels, and a positive fecal alpha-1 protease inhibitor
- Infiltrative bowel disease: diagnosed with intestinal biopsy
- Intestinal parasitism: flotation and cytologic examination of feces show parasites

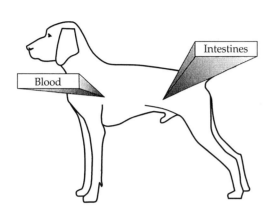

Signs
- Chronic diarrhea
- Weight loss
- Dehydration
- Ascites

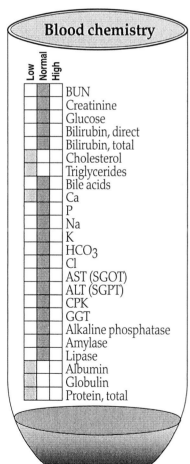

Blood chemistry

	Low	Normal	High	
				BUN
				Creatinine
				Glucose
				Bilirubin, direct
				Bilirubin, total
				Cholesterol
				Triglycerides
				Bile acids
				Ca
				P
				Na
				K
				HCO3
				Cl
				AST (SGOT)
				ALT (SGPT)
				CPK
				GGT
				Alkaline phosphatase
				Amylase
				Lipase
				Albumin
				Globulin
				Protein, total

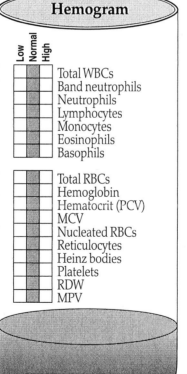

Hemogram

	Low	Normal	High	
				Total WBCs
				Band neutrophils
				Neutrophils
				Lymphocytes
				Monocytes
				Eosinophils
				Basophils

	Low	Normal	High	
				Total RBCs
				Hemoglobin
				Hematocrit (PCV)
				MCV
				Nucleated RBCs
				Reticulocytes
				Heinz bodies
				Platelets
				RDW
				MPV

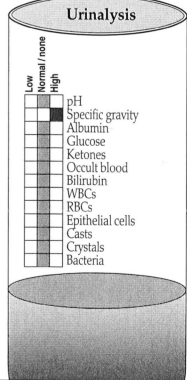

Urinalysis

	Low	Normal / none	High	
				pH
				Specific gravity
				Albumin
				Glucose
				Ketones
				Occult blood
				Bilirubin
				WBCs
				RBCs
				Epithelial cells
				Casts
				Crystals
				Bacteria

Special tests
- Fecal examination for common worms to determine if parasitic cause.
- Tests for malabsorption: xylose absorption (poor), cobalamine/folate.
- Tests for maldigestion: trypsinogen-like immunoreactivity (TLI).
- Increased T_4 level with hyperthyroidism.

Intestinal Bacterial Overgrowth

increased
numbers of small
bowel bacteria
break down bile
salts and cause
malabsorption

The small bowel microflora is normally sparse. When control mechanisms fail, bacteria proliferate, causing breakdown of bile salts and malabsorption. A more alkaline gastric pH, ileus, exocrine pancreatic insufficiency, or intestinal IgA deficiency can cause bacterial overgrowth.

Interpretation
A xylose absorption test can be used to screen for malabsorption caused by infiltrative bowel disease. Bacterial overgrowth causes decreased serum vitamin B_{12} levels and increased serum folate levels.

Normal trypsin-like immunoreactivity rules out pancreatic insufficiency. Radiographs may show intestinal stasis, and assays of gastric juice show an increased pH.

Differential Diagnoses
- Exocrine pancreatic insufficiency: decreased trypsin-like immunoreactivity
- Malabsorption: decreased xylose absorption
- Infiltrative disease of the ileum: diagnosed by intestinal biopsy
- Small intestinal villus atrophy: diagnosed by intestinal biopsy
- Achlorhydria: gastric pH increased

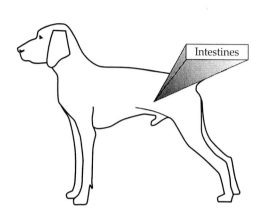

Intestines

Signs
- Weight loss
- Diarrhea
- Vomiting

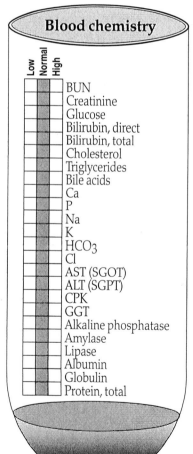

Blood chemistry

Low / Normal / High

- BUN
- Creatinine
- Glucose
- Bilirubin, direct
- Bilirubin, total
- Cholesterol
- Triglycerides
- Bile acids
- Ca
- P
- Na
- K
- HCO₃
- Cl
- AST (SGOT)
- ALT (SGPT)
- CPK
- GGT
- Alkaline phosphatase
- Amylase
- Lipase
- Albumin
- Globulin
- Protein, total

Hemogram

Low / Normal / High

- Total WBCs
- Band neutrophils
- Neutrophils
- Lymphocytes
- Monocytes
- Eosinophils
- Basophils

- Total RBCs
- Hemoglobin
- Hematocrit (PCV)
- MCV
- Nucleated RBCs
- Reticulocytes
- Heinz bodies
- Platelets
- RDW
- MPV

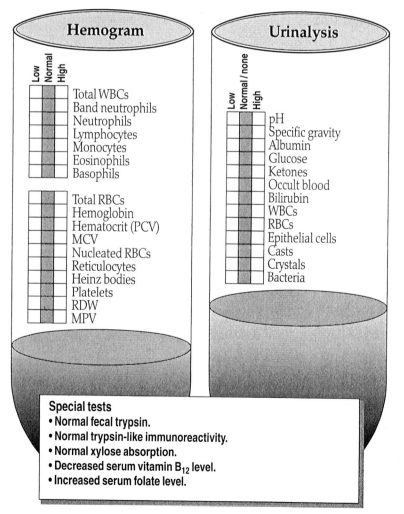

Urinalysis

Low / Normal / none / High

- pH
- Specific gravity
- Albumin
- Glucose
- Ketones
- Occult blood
- Bilirubin
- WBCs
- RBCs
- Epithelial cells
- Casts
- Crystals
- Bacteria

Special tests
- Normal fecal trypsin.
- Normal trypsin-like immunoreactivity.
- Normal xylose absorption.
- Decreased serum vitamin B₁₂ level.
- Increased serum folate level.

Intestinal Lymphangiectasia

increased levels of fecal alpha-1 protease inhibitor occur before decreases in serum albumin

Intestinal lymphangiectasia is a protein-losing enteropathy caused by dilatation of mesenteric lymph vessels. Lymphatic obstruction, infiltrative diseases of mesenteric lymph nodes, infiltrative intestinal disease, or heart failure may cause this condition, but most cases are idiopathic. Obstruction and rupture of intestinal lacteals cause leakage of lymph into the intestinal epithelium and lumen, resulting in hypoproteinemia. Leakage of lymphatic lipids into the intestinal wall causes granulomas that progressively obstruct more lacteals. Yorkshire Terriers and Soft-Coated Wheatons have a high incidence of this condition.

Interpretation
Early cases may show only increased amounts of fecal alpha-1 protease inhibitor. Lymphopenia, hypoalbuminemia, hypoglobulinemia, and hypocholesterolemia are found in advanced cases. Low serum calcium is secondary to low serum albumin.

Differential Diagnoses
- Heart failure: enlarged heart, negative fecal alpha-1 protease inhibitor
- Glomerulonephritis: increased urine albumin, increased protein:creatinine ratio
- Malabsorption: no hypoalbuminemia no fecal alpha-1 protease inhibitor

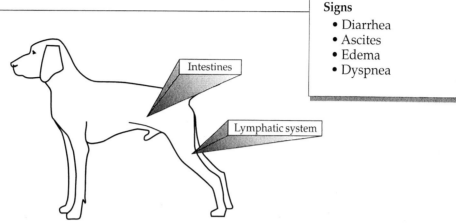

Signs
- Diarrhea
- Ascites
- Edema
- Dyspnea

Intestines

Lymphatic system

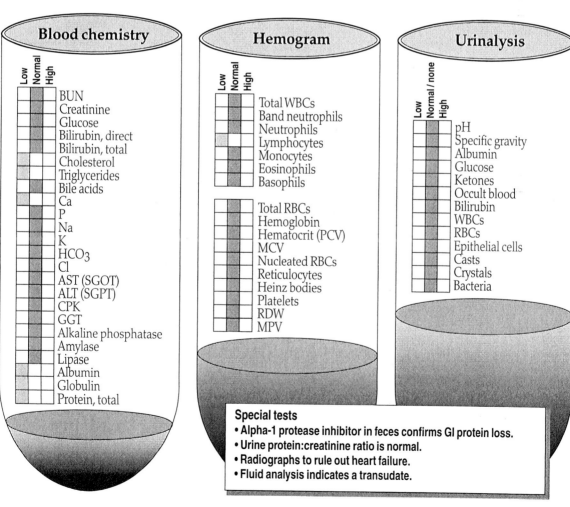

Blood chemistry

	Low	Normal	High	
				BUN
				Creatinine
				Glucose
				Bilirubin, direct
				Bilirubin, total
				Cholesterol
				Triglycerides
				Bile acids
				Ca
				P
				Na
				K
				HCO3
				Cl
				AST (SGOT)
				ALT (SGPT)
				CPK
				GGT
				Alkaline phosphatase
				Amylase
				Lipase
				Albumin
				Globulin
				Protein, total

Hemogram

	Low	Normal	High	
				Total WBCs
				Band neutrophils
				Neutrophils
				Lymphocytes
				Monocytes
				Eosinophils
				Basophils
				Total RBCs
				Hemoglobin
				Hematocrit (PCV)
				MCV
				Nucleated RBCs
				Reticulocytes
				Heinz bodies
				Platelets
				RDW
				MPV

Urinalysis

	Low	Normal / none	High	
				pH
				Specific gravity
				Albumin
				Glucose
				Ketones
				Occult blood
				Bilirubin
				WBCs
				RBCs
				Epithelial cells
				Casts
				Crystals
				Bacteria

Special tests
- Alpha-1 protease inhibitor in feces confirms GI protein loss.
- Urine protein:creatinine ratio is normal.
- Radiographs to rule out heart failure.
- Fluid analysis indicates a transudate.

Renal Disease from NSAID Use

antiprostaglan-
dins may cause
renal ischemia if
there is concur-
rent hypotension,
renal disease, or
vasoconstriction

Prostaglandins produced in the kidneys maintain renal blood flow, promote sodium and potassium excretion, and help control release of renin. Inhibition of prostaglandin production by nonsteroidal antiinflammatory drugs (NSAIDs), such as ibuprofen, flunixin meglumine, or aspirin, can cause renal ischemia if there is concurrent hypotension, renal disease, or vasoconstriction.

Animals are at risk if they have congestive heart failure, liver failure, dehydration, diabetes mellitus, renal disease, or urinary obstruction. The risk is also increased with concurrent administration of anesthetics, diuretics (furosemide), or angiotensin-converting enzyme inhibitors (enalapril, captopril).

Interpretation
Dehydration or azotemia can cause high BUN, creatinine, and phosphorus levels. High total plasma protein and albumin levels suggest dehydration. Low blood HCO_3 with an anion gap indicates acidosis. Platelet dysfunction caused by the antiprostaglandin increases bleeding time and inhibits clot retraction.

Normal to increased urine flow rules out postrenal causes of azotemia. The low urine specific gravity with cells, casts, and protein in the urine sediment suggests active kidney disease.

Differential Diagnoses
- Prerenal azotemia: corrected by rehydration, usually no casts or cells in urine sediment
- Postrenal azotemia: decreased urine production
- Glomerulonephritis: protein in the urine, high urine protein:creatinine ratio
- Pyelonephritis: protein, RBCs and WBCs in urine sediment, increased enzymuria
- Renal ischemia: distinguished by the history and physical examination

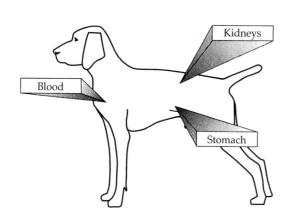

Signs
- Lethargy
- Anuria
- Anorexia
- Vomiting
- Diarrhea
- Anemia
- Melena

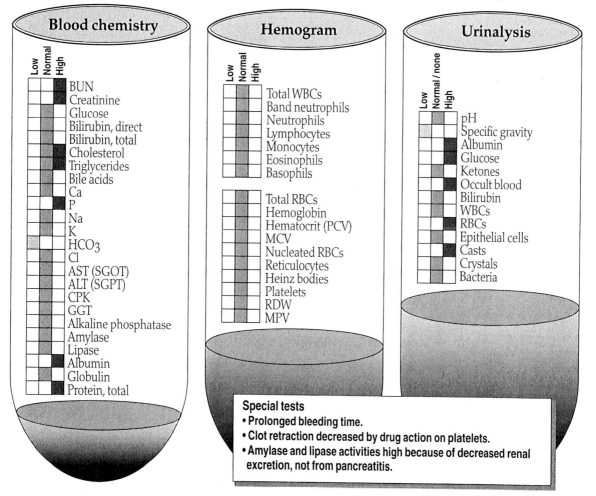

Blood chemistry

	Low	Normal	High	
BUN			■	
Creatinine			■	
Glucose		■		
Bilirubin, direct		■		
Bilirubin, total		■		
Cholesterol			■	
Triglycerides			■	
Bile acids		■		
Ca		■		
P			■	
Na		■		
K		■		
HCO₃	■			
Cl		■		
AST (SGOT)		■		
ALT (SGPT)		■		
CPK		■		
GGT		■		
Alkaline phosphatase		■		
Amylase			■	
Lipase			■	
Albumin		■		
Globulin		■		
Protein, total		■		

Hemogram

	Low	Normal	High
Total WBCs		■	
Band neutrophils		■	
Neutrophils		■	
Lymphocytes		■	
Monocytes		■	
Eosinophils		■	
Basophils		■	
Total RBCs	■		
Hemoglobin	■		
Hematocrit (PCV)	■		
MCV		■	
Nucleated RBCs		■	
Reticulocytes		■	
Heinz bodies		■	
Platelets		■	
RDW		■	
MPV		■	

Urinalysis

	Low	Normal / none	High
pH	■		
Specific gravity			■
Albumin			■
Glucose		■	
Ketones		■	
Occult blood			■
Bilirubin		■	
WBCs		■	
RBCs		■	
Epithelial cells		■	
Casts			■
Crystals		■	
Bacteria		■	

Special tests
- Prolonged bleeding time.
- Clot retraction decreased by drug action on platelets.
- Amylase and lipase activities high because of decreased renal excretion, not from pancreatitis.

Nephrogenic Diabetes Insipidus

decreased renal responsiveness to ADH may be caused by renal disease that affects the tubules and collecting ducts; hypercalcemia, hypokalemia, liver failure, and adrenal or thyroid dysfunction are common causes

Nephrogenic diabetes insipidus is a renal insensitivity to antidiuretic hormone (ADH, vasopressin). A number of systemic diseases can damage the ADH receptor sites in the distal convoluted tubules and collecting ducts of the kidney. Chronic renal failure, pyelonephritis, obstructive nephropathy, hypercalcemia, hepatic failure, pyometra, hypokalemia, and hyperadrenocorticism are common conditions causing this problem. Congenital dysfunction is rare.

Interpretation
The blood panel and hemogram can be used to rule out common causes of polydipsia such as uremia, liver disease, pyometra, and diabetes mellitus.

Special tests distinguish other causes of the very dilute urine. Water deprivation and salt administration are used to rule out psychogenic water consumption. The modified water deprivation test eliminates urinary washout as a cause. An exogenous vasopressin test distinguishes between central and nephrogenic diabetes insipidus. Negative results of vasopressin and repository vasopressin tests confirm nephrogenic diabetes insipidus.

Differential Diagnoses
- Diabetes mellitus: high blood glucose level, glycosuria
- Subclinical renal failure: slightly increased serum creatinine level
- Liver disease: usually low serum albumin level, high serum bile acid levels
- Hyperadrenocorticism: stress response on the hemogram, high serum alkaline phosphatase activity (in dogs)
- Psychogenic polydipsia: water deprivation increases urine specific gravity

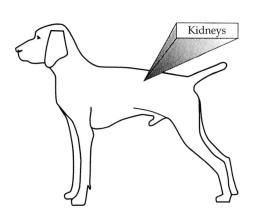

Kidneys

Signs
- Polyuria
- Polydipsia
- Dehydration

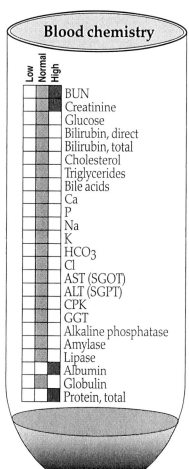

Blood chemistry

	Low	Normal	High	
				BUN
				Creatinine
				Glucose
				Bilirubin, direct
				Bilirubin, total
				Cholesterol
				Triglycerides
				Bile acids
				Ca
				P
				Na
				K
				HCO$_3$
				Cl
				AST (SGOT)
				ALT (SGPT)
				CPK
				GGT
				Alkaline phosphatase
				Amylase
				Lipase
				Albumin
				Globulin
				Protein, total

Hemogram

	Low	Normal	High	
				Total WBCs
				Band neutrophils
				Neutrophils
				Lymphocytes
				Monocytes
				Eosinophils
				Basophils

	Low	Normal	High	
				Total RBCs
				Hemoglobin
				Hematocrit (PCV)
				MCV
				Nucleated RBCs
				Reticulocytes
				Heinz bodies
				Platelets
				RDW
				MPV

Urinalysis

	Low	Normal / none	High	
				pH
				Specific gravity
				Albumin
				Glucose
				Ketones
				Occult blood
				Bilirubin
				WBCs
				RBCs
				Epithelial cells
				Casts
				Crystals
				Bacteria

Special tests
- Water deprivation, vasopressin, and repository vasopressin tests produce no increase in urine-specific gravity and no decrease in polyuria.
- Hickey-Hare test is negative for medullary washout.

Urate Uroliths in Non-Dalmatian Dogs

in most dogs, urate crystals in the urine are a sign of liver dysfunction

Dalmatians normally have high uric acid concentrations in their urine, but this is abnormal in other breeds. Hepatic dysfunction secondary to portal vascular shunts, hepatic cirrhosis, or protein-restricted diets causes uric aciduria in non-Dalmatians. High concentrations of urates in acidic urine can lead to formation of urate uroliths.

Interpretation
High serum GGT and alkaline phosphatase activities suggest biliary dysfunction from hepatic fibrosis. High serum bile acid and ammonia levels suggest shunting of blood from the portal circulation. Normal serum AST and ALT activities indicate no active liver necrosis. This pattern suggests chronic liver disease.

A low BUN level is common with marked liver fibrosis. A BUN:creatinine ratio <5 suggests decreased BUN production. A high uric acid level in urine is always abnormal in non-Dalmatian dogs. Urolith analysis, cold urine crystal precipitation, or amino acid electrophoresis of urine demonstrates high levels of uric acid in the urine.

Differential Diagnoses
- Hepatic cirrhosis: liver biopsy shows fibrosis
- Congenital hepatic shunts: usually a young animal, normal GGT and alkaline phosphatase
- Fanconi's syndrome: no increase in blood uric acid levels, multiple amino acids on urine electrophoresis

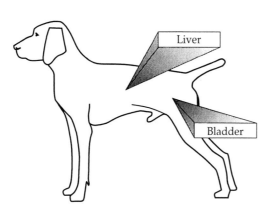

Liver

Bladder

Signs
- Depression
- Blindness
- Personality change
- Seizures or paresis
- Intolerance of tranquilizers and anesthetics
- Polydipsia
- Polyuria
- Dysuria

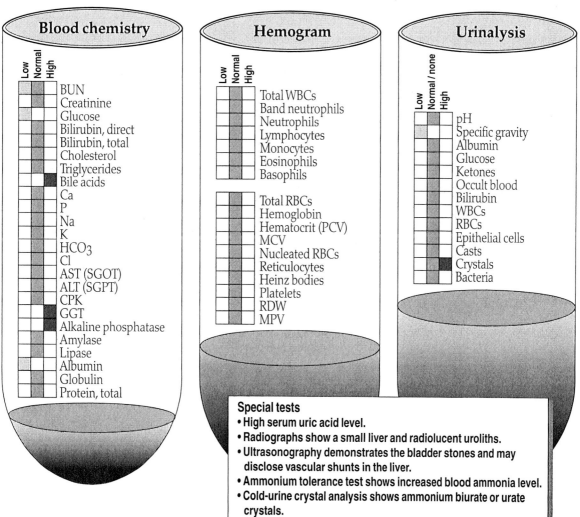

Blood chemistry

	Low	Normal	High	
BUN				
Creatinine				
Glucose				
Bilirubin, direct				
Bilirubin, total				
Cholesterol				
Triglycerides				
Bile acids				
Ca				
P				
Na				
K				
HCO$_3$				
Cl				
AST (SGOT)				
ALT (SGPT)				
CPK				
GGT				
Alkaline phosphatase				
Amylase				
Lipase				
Albumin				
Globulin				
Protein, total				

Hemogram

	Low	Normal	High	
Total WBCs				
Band neutrophils				
Neutrophils				
Lymphocytes				
Monocytes				
Eosinophils				
Basophils				
Total RBCs				
Hemoglobin				
Hematocrit (PCV)				
MCV				
Nucleated RBCs				
Reticulocytes				
Heinz bodies				
Platelets				
RDW				
MPV				

Urinalysis

	Low	Normal / none	High	
pH				
Specific gravity				
Albumin				
Glucose				
Ketones				
Occult blood				
Bilirubin				
WBCs				
RBCs				
Epithelial cells				
Casts				
Crystals				
Bacteria				

Special tests
- High serum uric acid level.
- Radiographs show a small liver and radiolucent uroliths.
- Ultrasonography demonstrates the bladder stones and may disclose vascular shunts in the liver.
- Ammonium tolerance test shows increased blood ammonia level.
- Cold-urine crystal analysis shows ammonium biurate or urate crystals.
- Decreased BUN:creatinine ratio <5.

Cystinuria

excretion of
cystine into
acidic urine can
cause urolith
formation

Cystinuria is caused by an inherited renal tubular defect that prevents the resorption of cystine. This inheritable defect is most common in male Dachshunds. The defect can involve transport of a single amino acid (cystine) or transport of several amino acids (cystine, ornithine, lysine, arginine). Serum cystine levels are normal in affected dogs.

The risk of cystine uroliths is greatest in acidic urine and least in alkaline urine.

Interpretation
Serum chemistry and hematologic findings are normal.

Urolith analysis, cold urine crystal precipitation, or amino acid electrophoresis of urine can be used to demonstrate cystinuria.

Differential Diagnoses
- Urolithiasis related to infection: usually triple phosphate crystals, positive urine culture

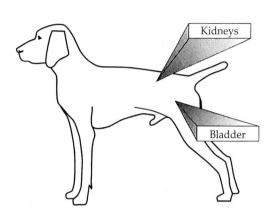

Kidneys

Bladder

Signs
- Dysuria
- Uroliths

Blood chemistry

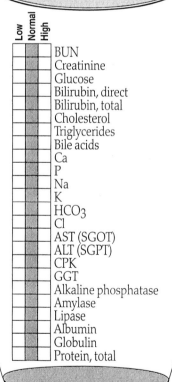

	Low	Normal	High	
				BUN
				Creatinine
				Glucose
				Bilirubin, direct
				Bilirubin, total
				Cholesterol
				Triglycerides
				Bile acids
				Ca
				P
				Na
				K
				HCO$_3$
				Cl
				AST (SGOT)
				ALT (SGPT)
				CPK
				GGT
				Alkaline phosphatase
				Amylase
				Lipase
				Albumin
				Globulin
				Protein, total

Hemogram

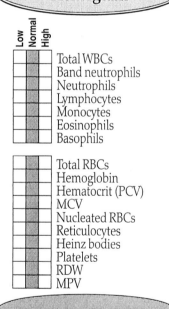

	Low	Normal	High	
				Total WBCs
				Band neutrophils
				Neutrophils
				Lymphocytes
				Monocytes
				Eosinophils
				Basophils
				Total RBCs
				Hemoglobin
				Hematocrit (PCV)
				MCV
				Nucleated RBCs
				Reticulocytes
				Heinz bodies
				Platelets
				RDW
				MPV

Urinalysis

	Low	Normal / none	High	
				pH
				Specific gravity
				Albumin
				Glucose
				Ketones
				Occult blood
				Bilirubin
				WBCs
				RBCs
				Epithelial cells
				Casts
				Crystals
				Bacteria

Special tests
- Double-contrast cystograms or ultrasonography shows the radiolucent uroliths.
- Cold-urine crystal precipitation shows cystine crystals (always abnormal).
- Amino acid electrophoresis of urine may show more than one amino acid.

Distal Renal Tubular Acidosis

failure of the distal renal tubules to fully acidify urine by excreting hydrogen ions causes metabolic acidosis

Renal tubular acidosis results from the kidneys' inability to secrete hydrogen ions. There are two types.

Type 1 is caused by a defect in the distal tubules that prevents urine acidification. It is usually an isolated defect that causes reduced hydrogen ion secretion.

Type 2 is a defect in the proximal tubules that causes excessive loss of bicarbonate. It is usually associated with other renal tubular defects, such as Fanconi's syndrome.

Interpretation

Persistently alkaline urine with a normal anion gap and metabolic acidosis suggests a distal renal tubular abnormality. Signs of active kidney disease, such as protein and casts in the urine and elevated BUN levels, could indicate an acquired lesion associated with acute nephritis.

Differential Diagnoses

- Fanconi's syndrome: acidosis, amino aciduria, glycosuria
- Bacterial cystitis: urine often alkaline, cytologic examination, and cultures of urine show bacteria
- Acute renal disease: casts, inflammatory cells, and protein in urine sediment

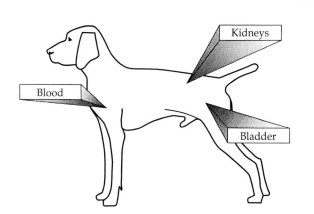

Signs
- Anorexia
- Polyuria
- Polydipsia
- Weight loss
- Weakness
- Uroliths

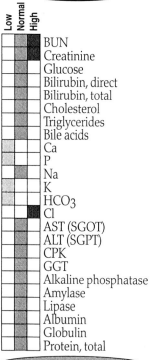

Blood chemistry

	Low	Normal	High	
BUN			■	
Creatinine		▨		
Glucose		▨		
Bilirubin, direct		▨		
Bilirubin, total		▨		
Cholesterol		▨		
Triglycerides		▨		
Bile acids		▨		
Ca	▨			
P		▨		
Na		▨		
K	▨			
HCO₃	▨			
Cl			■	
AST (SGOT)		▨		
ALT (SGPT)		▨		
CPK		▨		
GGT		▨		
Alkaline phosphatase		▨		
Amylase		▨		
Lipase		▨		
Albumin		▨		
Globulin		▨		
Protein, total		▨		

Hemogram

	Low	Normal	High	
Total WBCs		▨		
Band neutrophils		▨		
Neutrophils		▨		
Lymphocytes		▨		
Monocytes		▨		
Eosinophils		▨		
Basophils		▨		

	Low	Normal	High	
Total RBCs		▨		
Hemoglobin		▨		
Hematocrit (PCV)		▨		
MCV		▨		
Nucleated RBCs		▨		
Reticulocytes		▨		
Heinz bodies		▨		
Platelets		▨		
RDW		▨		
MPV		▨		

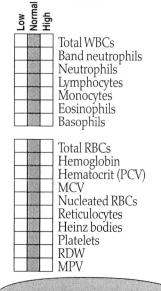
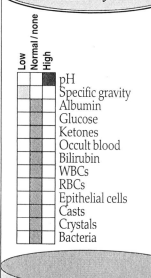

Urinalysis

	Low	Normal / none	High	
pH			■	
Specific gravity	▨			
Albumin		▨		
Glucose		▨		
Ketones		▨		
Occult blood		▨		
Bilirubin		▨		
WBCs		▨		
RBCs		▨		
Epithelial cells		▨		
Casts		▨		
Crystals		▨		
Bacteria		▨		

Special tests
- Radiographs show nephrocalcinosis and radiopaque uroliths.
- Urinalysis shows persistently alkaline urine.
- Normal anion gap indicates no retained acids.
- Urine culture shows no urea-splitting bacteria.
- Acid loading test fails to reduce the urine pH below 6.

Chronic Renal Failure

chronic renal failure leads to retention of nitrogenous waste; acid-base and water imbalances, anemia from lack of erythropoietin, and decreased calcium from decreased vitamin D activation contribute to the wasting signs of uremia

Various kidney problems can reduce the number of functioning nephrons by replacing active tissue with fibrous tissue. A 50% to 75% loss of nephrons impairs the kidney's ability to concentrate urine but does not result in azotemia unless renal perfusion is reduced, as in heart disease or dehydration.

When more than 75% of the nephrons are destroyed, the kidneys have difficulty conserving fluids and electrolytes, maintaining blood pH, excreting chemicals and hormones, or producing erythropoietin. At this point, clinical signs of uremia become evident. Phosphorus retention decreases ionized calcium, which stimulates the parathyroid. Increased levels of PTH cause progressive kidney damage.

Interpretation
High BUN, creatinine, and phosphorus levels indicate impaired renal function. Low blood HCO_3 with an anion gap indicates acidosis. Increased bleeding time and lack of clot retraction point to platelet dysfunction. A calcium × phosphorus product of >60 suggests an increased risk of dystrophic calcification. Increased fractional excretion of phosphorus when associated with normal serum levels of phosphorus suggests hyperparathyroidism.

Normal to increased urine flow rules out postrenal causes of renal failure. Low urine specific gravity and lack of cells or protein in the urine sediment suggest a chronic inactive kidney lesion. The depression anemia is caused by decreased levels of erythropoietin. High serum lipase and amylase activities are caused by decreased renal clearance, rather than by acute pancreatitis.

Differential Diagnoses
- Acute renal failure: casts and protein in urine sediment, no depression anemia
- Diabetes insipidus: polydipsia with no azotemia
- Liver failure: low serum albumin level, high serum bile acid levels, low BUN

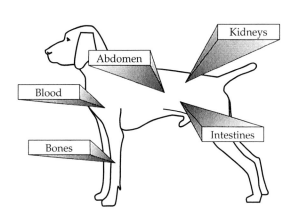

Signs
- Lethargy
- Anorexia
- Weight loss
- Polydipsia
- Polyuria
- Vomiting
- Diarrhea
- Anemia
- Bleeding tendency

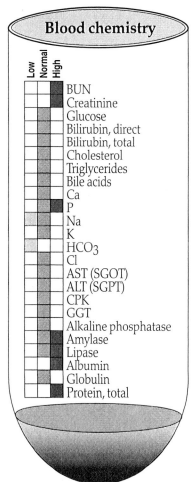

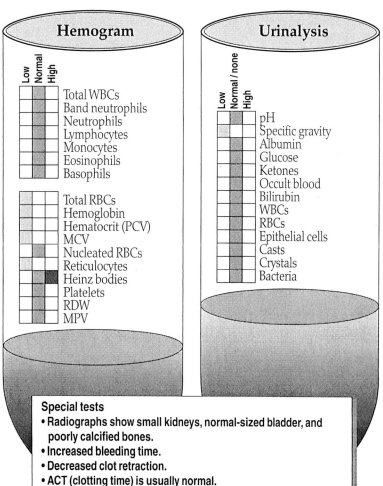

Special tests
- Radiographs show small kidneys, normal-sized bladder, and poorly calcified bones.
- Increased bleeding time.
- Decreased clot retraction.
- ACT (clotting time) is usually normal.
- Amylase and lipase activities are high because of decreased renal excretion.
- Increased FeP suggests hyperparathyroidism.

Fanconi's Syndrome

dysfunction of the proximal renal tubules causes excessive loss of glucose, amino acids, organic acids, minerals, and electrolytes

Fanconi's syndrome is a generalized disorder of the proximal renal tubular transport mechanisms, characterized by urinary loss of several amino acids, glucose, electrolytes, phosphates, bicarbonates, and organic acids. Some animals develop the syndrome after renal disease. A genetic form of the syndrome is found in Basenjis, Elkhounds, Schnauzers, and Shelties.

Interpretation
Polyuria and glycosuria with normal blood glucose levels suggest a renal tubular defect. Acidic urine and a normal anion gap with metabolic acidosis suggest a proximal renal tubular abnormality when diarrhea is not present. The condition is confirmed by detection of amino aciduria using electrophoresis or cold urine crystal precipitation.

Differential Diagnoses
- Distal renal tubular acidosis: no amino aciduria, no cystine or urate crystals in urine
- Diabetes mellitus: high blood glucose levels, glycosuria

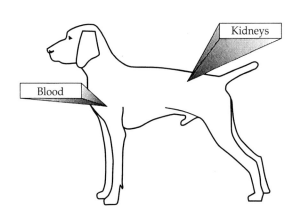

Kidneys

Blood

Signs
- Polyuria
- Polydipsia
- Weight loss
- Weakness

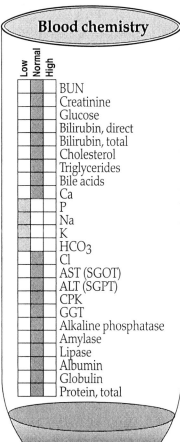

Blood chemistry

	Low	Normal	High	
BUN		■		
Creatinine		■		
Glucose		■		
Bilirubin, direct		■		
Bilirubin, total		■		
Cholesterol		■		
Triglycerides		■		
Bile acids		■		
Ca		■		
P	■			
Na	■			
K	■			
HCO₃	■			
Cl		■		
AST (SGOT)		■		
ALT (SGPT)		■		
CPK		■		
GGT		■		
Alkaline phosphatase		■		
Amylase		■		
Lipase		■		
Albumin		■		
Globulin		■		
Protein, total		■		

Hemogram

	Low	Normal	High
Total WBCs		■	
Band neutrophils		■	
Neutrophils		■	
Lymphocytes		■	
Monocytes		■	
Eosinophils		■	
Basophils		■	

	Low	Normal	High
Total RBCs		■	
Hemoglobin		■	
Hematocrit (PCV)		■	
MCV		■	
Nucleated RBCs		■	
Reticulocytes		■	
Heinz bodies		■	
Platelets		■	
RDW		■	
MPV		■	

Urinalysis

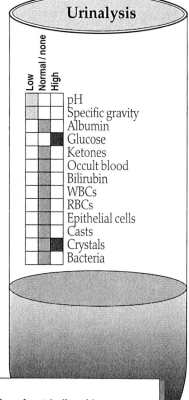

	Low	Normal / none	High
pH	■		
Specific gravity	■		
Albumin			■
Glucose			■
Ketones		■	
Occult blood		■	
Bilirubin		■	
WBCs		■	
RBCs		■	
Epithelial cells		■	
Casts		■	
Crystals			■
Bacteria		■	

Special tests
- Anion gap is normal if no retention of metabolic acids.
- Urine electrophoresis/chromatographs show amino acids.
- Cold urine crystal precipitation shows amino acid crystals (cystine or urates).

Juvenile Renal Disease

juvenile renal disease can be an inherited or acquired disease that decreases the functional nephrons in the neonatal kidney; environmental factors may affect a whole litter, mimicking a genetic disease

The kidneys of neonatal dogs and cats are not fully developed at birth. For several weeks after birth, neonates are very susceptible to hypoxia, dehydration, and environmental temperature changes.

Although renal dysplasia can be an inherited defect, it also can follow hypoperfusion induced by environmental factors (hypothermia, dehydration). Because the renal problem is usually not diagnosed until the animal is more than 6 months old and in renal failure, the cause is difficult to determine.

Interpretation

Depression anemia with high BUN, creatinine, and phosphorus levels are characteristic of chronic renal failure. Low blood HCO_3 tension with an anion gap indicates acidosis. If the serum calcium $\times$ phosphorus product is >60, there is danger of dystrophic calcification.

Low urine specific gravity indicates chronic kidney disease. Casts in the urine sediment indicate active kidney disease.

Differential Diagnoses
- Congenital renal dysplasia:
    Doberman Pinscher—glomerulonephritis
    Cocker Spaniel—renal cortical hypoplasia
    Norwegian Elkhound—glomerular lesion
    Lhasa Apso or Shih Tzu—cortical degeneration and
      dysplasia
    Basenji—tubular dysfunction and tubular cell karyomegaly
    Samoyed—glomerular disease
    Cairn Terrier—polycystic kidneys
    Welsh Corgi—telangiectasis and hydronephrosis
    Wheaten Terrier—cortical fibrosis and renal dysplasia
    Bull Terrier—glomerular lesions

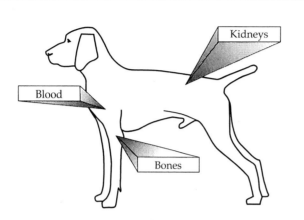

Signs
- Anorexia
- Lethargy
- Stunted growth
- Weight loss
- Polyuria
- Polydipsia
- Vomiting
- Poorly calcified bones

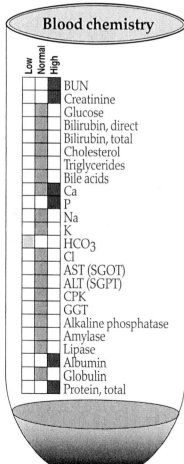

Blood chemistry

	Low	Normal	High
BUN			
Creatinine			
Glucose			
Bilirubin, direct			
Bilirubin, total			
Cholesterol			
Triglycerides			
Bile acids			
Ca			
P			
Na			
K			
HCO$_3$			
Cl			
AST (SGOT)			
ALT (SGPT)			
CPK			
GGT			
Alkaline phosphatase			
Amylase			
Lipase			
Albumin			
Globulin			
Protein, total			

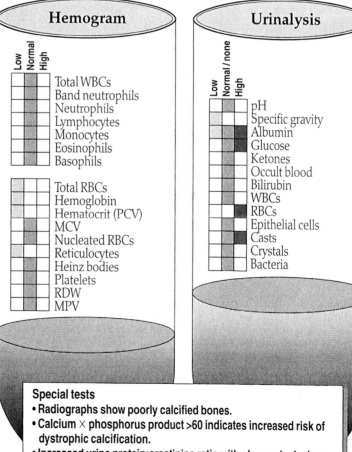

Hemogram

	Low	Normal	High
Total WBCs			
Band neutrophils			
Neutrophils			
Lymphocytes			
Monocytes			
Eosinophils			
Basophils			
Total RBCs			
Hemoglobin			
Hematocrit (PCV)			
MCV			
Nucleated RBCs			
Reticulocytes			
Heinz bodies			
Platelets			
RDW			
MPV			

Urinalysis

	Low	Normal / none	High
pH			
Specific gravity			
Albumin			
Glucose			
Ketones			
Occult blood			
Bilirubin			
WBCs			
RBCs			
Epithelial cells			
Casts			
Crystals			
Bacteria			

Special tests
- Radiographs show poorly calcified bones.
- Calcium × phosphorus product >60 indicates increased risk of dystrophic calcification.
- Increased urine protein:creatinine ratio with glomerular lesions.
- Anion gap >20 indicates metabolic acidosis.
- Reticulocyte production index <2 indicates depression anemia.
- Renal biopsy is needed to determine the type of kidney lesion.

Postrenal Uremia from Obstruction

urethral obstruction causes reflux of urine into the renal pelvis, leading to pyelo-nephritis

Obstructed passage of urine from the body causes postrenal azotemia. With urinary tract obstruction, the kidneys are initially normal, but increased renal tubular pressure leads to renal failure. The obstruction can occur anywhere from the renal pelvis to the urethra, but both kidneys must be affected by the obstruction before uremia becomes evident.

Interpretation
Dehydration and poor renal perfusion cause high BUN, creatinine, and phosphorus levels. An elevated PCV and high total plasma protein and albumin levels suggest dehydration. Low blood HCO_3 with an anion gap indicates acidosis. Platelet dysfunction causes increased bleeding time and lack of clot retraction. Reduced renal clearance causes high serum lipase and amylase activities. Urinary obstruction can be distinguished from the anuric phase of acute renal failure by the lack of casts and the enlarged bladder.

Differential Diagnoses
- Anuric renal failure: casts and protein in the urine sediment, normal urine protein:creatinine ratio
- Uroabdomen: normal urine, abdominocentesis yields urine
- Urinary calculi: visible on radiographs or ultrasonograms

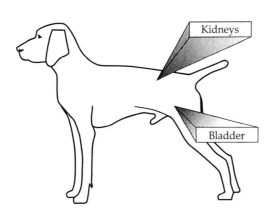

Signs
- Vomiting
- Depression
- Oliguria
- Enlarged bladder

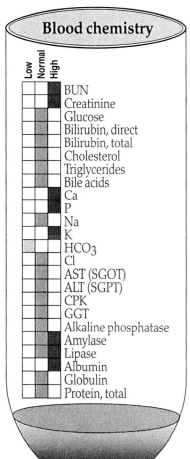

Blood chemistry

	Low	Normal	High	
				BUN
				Creatinine
				Glucose
				Bilirubin, direct
				Bilirubin, total
				Cholesterol
				Triglycerides
				Bile acids
				Ca
				P
				Na
				K
				HCO₃
				Cl
				AST (SGOT)
				ALT (SGPT)
				CPK
				GGT
				Alkaline phosphatase
				Amylase
				Lipase
				Albumin
				Globulin
				Protein, total

Hemogram

	Low	Normal	High	
				Total WBCs
				Band neutrophils
				Neutrophils
				Lymphocytes
				Monocytes
				Eosinophils
				Basophils

	Low	Normal	High	
				Total RBCs
				Hemoglobin
				Hematocrit (PCV)
				MCV
				Nucleated RBCs
				Reticulocytes
				Heinz bodies
				Platelets
				RDW
				MPV

Urinalysis

	Low	Normal / none	High	
				pH
				Specific gravity
				Albumin
				Glucose
				Ketones
				Occult blood
				Bilirubin
				WBCs
				RBCs
				Epithelial cells
				Casts
				Crystals
				Bacteria

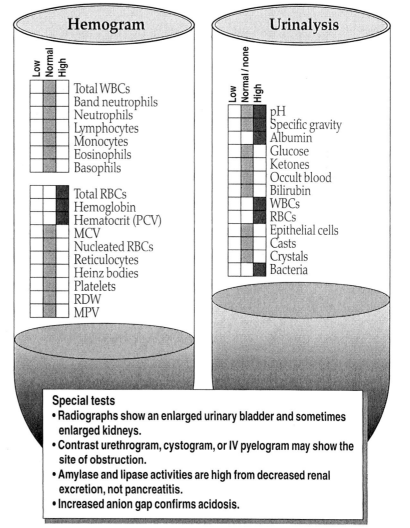

Special tests
- Radiographs show an enlarged urinary bladder and sometimes enlarged kidneys.
- Contrast urethrogram, cystogram, or IV pyelogram may show the site of obstruction.
- Amylase and lipase activities are high from decreased renal excretion, not pancreatitis.
- Increased anion gap confirms acidosis.

Postrenal Uremia from Uroabdomen

intraabdominal
urine leakage
can cause
chemical
peritonitis and
systemic signs of
uremia

Rupture of the kidney, ureter, urinary bladder, or urethra causes urine leakage into the abdomen with resorption of nitrogenous waste products into the systemic circulation. The rupture may arise from urinary tract trauma, obstruction, or neoplasia.

Interpretation
Resorption of urine causes high BUN, creatinine, and phosphorus levels. The high WBC count is related to peritonitis. High plasma protein levels and a high hematocrit indicate dehydration.

Low blood HCO_3 with an anion gap indicates acidosis. High serum lipase and amylase activates are from lack of kidney clearance and not from acute pancreatitis.

Analysis of the abdominal fluid shows an exudate with a high BUN and creatinine.

Differential Diagnoses
- Anuric renal failure: casts and protein in the urine, normal urine protein:creatinine ratio
- Urethral obstruction: enlarged bladder, no casts in the urine
- Urolithiasis: usually visible on radiographs or sonograms

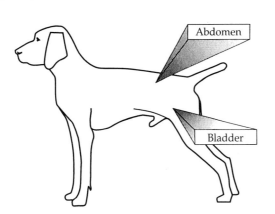

Signs
- Vomiting
- Depression
- Oliguria
- ±Anuria

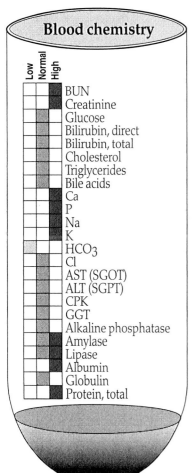

Blood chemistry

	Low	Normal	High	
				BUN
				Creatinine
				Glucose
				Bilirubin, direct
				Bilirubin, total
				Cholesterol
				Triglycerides
				Bile acids
				Ca
				P
				Na
				K
				HCO3
				Cl
				AST (SGOT)
				ALT (SGPT)
				CPK
				GGT
				Alkaline phosphatase
				Amylase
				Lipase
				Albumin
				Globulin
				Protein, total

Hemogram

	Low	Normal	High	
				Total WBCs
				Band neutrophils
				Neutrophils
				Lymphocytes
				Monocytes
				Eosinophils
				Basophils

	Low	Normal	High	
				Total RBCs
				Hemoglobin
				Hematocrit (PCV)
				MCV
				Nucleated RBCs
				Reticulocytes
				Heinz bodies
				Platelets
				RDW
				MPV

Urinalysis

	Low	Normal / none	High	
				pH
				Specific gravity
				Albumin
				Glucose
				Ketones
				Occult blood
				Bilirubin
				WBCs
				RBCs
				Epithelial cells
				Casts
				Crystals
				Bacteria

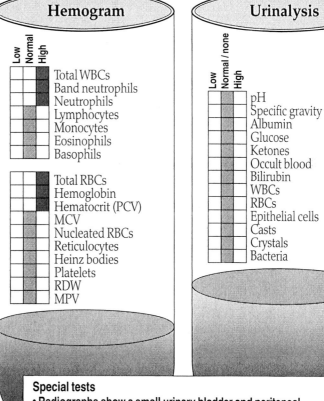

Special tests
- Radiographs show a small urinary bladder and peritoneal effusion.
- IV pyelogram, contrast urethrogram, or cystogram demonstrates the site of leakage.
- Analysis of the effusion shows an exudate with a very high urea nitrogen level.
- Amylase and lipase activities are high because of decreased renal excretion.

Pyelonephritis

renal infections
are usually
caused by
bacteria
ascending from
the lower urinary
tract

Pyelonephritis is a bacterial infection of the kidney. Bacteria ascending from the lower urinary tract are the usual source of infection. The chance of infection increases with urine stasis and cystitis. Infections elsewhere in the body may occasionally cause septicemia and kidney infection. Trauma, nephroliths, diabetes mellitus, and immunosuppression increase the risk of kidney infection. Pyelonephritis causes bacteriuria, bacteremia, nephrolithiasis, and renal failure.

Interpretation
Not all affected animals are azotemic, but when 75% or more of the kidney is damaged, BUN, creatinine, and phosphorus levels increase. Serum globulin levels increase in chronic infections. The WBCs, RBCs, casts, and bacteria in urine samples suggest kidney infection. The presence of casts distinguishes a kidney lesion from a lower urinary tract lesion.

Differential Diagnoses
- Nephrolithiasis: nephroliths visible on radiographs, pyelograms, or monograms
- Lower urinary tract infection: usually *no casts* in urine sediment

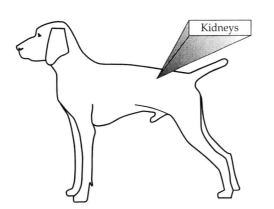

Signs
- Fever
- Depression
- Lumbar pain
- Vomiting
- Polydipsia
- Polyuria

Kidneys

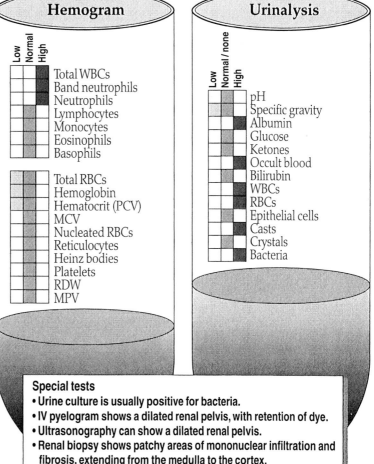

Blood chemistry

	Low	Normal	High	
			■	BUN
			■	Creatinine
		▨		Glucose
		▨		Bilirubin, direct
		▨		Bilirubin, total
		▨		Cholesterol
		▨		Triglycerides
		▨		Bile acids
		▨		Ca
	▨		■	P
		▨		Na
		▨		K
		▨		HCO₃
		▨		Cl
		▨		AST (SGOT)
		▨		ALT (SGPT)
		▨		CPK
		▨		GGT
		▨		Alkaline phosphatase
		▨		Amylase
		▨		Lipase
		▨		Albumin
		■		Globulin
		▨		Protein, total

Hemogram

	Low	Normal	High	
			■	Total WBCs
			■	Band neutrophils
			■	Neutrophils
		▨		Lymphocytes
		▨		Monocytes
		▨		Eosinophils
		▨		Basophils
	▨			Total RBCs
	▨			Hemoglobin
	▨			Hematocrit (PCV)
		▨		MCV
		▨		Nucleated RBCs
		▨		Reticulocytes
		▨		Heinz bodies
		▨		Platelets
		▨		RDW
	▨			MPV

Urinalysis

	Low	Normal / none	High	
		▨		pH
	▨			Specific gravity
			■	Albumin
		▨		Glucose
		▨		Ketones
			■	Occult blood
		▨		Bilirubin
			■	WBCs
			■	RBCs
		▨		Epithelial cells
			■	Casts
		▨		Crystals
			■	Bacteria

Special tests
- Urine culture is usually positive for bacteria.
- IV pyelogram shows a dilated renal pelvis, with retention of dye.
- Ultrasonography can show a dilated renal pelvis.
- Renal biopsy shows patchy areas of mononuclear infiltration and fibrosis, extending from the medulla to the cortex.
- Ultrasound can show dilated renal pelvis, dilated ureters, and hyperechoic pelvis.

Renal Amyloidosis

renal amyloidosis causes severe protein loss and results in edema, ascites, and renal failure

Reactive amyloidosis is caused by macrophage-induced cytokines that stimulate hepatocytes to produce amyloid A protein. This insoluble protein is deposited in the kidney glomeruli as well as in other organs. Although many chronic inflammatory diseases are associated with reactive amyloidosis, most cases occur without a discernible cause. Shar peis and Beagles have a familial form of reactive amyloidosis. Amyloid deposits in the glomeruli cause proteinuria. This may progress to chronic end stage renal failure as the glomerular blood flow is impaired.

Interpretation
Other abnormalities may be caused by the primary problem. When the kidney is affected, the disease is progressive. The main sign is marked proteinuria. Serum albumin decreases, and fibrinogen increases. Increased cholesterol and serum lipids are caused by inactivation of lipoprotein lipase.

Differential Diagnoses
- Glomerulonephritis: differentiated by renal biopsy; proteinuria less severe
- Protein-losing enteropathy: positive fecal alpha protease, negative urinary protein

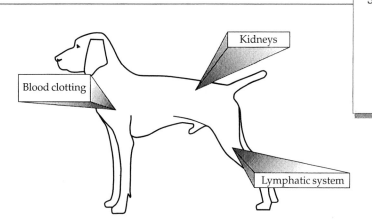

Signs
- Edema/ascites
- Vomiting
- Polydipsia
- Polyuria
- Anemia
- ±Dyspnea

Kidneys

Blood clotting

Lymphatic system

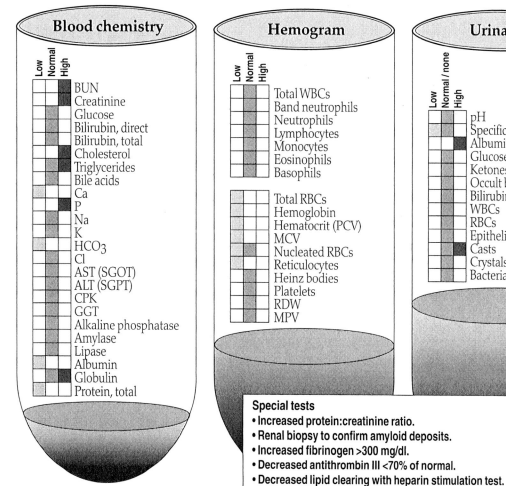

Blood chemistry

	Low	Normal	High	
				BUN
				Creatinine
				Glucose
				Bilirubin, direct
				Bilirubin, total
				Cholesterol
				Triglycerides
				Bile acids
				Ca
				P
				Na
				K
				HCO3
				Cl
				AST (SGOT)
				ALT (SGPT)
				CPK
				GGT
				Alkaline phosphatase
				Amylase
				Lipase
				Albumin
				Globulin
				Protein, total

Hemogram

	Low	Normal	High	
				Total WBCs
				Band neutrophils
				Neutrophils
				Lymphocytes
				Monocytes
				Eosinophils
				Basophils
				Total RBCs
				Hemoglobin
				Hematocrit (PCV)
				MCV
				Nucleated RBCs
				Reticulocytes
				Heinz bodies
				Platelets
				RDW
				MPV

Urinalysis

	Low	Normal / none	High	
				pH
				Specific gravity
				Albumin
				Glucose
				Ketones
				Occult blood
				Bilirubin
				WBCs
				RBCs
				Epithelial cells
				Casts
				Crystals
				Bacteria

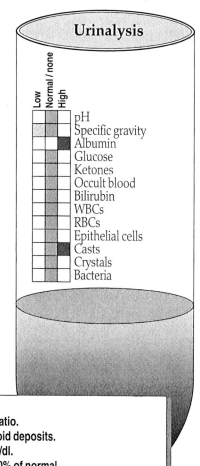

Special tests
- Increased protein:creatinine ratio.
- Renal biopsy to confirm amyloid deposits.
- Increased fibrinogen >300 mg/dl.
- Decreased antithrombin III <70% of normal.
- Decreased lipid clearing with heparin stimulation test.

Anuric Renal Failure

renal ischemia or a toxic reaction causes tubular necrosis; the lumen becomes occluded by cellular debris or protein exudation, and urine production markedly decreases

Acute anuric renal failure is caused by ischemia and necrosis of the renal tubules. Ischemia can be caused by shock, heart disease, or low blood pressure. Tubular necrosis can be caused by bacteria, viruses, nephrotoxic chemicals, trauma, or obstructive uropathy.

Initially a small volume of dilute urine is produced. This stage can last 7 to 12 days.

Interpretation
Dehydration and nephritis cause high BUN, creatinine, and phosphorus levels. Dehydration is suggested by high total plasma protein and albumin levels. Low urine specific gravity with cells, casts, protein, and a normal protein/creatinine ratio suggests active tubular lesions, rather than glomerulonephritis.

Low blood HCO_3 with an anion gap indicates acidosis. Platelet dysfunction causes increased bleeding time and lack of clot retraction. High serum lipase and amylase activities are caused by decreased kidney excretion and not by acute pancreatitis.

Differential Diagnoses
• Prerenal azotemia: responds to rehydration
• Postrenal azotemia: normal to increased urine flow after correction of urinary obstruction

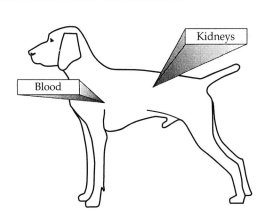

Kidneys

Blood

Signs
- Lethargy
- Anuria
- Anorexia
- Vomiting
- Diarrhea
- Anemia
- Melena

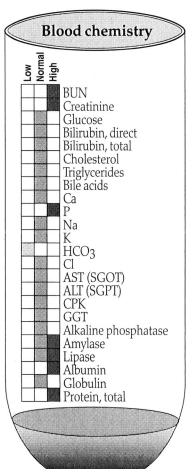

Blood chemistry

	Low	Normal	High	
				BUN
				Creatinine
				Glucose
				Bilirubin, direct
				Bilirubin, total
				Cholesterol
				Triglycerides
				Bile acids
				Ca
				P
				Na
				K
				HCO₃
				Cl
				AST (SGOT)
				ALT (SGPT)
				CPK
				GGT
				Alkaline phosphatase
				Amylase
				Lipase
				Albumin
				Globulin
				Protein, total

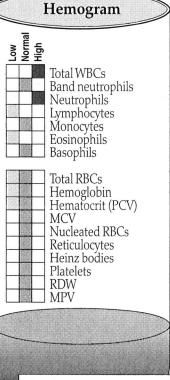

Hemogram

	Low	Normal	High	
				Total WBCs
				Band neutrophils
				Neutrophils
				Lymphocytes
				Monocytes
				Eosinophils
				Basophils
				Total RBCs
				Hemoglobin
				Hematocrit (PCV)
				MCV
				Nucleated RBCs
				Reticulocytes
				Heinz bodies
				Platelets
				RDW
				MPV

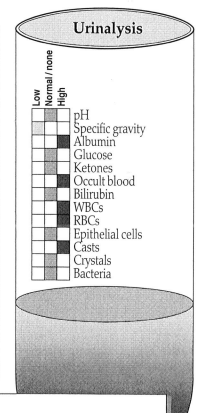

Urinalysis

	Low	Normal / none	High	
				pH
				Specific gravity
				Albumin
				Glucose
				Ketones
				Occult blood
				Bilirubin
				WBCs
				RBCs
				Epithelial cells
				Casts
				Crystals
				Bacteria

Special tests
- Radiographs show a small urinary bladder and normal to enlarged kidneys. IV pyelogram shows decreased renal perfusion.
- Normal calcium × phosphorus product.
- Bleeding time is increased from platelet dysfunction.
- Clot retraction delayed from platelet dysfunction.

Diuretic Renal Failure

this is the recovery stage of acute renal failure in which the kidneys are unable to concentrate urine; volume depletion must be controlled

If a patient survives the anuric phase of acute renal failure, kidney function can return within 10 days despite loss of some nephrons. During recovery, the kidney produces large volumes of urine with a low specific gravity. In this *diuretic phase,* the most serious problems are hypovolemia and dehydration. If more than 25% of kidney function remains, water balance and blood levels of nitrogenous waste return to normal.

Interpretation
High BUN, creatinine, and phosphorus levels are characteristic of acute renal failure. Low blood HCO_3, with an anion gap indicates acidosis. A calcium $\times$ phosphorus product of <60 indicates little danger of dystrophic calcification. Glycosuria may be caused by an acute renal tubular defect.

Platelet dysfunction causes increased bleeding time and lack of clot retraction. High serum lipase and amylase activities are caused by lack of kidney clearance rather than by acute pancreatitis.

Normal to increased urine flow rules out postrenal causes. Low urine specific gravity dilutes cells and protein, and can mask an active kidney lesion. Poor tubular function prevents glucose resorption. If kidney function has been marginal for a long time, depression anemia can be present. This could be masked by concurrent dehydration.

Differential Diagnoses
• Chronic renal failure: usually produces nonregenerative anemia

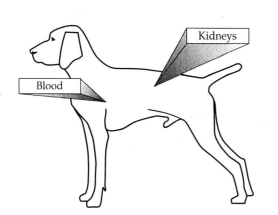

Signs
- Lethargy
- Anorexia
- Weight loss
- Polydipsia
- Polyuria
- Vomiting
- Diarrhea
- Anemia
- Bleeding tendency

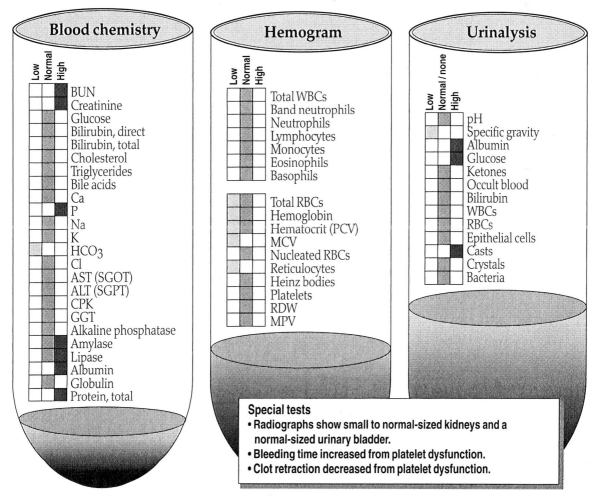

Blood chemistry

Low / Normal / High

BUN
Creatinine
Glucose
Bilirubin, direct
Bilirubin, total
Cholesterol
Triglycerides
Bile acids
Ca
P
Na
K
HCO₃
Cl
AST (SGOT)
ALT (SGPT)
CPK
GGT
Alkaline phosphatase
Amylase
Lipase
Albumin
Globulin
Protein, total

Hemogram

Low / Normal / High

Total WBCs
Band neutrophils
Neutrophils
Lymphocytes
Monocytes
Eosinophils
Basophils

Total RBCs
Hemoglobin
Hematocrit (PCV)
MCV
Nucleated RBCs
Reticulocytes
Heinz bodies
Platelets
RDW
MPV

Urinalysis

Low / Normal / none / High

pH
Specific gravity
Albumin
Glucose
Ketones
Occult blood
Bilirubin
WBCs
RBCs
Epithelial cells
Casts
Crystals
Bacteria

Special tests
- Radiographs show small to normal-sized kidneys and a normal-sized urinary bladder.
- Bleeding time increased from platelet dysfunction.
- Clot retraction decreased from platelet dysfunction.

Glomerulonephritis, Immune Complex

glomerulonephritis is usually caused by deposition of immune complexes secondary to an antigen-antibody reaction

Glomerulonephritis is a protein-losing nephropathy caused by reactions to immune complexes in the blood that indirectly damage the kidney. These antigen-antibody complexes are deposited in the small blood vessels of the renal glomeruli. The antigen can consist of nuclear material, virus particles, bacteria, microfilaria, or debris from inflammation of any organ. Clinical signs are related to loss of serum albumin and, rarely, uremia.

Interpretation
Glomerular leakage is the usual cause of proteinuria without hemorrhage or pyuria. The amount of protein loss can be estimated by the urine protein:creatinine ratio. Low albumen with normal serum globulin levels suggest renal loss rather than intestinal or exudative loss.

As the condition worsens and edema develops, the serum cholesterol level rises and the animal becomes hypertensive. Kidney biopsy confirms the diagnosis.

Differential Diagnoses
- Amyloidosis: demonstrated with special staining of kidney biopsies
- Urinary tract infection: positive urine cultures, WBCs in urine
- Hepatic insufficiency: no significant urine protein, high serum bile acid levels, low BUN level
- Malnutrition: very thin animal, anorexia, no urine protein loss
- Protein-losing enteropathy: no urine protein loss, low serum globulin level, increased fecal alpha-1 protease inhibitor
- Chronic hemorrhage: anemia, low serum globulin level, proteinuria from hemorrhage

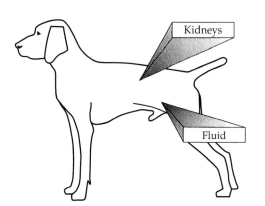

Signs
- Weight loss
- Ascites
- Peripheral edema
- ±Dyspnea

Kidneys

Fluid

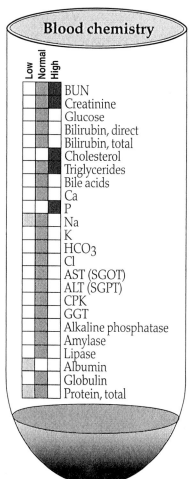

Blood chemistry

	Low	Normal	High	
				BUN
				Creatinine
				Glucose
				Bilirubin, direct
				Bilirubin, total
				Cholesterol
				Triglycerides
				Bile acids
				Ca
				P
				Na
				K
				HCO3
				Cl
				AST (SGOT)
				ALT (SGPT)
				CPK
				GGT
				Alkaline phosphatase
				Amylase
				Lipase
				Albumin
				Globulin
				Protein, total

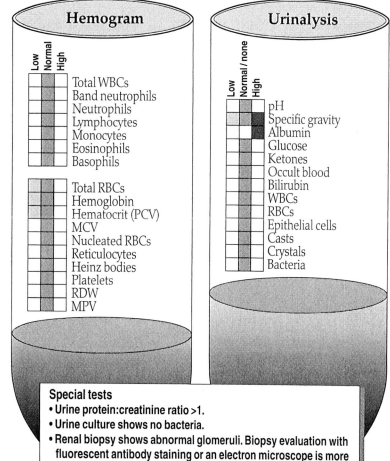

Hemogram

	Low	Normal	High	
				Total WBCs
				Band neutrophils
				Neutrophils
				Lymphocytes
				Monocytes
				Eosinophils
				Basophils
				Total RBCs
				Hemoglobin
				Hematocrit (PCV)
				MCV
				Nucleated RBCs
				Reticulocytes
				Heinz bodies
				Platelets
				RDW
				MPV

Urinalysis

	Low	Normal / none	High	
				pH
				Specific gravity
				Albumin
				Glucose
				Ketones
				Occult blood
				Bilirubin
				WBCs
				RBCs
				Epithelial cells
				Casts
				Crystals
				Bacteria

Special tests
- Urine protein:creatinine ratio >1.
- Urine culture shows no bacteria.
- Renal biopsy shows abnormal glomeruli. Biopsy evaluation with fluorescent antibody staining or an electron microscope is more diagnostic than with a light microscope.

Acute Renal Failure, Induction Stage

recognition of the induction stage of acute failure and early treatment can prevent loss of nephrons

changes are detected by sequential urinalyses, enzymuria, and increased fractional excretion of sodium

Early kidney damage from infections, immune complexes, ischemia, or toxins is difficult to diagnose. Often the only clinical sign is listlessness and polyuria without polydipsia. This nonuremic or latent phase of renal failure shows few clinical signs but is important to diagnose because early intervention can prevent nephron loss and permanent kidney damage.

Progressive changes can be detected by serial laboratory tests. The urine specific gravity gradually decreases. When the urine sediment contains casts and protein, and the serum creatinine level rises to 2 or 3 mg/dl, the maintenance stage has been entered.

Interpretation
Often the only abnormalities are an increased cholesterol, a lipemic plasma, and a dilute urine. Blood urea nitrogen and creatinine levels gradually increase in serial samples, while urine specific gravity decreases. This pattern suggests gradual loss of kidney function. Increases in the urine protein, glucose, and occult blood suggest renal tubular damage. The GGT:creatinine ratio screens for destruction of the renal tubular epithelial cells. Increases in the fractional excretion of sodium (FeNa) screens for destruction of the tight junctions between the epithelial cells. Changes in these tests appear before casts are formed.

Differential Diagnoses
• Glomerulonephritis: protein in the urine, high urine protein:creatinine ratio
• Pyelonephritis: protein, RBCs, and WBCs in urine sediment

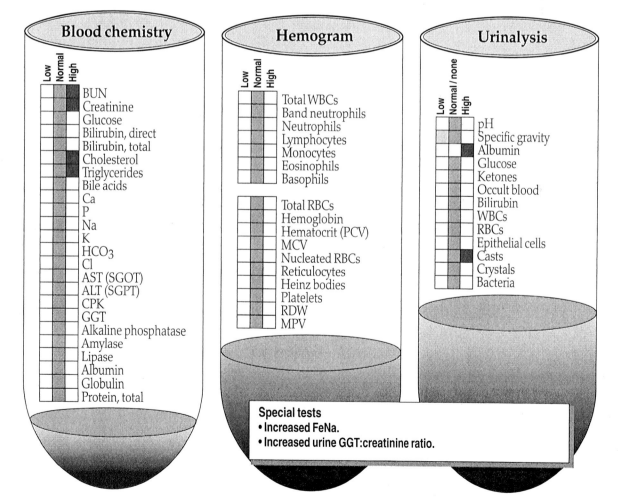

Signs
- Polyuria
- Listlessness
- Anorexia

Kidneys

Blood chemistry

	Low	Normal	High	
				BUN
				Creatinine
				Glucose
				Bilirubin, direct
				Bilirubin, total
				Cholesterol
				Triglycerides
				Bile acids
				Ca
				P
				Na
				K
				HCO$_3$
				Cl
				AST (SGOT)
				ALT (SGPT)
				CPK
				GGT
				Alkaline phosphatase
				Amylase
				Lipase
				Albumin
				Globulin
				Protein, total

Hemogram

	Low	Normal	High	
				Total WBCs
				Band neutrophils
				Neutrophils
				Lymphocytes
				Monocytes
				Eosinophils
				Basophils

	Low	Normal	High	
				Total RBCs
				Hemoglobin
				Hematocrit (PCV)
				MCV
				Nucleated RBCs
				Reticulocytes
				Heinz bodies
				Platelets
				RDW
				MPV

Urinalysis

	Low	Normal / none	High	
				pH
				Specific gravity
				Albumin
				Glucose
				Ketones
				Occult blood
				Bilirubin
				WBCs
				RBCs
				Epithelial cells
				Casts
				Crystals
				Bacteria

Special tests
- Increased FeNa.
- Increased urine GGT:creatinine ratio.

Nephrotoxicosis

nephrotoxicity can occur through many mechanisms; aminoglycosides inhibit lysosomes, chemotherapy drugs cause direct tubular damage, ethylene glycol causes tubular obstruction, and NSAIDs cause hypoxia

Aminoglycoside antibiotics, ethylene glycol (antifreeze), acetaminophen, cisplatin, ACE inhibitors, and antiprostaglandins can be toxic to the renal tubules. Toxicity increases with impaired renal blood flow, so heart failure, dehydration, or hypotension increases the risk of kidney damage from nephrotoxins. These toxins cause tubular dysfunction, tubular necrosis, tubule lumen obstruction, and acute renal failure. The duration of exposure and the type and amount of nephrotoxin influence the reversibility of renal failure. Monitoring with urine enzyme tests and fractional excretion of electrolytes makes it possible to detect this injury before irreversible kidney damage is done.

Interpretation
Increased urinary GGT:creatinine indicates renal tubular cell damage. Increased fractional excretion of sodium (FeNa) indicates damage to the tight junctions between the tubular cells. The earliest screening test abnormalities may be increased cholesterol and triglycerides from deficient lipoprotein lipase. Blood urea nitrogen, creatinine, and phosphorus levels rise because of dehydration and loss of nephrons. High total plasma protein and albumin levels suggest prerenal dehydration. Low blood HCO_3 with an anion gap indicates acidosis. Platelet dysfunction causes increased bleeding time and decreased clot retraction. Normal to low urine specific gravity with casts, cells, and protein in urine sediment indicates an advanced active kidney lesion.

Differential Diagnoses
- Prerenal azotemia: corrected by rehydration, usually no cells or casts in urine sediment
- Postrenal azotemia: decreased urine excretion
- Glomerulonephritis: protein in urine, high urine protein:creatinine ratio
- Pyelonephritis: casts, protein, RBCs, and WBCs in urine sediment; positive urine culture
- Renal ischemia: distinguished by the history and physical examination

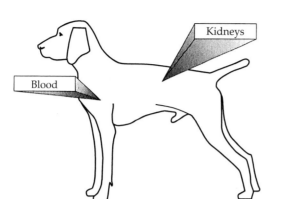

Signs
- Lethargy
- Anuria
- Anorexia
- Vomiting
- Diarrhea
- Anemia
- Melena

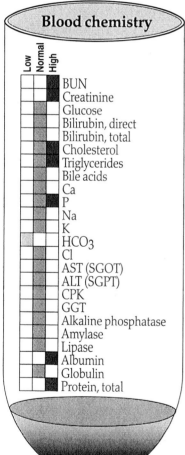

Blood chemistry

	Low	Normal	High	
				BUN
				Creatinine
				Glucose
				Bilirubin, direct
				Bilirubin, total
				Cholesterol
				Triglycerides
				Bile acids
				Ca
				P
				Na
				K
				HCO₃
				Cl
				AST (SGOT)
				ALT (SGPT)
				CPK
				GGT
				Alkaline phosphatase
				Amylase
				Lipase
				Albumin
				Globulin
				Protein, total

Hemogram

	Low	Normal	High	
				Total WBCs
				Band neutrophils
				Neutrophils
				Lymphocytes
				Monocytes
				Eosinophils
				Basophils

	Low	Normal	High	
				Total RBCs
				Hemoglobin
				Hematocrit (PCV)
				MCV
				Nucleated RBCs
				Reticulocytes
				Heinz bodies
				Platelets
				RDW
				MPV

Urinalysis

	Low	Normal / none	High	
				pH
				Specific gravity
				Albumin
				Glucose
				Ketones
				Occult blood
				Bilirubin
				WBCs
				RBCs
				Epithelial cells
				Casts
				Crystals
				Bacteria

Special tests
- Radiographs show kidneys of normal size and a small to normal-sized urinary bladder.
- Bleeding time increased from platelet dysfunction.
- Clot retraction decreased from platelet dysfunction.
- Increased GGT:creatinine ratio.
- Increased FeNa.
- Decreased response to heparin stimulation test.

Systemic Lupus Erythematosus (SLE)

SLE is an immune complex disease that requires a positive ANA test plus two to three other signs

SLE is a disorder of immunologic regulation resulting in autoimmune reactions against DNA and a variety of other host tissue. These reactions cause immune complexes, inflammation, and damage to blood vessels and other tissues. The etiology is unknown, but there is evidence supporting excessive B-cell activation triggered by chemicals, drugs, viruses, or bacterial antigens. Blood cells are directly damaged, causing an anemia and a thrombocytopenia. Other organs such as the kidneys, joints, and skin are damaged by immune complex deposition.

Major signs consists of polyarthritis, glomerulonephritis, dermatitis, Coombs'-positive anemia, and thrombocytopenia. Minor signs are fever, pleuritis, neuropathy, myocarditis, pericarditis, and myositis. Other signs such as lymphadenopathy, leukocytosis, splenomegaly, or hepatomegaly may also be present. Because several tissues are affected, SLE can mimic many chronic inflammatory, infectious, and neoplastic conditions.

Interpretation
Usually a complex of abnormalities is needed to suggest SLE. A positive ANA test in combination with at least two major or one major and two minor signs are required for a positive diagnosis.

Differential Diagnoses
• Immune anemia: positive Coombs' test with negative ANA
• Glomerulonephritis: negative Coombs' test, depression anemia
• Infective or immune thrombocytopenia: normal urine protein:creatinine ratio

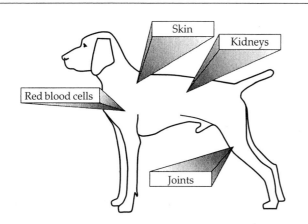

Signs
- Swollen joints
- Skin lesions
- Fever
- Enlarged lymph nodes
- Pleuritis
- Pericarditis

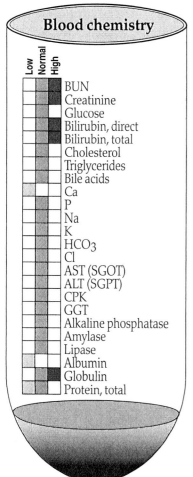

Blood chemistry

	Low	Normal	High	
				BUN
				Creatinine
				Glucose
				Bilirubin, direct
				Bilirubin, total
				Cholesterol
				Triglycerides
				Bile acids
				Ca
				P
				Na
				K
				HCO$_3$
				Cl
				AST (SGOT)
				ALT (SGPT)
				CPK
				GGT
				Alkaline phosphatase
				Amylase
				Lipase
				Albumin
				Globulin
				Protein, total

Hemogram

	Low	Normal	High	
				Total WBCs
				Band neutrophils
				Neutrophils
				Lymphocytes
				Monocytes
				Eosinophils
				Basophils
				Total RBCs
				Hemoglobin
				Hematocrit (PCV)
				MCV
				Nucleated RBCs
				Reticulocytes
				Heinz bodies
				Platelets
				RDW
				MPV

Urinalysis

	Low	Normal / none	High	
				pH
				Specific gravity
				Albumin
				Glucose
				Ketones
				Occult blood
				Bilirubin
				WBCs
				RBCs
				Epithelial cells
				Casts
				Crystals
				Bacteria

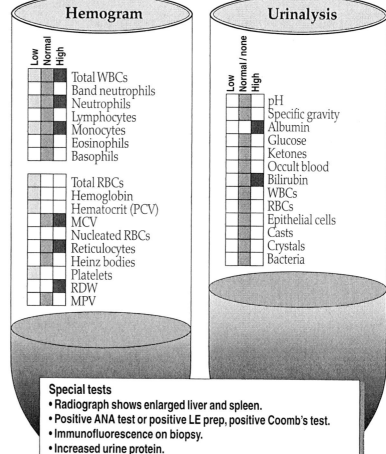

Special tests
- Radiograph shows enlarged liver and spleen.
- Positive ANA test or positive LE prep, positive Coomb's test.
- Immunofluorescence on biopsy.
- Increased urine protein.
- Increased protein:creatinine ratio.
- Joint fluid shows increased protein, WBCs, and monocytes.

Immune-Mediated Vasculitis

inflammation of arterioles, venules, and capillaries is often secondary to immune-complex disease

Soluble antigen-antibody complexes adhering to vessel walls disrupt the endothelium causing platelet adhesion and inflammatory infiltration. Secondary ischemic lesions occur in peripheral nerves, joints, kidneys, intestine, coronary arteries, CNS, eyes, and skin. Infectious, parasitic, and immune-mediated diseases that produce soluble immune complexes cause these vascular lesions.

Interpretation
A high serum globulin indicates chronic inflammation. Proteinuria and low serum albumin suggest glomerular lesions. The low platelet count could be the result of hemorrhage or intravascular coagulation. High serum ALT indicates liver necrosis. Neutrophilia with lymphopenia and eosinopenia indicates systemic stress.

Special tests, such as the Coombs' test or heartworm antigen test, may disclose the underlying antigen source. A high serum triglyceride level indicates a defect in endothelial lipoprotein lipase from vascular lesions.

Differential Diagnoses
- Infectious vasculitis: positive serologic tests for rickettsiae
- Lupus erythematosus: positive antinuclear (ANA) test
- Heartworm infection: microfilariae found or positive heartworm antigen test
- Disseminated intravascular coagulation: fibrin degradation products, increased clot lysis
- Primary thrombocytopenia: bone marrow examination, positive platelet factor III test, positive platelet antibody test

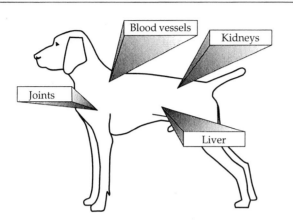

Signs
- Lethargy
- Anorexia
- Polydipsia
- Polyuria
- Lameness
- Weakness
- Pain
- Cutaneous and subcutaneous petechia and ecchymoses

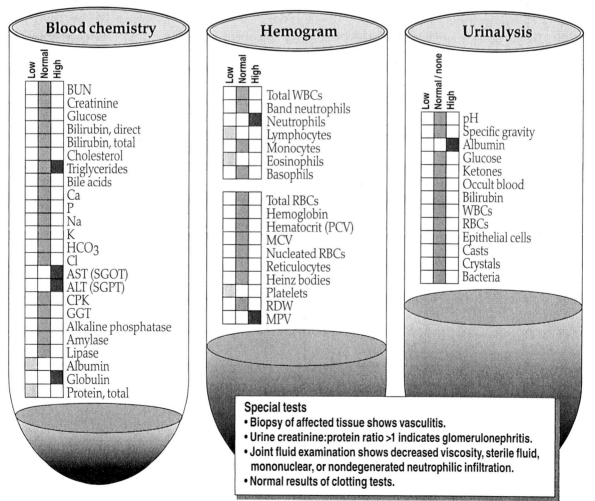

Blood chemistry	Low	Normal	High
BUN		▓	
Creatinine		▓	
Glucose		▓	
Bilirubin, direct		▓	
Bilirubin, total		▓	
Cholesterol		▓	
Triglycerides			▓
Bile acids		▓	
Ca		▓	
P		▓	
Na		▓	
K		▓	
HCO3		▓	
Cl		▓	
AST (SGOT)			▓
ALT (SGPT)		▓	
CPK		▓	
GGT		▓	
Alkaline phosphatase		▓	
Amylase		▓	
Lipase		▓	
Albumin	▓		
Globulin			▓
Protein, total	▓		

Hemogram	Low	Normal	High
Total WBCs		▓	
Band neutrophils		▓	
Neutrophils			▓
Lymphocytes	▓		
Monocytes		▓	
Eosinophils		▓	
Basophils		▓	

Hemogram	Low	Normal	High
Total RBCs		▓	
Hemoglobin		▓	
Hematocrit (PCV)		▓	
MCV		▓	
Nucleated RBCs		▓	
Reticulocytes		▓	
Heinz bodies		▓	
Platelets	▓		
RDW		▓	
MPV			▓

Urinalysis	Low	Normal / none	High
pH		▓	
Specific gravity		▓	
Albumin			▓
Glucose		▓	
Ketones		▓	
Occult blood		▓	
Bilirubin		▓	
WBCs		▓	
RBCs		▓	
Epithelial cells		▓	
Casts		▓	
Crystals		▓	
Bacteria		▓	

Special tests
- Biopsy of affected tissue shows vasculitis.
- Urine creatinine:protein ratio >1 indicates glomerulonephritis.
- Joint fluid examination shows decreased viscosity, sterile fluid, mononuclear, or nondegenerated neutrophilic infiltration.
- Normal results of clotting tests.

Heartworm Disease (Dirofilariasis)

in the United States heart worm disease has been detected in every state

adult heartworms and their microfilaria cause pulmonary hypertension, right heart failure, and immune-complex disease

Heartworms cause valvular heart disease, hepatic congestion, poor renal perfusion, and immune-complex disease. Signs of heart failure are related to the number of adult worms in the heart and great vessels. Antibody-antigen reactions cause kidney disease and arteritis. Emboli can cause lesions in the lungs, kidneys, or brain.

Interpretation
Allergic reaction to the parasite produces eosinophilia and basophilia. Mechanical destruction of RBCs causes anemia, hemoglobinemia, and hemoglobinuria. High serum ALT and AST activities indicate liver necrosis from increased portal pressure.

Decreased renal blood flow increases the BUN. This azotemia is classified as *prerenal azotemia.* Proteinuria and hypoalbuminemia suggest concurrent glomerulonephritis.

Heartworm disease is diagnosed by finding circulating microfilariae or a positive heartworm antigen test.

Differential Diagnoses
- Mitral valve disease: no eosinophilia or basophilia
- Chronic renal disease: low urine specific gravity, no marked albuminuria
- Cholangiohepatitis: elevated serum bilirubin level

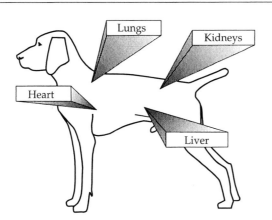

Signs
- Heart murmur
- Cough
- Respiratory sounds
- Weight loss

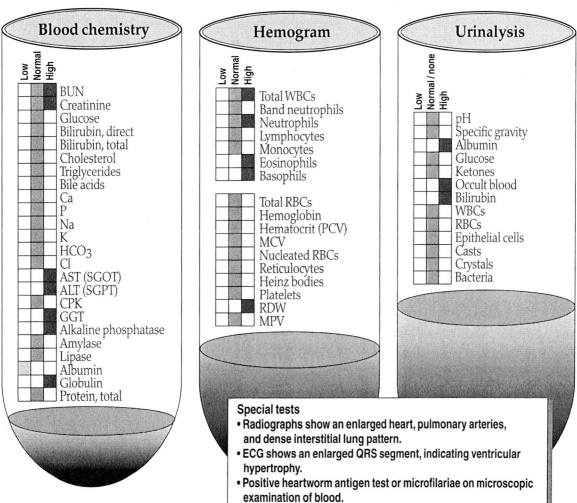

Blood chemistry

	Low	Normal	High	
				BUN
				Creatinine
				Glucose
				Bilirubin, direct
				Bilirubin, total
				Cholesterol
				Triglycerides
				Bile acids
				Ca
				P
				Na
				K
				HCO₃
				Cl
				AST (SGOT)
				ALT (SGPT)
				CPK
				GGT
				Alkaline phosphatase
				Amylase
				Lipase
				Albumin
				Globulin
				Protein, total

Hemogram

	Low	Normal	High	
				Total WBCs
				Band neutrophils
				Neutrophils
				Lymphocytes
				Monocytes
				Eosinophils
				Basophils

	Low	Normal	High	
				Total RBCs
				Hemoglobin
				Hematocrit (PCV)
				MCV
				Nucleated RBCs
				Reticulocytes
				Heinz bodies
				Platelets
				RDW
				MPV

Urinalysis

	Low	Normal / none	High	
				pH
				Specific gravity
				Albumin
				Glucose
				Ketones
				Occult blood
				Bilirubin
				WBCs
				RBCs
				Epithelial cells
				Casts
				Crystals
				Bacteria

Special tests
- Radiographs show an enlarged heart, pulmonary arteries, and dense interstitial lung pattern.
- ECG shows an enlarged QRS segment, indicating ventricular hypertrophy.
- Positive heartworm antigen test or microfilariae on microscopic examination of blood.

Acute Babesiosis

Babesia causes regenerative anemia; organisms may be observed on RBCs of capillary blood

Babesia is a tick-borne parasite that infects red blood cells, causing hemolytic anemia, thrombocytopenia, and fever. Animals that survive the acute disease become clinically normal carriers. These carriers usually cannot be distinguished from normal animals.

Interpretation
The primary abnormality is regenerative hemolytic anemia. High serum AST and ALT activities indicate liver necrosis. Increased hemolysis and secondary liver damage from hypoxia cause bilirubinemia and bilirubinuria.

Microvascular stasis results in renal lesions and disseminated intravascular coagulation. *Babesia-specific* antibody coating of parasitized red blood cells produces a positive Coombs' test. Despite the reticulocytosis, the MCV is low because of the spherocytosis induced by the globulin coating the red cells. The blood smear shows marked anisocytosis. This is indicated by a high red cell distribution width (RDW).

Differential Diagnoses
- Other causes of regenerative anemia: no *Babesia* organisms on RBCs
- Extravascular hemolysis (IgG immune-mediated anemia): no bilirubinemia
- Intravascular hemolysis (IgM immune-mediated anemia, Heinz-body anemia, leptospirosis, microangiopathy): no *Babesia* organisms on RBCs

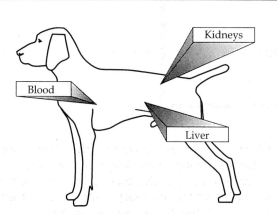

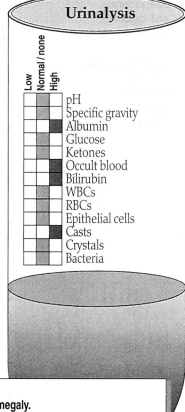

Signs
- Anorexia
- Anemia
- Depression
- Fever
- Hemoglobinuria
- Splenomegaly
- Hepatomegaly
- Lymphadenopathy
- Petechial and ecchymotic hemorrhage

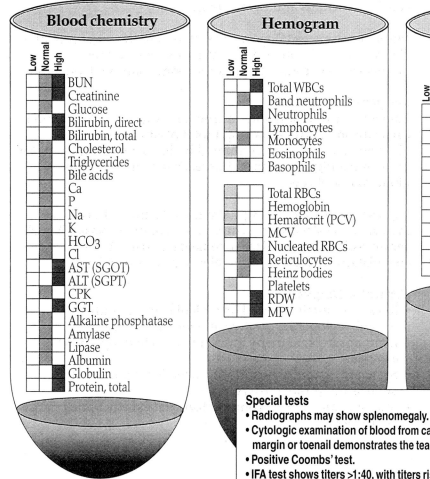

Blood chemistry

	Low	Normal	High
BUN			
Creatinine			
Glucose			
Bilirubin, direct			
Bilirubin, total			
Cholesterol			
Triglycerides			
Bile acids			
Ca			
P			
Na			
K			
HCO$_3$			
Cl			
AST (SGOT)			
ALT (SGPT)			
CPK			
GGT			
Alkaline phosphatase			
Amylase			
Lipase			
Albumin			
Globulin			
Protein, total			

Hemogram

	Low	Normal	High
Total WBCs			
Band neutrophils			
Neutrophils			
Lymphocytes			
Monocytes			
Eosinophils			
Basophils			
Total RBCs			
Hemoglobin			
Hematocrit (PCV)			
MCV			
Nucleated RBCs			
Reticulocytes			
Heinz bodies			
Platelets			
RDW			
MPV			

Urinalysis

	Low	Normal / none	High
pH			
Specific gravity			
Albumin			
Glucose			
Ketones			
Occult blood			
Bilirubin			
WBCs			
RBCs			
Epithelial cells			
Casts			
Crystals			
Bacteria			

Special tests
- Radiographs may show splenomegaly.
- Cytologic examination of blood from capillaries of the pinna margin or toenail demonstrates the tear-shaped *Babesia* organism.
- Positive Coombs' test.
- IFA test shows titers >1:40, with titers rising 3 weeks after infection and persisting for at least 6 months.
- Increased PTT, PT, ACT, and positive fibrin degradation in some animals.
- Increase red cell distribution width (RDW).

Ehrlichiosis

Ehrlichia canis replicates in mononuclear cells, causing lymphade-nopathy, splenomegaly, and hepato-megaly

thrombocytopenia is due to peripheral destruction of platelets

Ehrlichia canis is transmitted by the brown dog tick, *Rhipicephalus sanguineus*. The rickettsia replicates within mononuclear cells in the blood, spleen, liver, and lymph nodes, causing organ enlargement from lymphoreticular hyperplasia. Infected monocytes attach to small vessels, causing vasculitis and hemorrhage.

Immunocompetent dogs usually eliminate the organism after clinical illness. In other dogs, such as some German Shepherds, a chronic phase causes bone marrow depression.

Interpretation
Platelet consumption and destruction by antiplatelet antibody cause thrombocytopenia. High total plasma protein and globulin levels suggest immunoglobulin excess. Protein in the urine and a high urine protein:creatinine ratio indicate glomerulonephritis.

High serum alkaline phosphatase, GGT, and bilirubin values indicate cholestasis from lymphoreticular hyperplasia. A high serum ALT activity indicates hepatic necrosis. Altered coagulation tests and low platelets cause hemorrhage.

Differential Diagnoses
• Rocky Mountain spotted fever: leukocytosis with thrombocytopenia, positive antigen or antibody test
• Lymphosarcoma: many immature cells in lymph node aspirates
• Systemic lupus erythematosus: usually no bone marrow depression, positive ANA test
• Immune-mediated thrombocytopenia: usually bone marrow depression

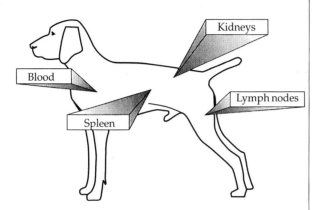

Signs of Acute Infection
- Fever
- Lymphadenopathy
- Splenomegaly
- Depression

Signs of Chronic Infection
- Anemia
- Weakness
- Weight loss
- Petechial and ecchymotic hemorrhage
- Ocular discharge
- Epistaxis
- Hematuria
- Melena
- Neurologic signs
- Renal failure
- Lameness

Blood chemistry

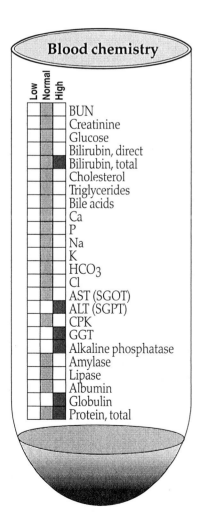

	Low	Normal	High
BUN			
Creatinine			
Glucose			
Bilirubin, direct			
Bilirubin, total			
Cholesterol			
Triglycerides			
Bile acids			
Ca			
P			
Na			
K			
HCO3			
Cl			
AST (SGOT)			
ALT (SGPT)			
CPK			
GGT			
Alkaline phosphatase			
Amylase			
Lipase			
Albumin			
Globulin			
Protein, total			

Hemogram

	Low	Normal	High
Total WBCs			
Band neutrophils			
Neutrophils			
Lymphocytes			
Monocytes			
Eosinophils			
Basophils			
Total RBCs			
Hemoglobin			
Hematocrit (PCV)			
MCV			
Nucleated RBCs			
Reticulocytes			
Heinz bodies			
Platelets			
RDW			
MPV			

Urinalysis

	Low	Normal / none	High
pH			
Specific gravity			
Albumin			
Glucose			
Ketones			
Occult blood			
Bilirubin			
WBCs			
RBCs			
Epithelial cells			
Casts			
Crystals			
Bacteria			

Special tests
- Radiographs/ultrasound show large spleen and liver.
- Urine protein:creatinine ratio >1 indicates protein loss from glomerulonephritis.
- Antiplatelet antibody and ANA tests may be positive.
- IFA titer >1:10 is diagnostic.
- Cytologic examination of buffy coat or blood from marginal ear vein for morulae (organisms within monocytes and neutrophils).
- Cytologic examination of bone marrow shows pancytopenia.
- IFA >1:20 or rising titer, positive Western blot, positive PCR.
- Increased ACT, PTT, PT, and FDPs.

Infectious Canine Hepatitis

acute adenovirus infections cause hepatic necrosis; dogs with partial immunity may have a persistent infection, leading to chronic active hepatitis

Adenovirus type I causes hepatitis in young, unvaccinated dogs. The virus infects liver parenchymal cells and vascular endothelium, causing liver necrosis, immune-complex uveitis, glomerulonephritis, and hemorrhages from vascular damage, disseminated intravascular coagulation, and reduced numbers of marrow megakaryocytes. The disease is diagnosed at necropsy by finding intranuclear inclusions in liver cells.

Interpretation
The low WBC and platelet counts reflect bone marrow depression. High serum ALT activity indicates liver necrosis, while high serum alkaline phosphatase and GGT activities indicate biliary stasis from cholangitis.

Clotting tests are prolonged because of disseminated intravascular coagulation. Rapid clot lysis also suggests disseminated intravascular coagulation. Urinary protein loss is related to glomerulonephritis. Bilirubinuria suggests preclinical icterus.

Differential Diagnoses
- Poison: clinical history, toxicologic tests
- Leptospirosis: leukocytosis, high BUN level, elevated activity of muscle-derived enzymes

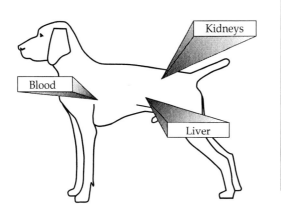

Kidneys

Blood

Liver

Signs
- Vomiting
- Diarrhea
- Abdominal pain
- Fever
- Tonsillar enlargement
- Cough
- Edema of head and neck
- Petechial and ecchymotic hemorrhage
- Epistaxis
- Corneal edema later in recovered animal

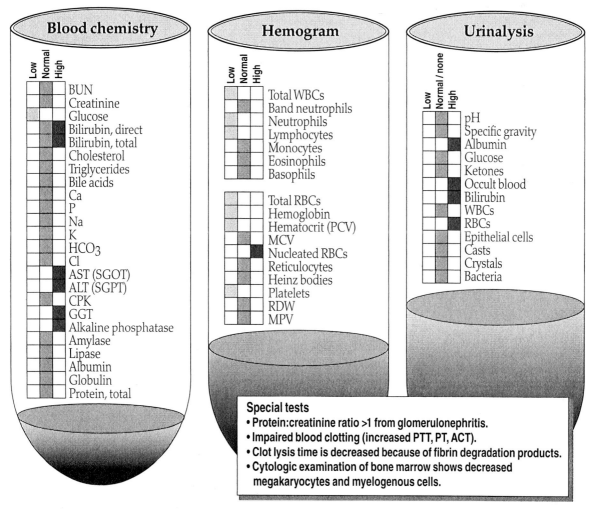

Blood chemistry

Low / Normal / High

- BUN
- Creatinine
- Glucose
- Bilirubin, direct
- Bilirubin, total
- Cholesterol
- Triglycerides
- Bile acids
- Ca
- P
- Na
- K
- HCO3
- Cl
- AST (SGOT)
- ALT (SGPT)
- CPK
- GGT
- Alkaline phosphatase
- Amylase
- Lipase
- Albumin
- Globulin
- Protein, total

Hemogram

Low / Normal / High

- Total WBCs
- Band neutrophils
- Neutrophils
- Lymphocytes
- Monocytes
- Eosinophils
- Basophils

- Total RBCs
- Hemoglobin
- Hematocrit (PCV)
- MCV
- Nucleated RBCs
- Reticulocytes
- Heinz bodies
- Platelets
- RDW
- MPV

Urinalysis

Low / Normal / none / High

- pH
- Specific gravity
- Albumin
- Glucose
- Ketones
- Occult blood
- Bilirubin
- WBCs
- RBCs
- Epithelial cells
- Casts
- Crystals
- Bacteria

Special tests
- Protein:creatinine ratio >1 from glomerulonephritis.
- Impaired blood clotting (increased PTT, PT, ACT).
- Clot lysis time is decreased because of fibrin degradation products.
- Cytologic examination of bone marrow shows decreased megakaryocytes and myelogenous cells.

Leptospirosis

Leptospira primarily affects the liver and kidneys

Leptospirosis is most common in unvaccinated male dogs in rural areas. Infection occurs through mucous membranes or abraded skin following contact with an infected animal, or by ingestion of contaminated food or water.

Leptospirosis affects the liver, kidney, and red blood cells. Peracute infections cause vascular collapse without renal and hepatic damage. Subacute infections cause vascular damage, coagulation defects, and subsequent renal and liver disease.

Interpretation
A high WBC count suggests bacterial infection. Increased BUN and creatinine levels reflect kidney damage. Increased serum ALT and bilirubin values with high serum alkaline phosphatase activity indicate biliary disease and liver necrosis. Increased serum CPK and AST activities reflect muscle necrosis.

Hypocalcemia is related to hypoalbuminemia and has no significance. Electrolyte abnormalities are caused by loss through the gastrointestinal tract. Clotting tests are altered because of disseminated intravascular coagulation and uremia.

Differential Diagnoses
- Viral hepatitis: leukopenia, viral inclusions
- Acute toxic hepatitis: normal WBC count, normal serum CPK activity
- Pyelonephritis: casts and WBCs in urine sediment, bacteria on urine culture, usually no bilirubinemia or bilirubinuria
- Ehrlichiosis: leukopenia, neutropenia, high serum globulin level, nonregenerative anemia
- Ethylene glycol toxicity: no leukocytosis, no icterus, no liver or muscle necrosis
- Infectious canine hepatitis: usually low WBC count

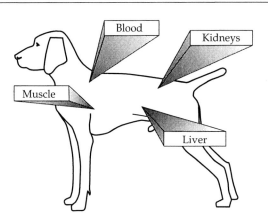

Signs
- Fever
- Polydipsia
- Anorexia
- Vomiting
- Dehydration
- Petechial and ecchymotic hemorrhage
- Conjunctivitis
- Rhinitis
- Tonsillitis
- Dyspnea
- Icterus
- Muscle pain

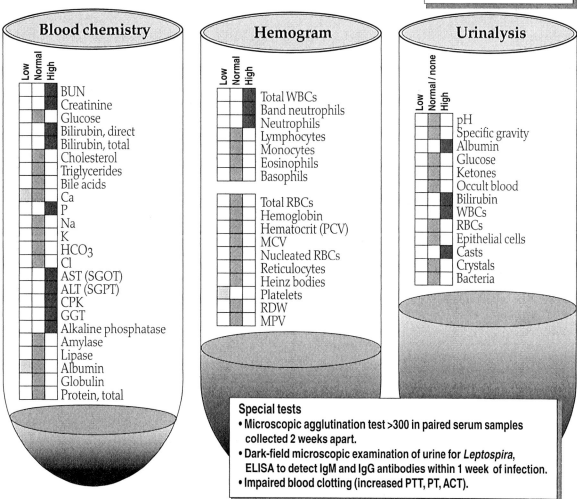

Blood chemistry

Low / Normal / High

BUN
Creatinine
Glucose
Bilirubin, direct
Bilirubin, total
Cholesterol
Triglycerides
Bile acids
Ca
P
Na
K
HCO$_3$
Cl
AST (SGOT)
ALT (SGPT)
CPK
GGT
Alkaline phosphatase
Amylase
Lipase
Albumin
Globulin
Protein, total

Hemogram

Low / Normal / High

Total WBCs
Band neutrophils
Neutrophils
Lymphocytes
Monocytes
Eosinophils
Basophils

Total RBCs
Hemoglobin
Hematocrit (PCV)
MCV
Nucleated RBCs
Reticulocytes
Heinz bodies
Platelets
RDW
MPV

Urinalysis

Low / Normal / none / High

pH
Specific gravity
Albumin
Glucose
Ketones
Occult blood
Bilirubin
WBCs
RBCs
Epithelial cells
Casts
Crystals
Bacteria

Special tests
- Microscopic agglutination test >300 in paired serum samples collected 2 weeks apart.
- Dark-field microscopic examination of urine for *Leptospira*, ELISA to detect IgM and IgG antibodies within 1 week of infection.
- Impaired blood clotting (increased PTT, PT, ACT).

Rocky Mountain Spotted Fever

rickettsia organisms inoculated by ticks replicate in the vascular endothelium; widespread vasculitis causes platelet aggregation and DIC

Rocky Mountain spotted fever is a tick-transmitted disease caused by *Rickettsia rickettsia*. The primary lesion is vasculitis that causes hemorrhage in the skin, retina, GI tract, muscles, urinary bladder, and heart. The lymph nodes and spleen become enlarged and hemorrhagic.

Interpretation
Although the WBC count may initially be low, infected dogs usually have leukocytosis when presented. High serum ALT and bilirubin values reflect acute liver necrosis. High serum CPK and AST activities indicate acute muscle necrosis.

Tests for autoimmune diseases are negative. The disease is diagnosed by fluorescent antibody staining of skin biopsies, IgM antibody titers, or rising titers of IgG.

Differential Diagnoses
- Ehrlichiosis: decreased WBC count with thrombocytopenia, positive antigen or antibody test
- Canine distemper: inclusion bodies
- Immune thrombocytopenia: positive platelet-bound antibody test, increased platelet factor III

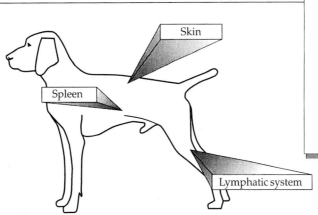

Signs
- Fever
- Splenomegaly
- Lymphadenopathy
- Anorexia
- Petechiae
- Edema of limbs, prepuce, scrotum, ears, and ventral abdomen

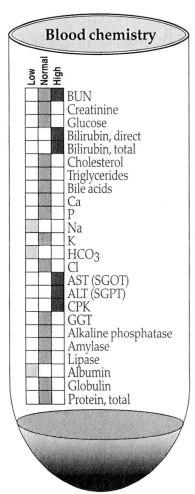

Blood chemistry

	Low	Normal	High	
				BUN
				Creatinine
				Glucose
				Bilirubin, direct
				Bilirubin, total
				Cholesterol
				Triglycerides
				Bile acids
				Ca
				P
				Na
				K
				HCO3
				Cl
				AST (SGOT)
				ALT (SGPT)
				CPK
				GGT
				Alkaline phosphatase
				Amylase
				Lipase
				Albumin
				Globulin
				Protein, total

Hemogram

	Low	Normal	High	
				Total WBCs
				Band neutrophils
				Neutrophils
				Lymphocytes
				Monocytes
				Eosinophils
				Basophils
				Total RBCs
				Hemoglobin
				Hematocrit (PCV)
				MCV
				Nucleated RBCs
				Reticulocytes
				Heinz bodies
				Platelets
				RDW
				MPV

Urinalysis

	Low	Normal / none	High	
				pH
				Specific gravity
				Albumin
				Glucose
				Ketones
				Occult blood
				Bilirubin
				WBCs
				RBCs
				Epithelial cells
				Casts
				Crystals
				Bacteria

Special tests
- Indirect microimmunofluorescence for IgG/rising titer.
- Indirect microimmunofluorescence for IgM single high titer.
- Negative LE cell, ANA, Coombs' test, platelet antibody test, blood culture.
- IgG titer >1:64 or IgM titer >1.
- Skin biopsies show positive flourescent antibody staining 75% of the time.

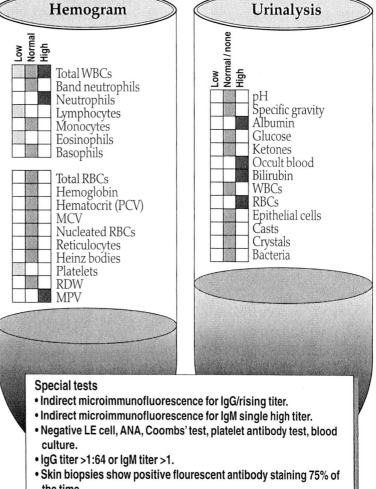

Aflatoxins

moldy grains
produce an
aflatoxin that
causes liver
necrosis

Aflatoxins are produced by *Aspergillus* sp. in moldy grains. Dogs fed poor-quality foods produced from moldy grains are at risk. High doses cause hepatosis, immune suppression, hemorrhage, and gastrointestinal congestion.

Interpretation
Early cases may present with polycythemia secondary to hemorrhagic gastroenteritis. Later this may progress to anemia from intestinal blood loss. The rise in liver enzymes indicates cholangitis and parenchymal necrosis. Increased bile acids may occur before hyperbilirubinemia. The hypoproteinemia is secondary to intestinal blood loss. The abnormal bleeding tests suggest DIC. Rises in the BUN and creatinine may be due to acute nephrosis or prerenal conditions. Diagnosis is based on history of exposure.

Differential Diagnoses
• Hemorrhagic gastroenteritis: normal BUN, no progressive liver disease
• Warfarin toxicity: normal BUN, no liver disease
• Other causes of chronic liver disease

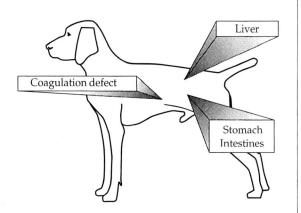

Signs
- Vomiting
- Jaundice
- Weakness
- Petechia
- Bloody diarrhea
- Oliguria
- Dehydration
- Muscle tremors
- Seizures
- Weight loss
- Ascites
- Hepatomegaly
- Liver necrosis
- Disseminated intravascular coagulation
- Hemorrhagic gastroenteritis

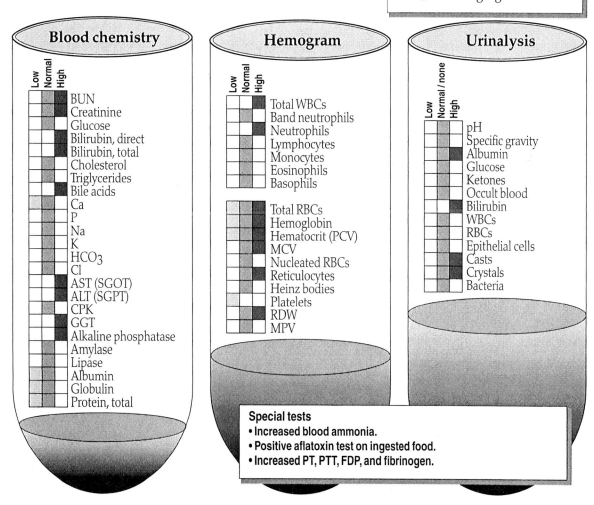

Blood chemistry

	Low	Normal	High	
				BUN
				Creatinine
				Glucose
				Bilirubin, direct
				Bilirubin, total
				Cholesterol
				Triglycerides
				Bile acids
				Ca
				P
				Na
				K
				HCO₃
				Cl
				AST (SGOT)
				ALT (SGPT)
				CPK
				GGT
				Alkaline phosphatase
				Amylase
				Lipase
				Albumin
				Globulin
				Protein, total

Hemogram

	Low	Normal	High	
				Total WBCs
				Band neutrophils
				Neutrophils
				Lymphocytes
				Monocytes
				Eosinophils
				Basophils
				Total RBCs
				Hemoglobin
				Hematocrit (PCV)
				MCV
				Nucleated RBCs
				Reticulocytes
				Heinz bodies
				Platelets
				RDW
				MPV

Urinalysis

	Low	Normal / none	High	
				pH
				Specific gravity
				Albumin
				Glucose
				Ketones
				Occult blood
				Bilirubin
				WBCs
				RBCs
				Epithelial cells
				Casts
				Crystals
				Bacteria

Special tests
- Increased blood ammonia.
- Positive aflatoxin test on ingested food.
- Increased PT, PTT, FDP, and fibrinogen.

Mushroom Poisoning

mushroom toxins
cause liver and
renal necrosis

Mushrooms contain several types of poisons. Of the many cytotoxins produced by mushrooms, the most important is anatoxin, which is found in the genera *Amanita* and *Galerina*. Very small doses of this toxin cause lethal hepatic and renal tubule destruction. Phalloidin, a toxin that accompanies anatoxin, is probably responsible for the initial gastrointestinal symptoms. The clinical course depends on the type of mushroom.

Interpretation
Within 48 hours of ingestion, marked increases in liver enzymes and bilirubin point to acute liver necrosis. A rise in BUN and creatinine with casts and an increased urine GGT:creatinine ratio indicate acute nephrosis.

Differential Diagnoses
• Diagnosis usually depends on owner observation of mushroom ingestion

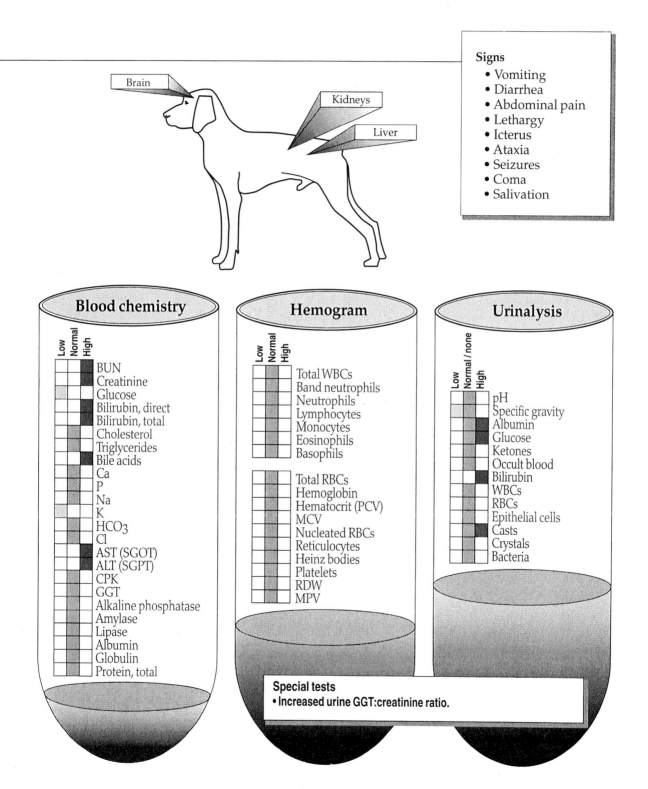

Signs
- Vomiting
- Diarrhea
- Abdominal pain
- Lethargy
- Icterus
- Ataxia
- Seizures
- Coma
- Salivation

Blood chemistry

	Low	Normal	High	
				BUN
				Creatinine
				Glucose
				Bilirubin, direct
				Bilirubin, total
				Cholesterol
				Triglycerides
				Bile acids
				Ca
				P
				Na
				K
				HCO3
				Cl
				AST (SGOT)
				ALT (SGPT)
				CPK
				GGT
				Alkaline phosphatase
				Amylase
				Lipase
				Albumin
				Globulin
				Protein, total

Hemogram

	Low	Normal	High	
				Total WBCs
				Band neutrophils
				Neutrophils
				Lymphocytes
				Monocytes
				Eosinophils
				Basophils
				Total RBCs
				Hemoglobin
				Hematocrit (PCV)
				MCV
				Nucleated RBCs
				Reticulocytes
				Heinz bodies
				Platelets
				RDW
				MPV

Urinalysis

	Low	Normal / none	High	
				pH
				Specific gravity
				Albumin
				Glucose
				Ketones
				Occult blood
				Bilirubin
				WBCs
				RBCs
				Epithelial cells
				Casts
				Crystals
				Bacteria

Special tests
- Increased urine GGT:creatinine ratio.

Ethylene Glycol Poisoning (Antifreeze Poisoning)

ultraviolet light screening of urine may detect the fluorescein marker of many antifreeze preparations

Ethylene glycol, a component of many antifreeze preparations, is rapidly absorbed after ingestion. It is metabolized to substances that cause metabolic acidosis and renal epithelial damage. CNS signs are caused by direct effects of ethylene glycol and its metabolites, as well as the secondary effects of acidosis and hyperosmolarity. Metabolites are toxic to renal tubules resulting in renal failure. This is complicated by precipitation of calcium oxalate crystals in the lumen of the renal tubules.

For treatment to be effective, it must start before the ethylene glycol has been metabolized and induced fatal kidney disease.

Interpretation
Ultraviolet light screening of urine may detect the fluorescein marker that is placed in many antifreeze preparations. Propylene glycol may be detected in the urine and serum up to 72 hours after ingestion. Later indications of nephrosis start with increased GGT and Na in the urine and progress to casts and oxalate crystals. Uremic cases are usually fatal. High blood sugar and urinary sugar mimic diabetes mellitus.

Differential Diagnoses
• Alcohol toxicosis: usually based on history
• Ketotic diabetes mellitus: ketone bodies are present
• Acute kidney failure: rule out other causes

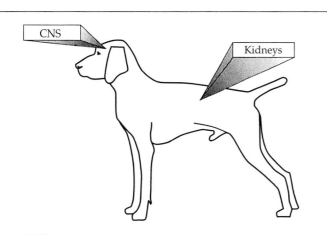

Signs
- History of antifreeze ingestion

Early
- Ataxia
- Nystagmus
- Depression

Late
- Polyuria
- Vomiting

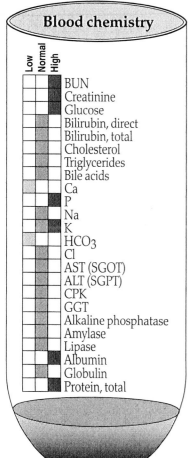

Blood chemistry

	Low	Normal	High	
				BUN
				Creatinine
				Glucose
				Bilirubin, direct
				Bilirubin, total
				Cholesterol
				Triglycerides
				Bile acids
				Ca
				P
				Na
				K
				HCO3
				Cl
				AST (SGOT)
				ALT (SGPT)
				CPK
				GGT
				Alkaline phosphatase
				Amylase
				Lipase
				Albumin
				Globulin
				Protein, total

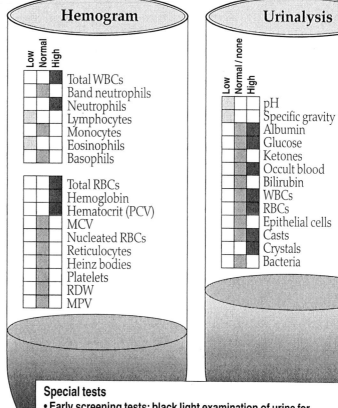

Hemogram

	Low	Normal	High	
				Total WBCs
				Band neutrophils
				Neutrophils
				Lymphocytes
				Monocytes
				Eosinophils
				Basophils
				Total RBCs
				Hemoglobin
				Hematocrit (PCV)
				MCV
				Nucleated RBCs
				Reticulocytes
				Heinz bodies
				Platelets
				RDW
				MPV

Urinalysis

	Low	Normal / none	High	
				pH
				Specific gravity
				Albumin
				Glucose
				Ketones
				Occult blood
				Bilirubin
				WBCs
				RBCs
				Epithelial cells
				Casts
				Crystals
				Bacteria

Special tests
- Early screening tests: black light examination of urine for fluorescence and urine propylene glycol.
- Increased anion gap and serum osmolarity.
- CaOxalate crystals in urine.
- Increased GGT:creatinine ratio and fractional excretion of sodium.
- Increased serum or urine ethylene glycol levels.

Lead Poisoning

nucleated RBCs
and reticulocyto-
sis without a
severe anemia is
common

Lead poisoning is often a problem of inner cities where an animal may ingest material from an old building such as linoleum, lead paints, or other lead-containing objects such as solder, batteries, or weights. This is usually seen in young dogs.

Interpretation
The key abnormality is a normal RBC count or a mild anemia with an intense bone marrow response consisting of many nucleated RBCs and reticulocytes. Basophilic stippling occurs in <25% of the cases. In early cases the abnormal red cell response may not be present. A neutrophilic leukocytosis is common. The albumin, glucose, casts, and increased GGT:creatinine ratio indicate active kidney damage.

Differential Diagnoses
• Viral disease: infectious canine hepatitis
• Canine distemper: normal RBCs
• Epilepsy: normal hemogram
• Acute pancreatitis: high lipase and TLI

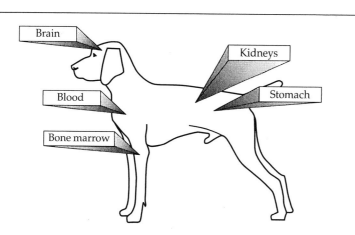

Signs
- Vomiting
- Diarrhea
- Abdominal pain
- Seizure
- Lethargy
- Blindness
- Hysteria

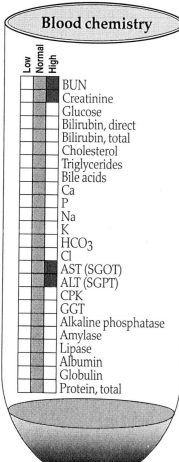

Blood chemistry

	Low	Normal	High	
			■	BUN
			■	Creatinine
		■		Glucose
		■		Bilirubin, direct
		■		Bilirubin, total
		■		Cholesterol
		■		Triglycerides
		■		Bile acids
		■		Ca
		■		P
		■		Na
		■		K
		■		HCO3
		■		Cl
			■	AST (SGOT)
			■	ALT (SGPT)
		■		CPK
		■		GGT
		■		Alkaline phosphatase
		■		Amylase
		■		Lipase
		■		Albumin
		■		Globulin
		■		Protein, total

Hemogram

	Low	Normal	High	
			■	Total WBCs
			■	Band neutrophils
			■	Neutrophils
		■		Lymphocytes
		■		Monocytes
		■		Eosinophils
		■		Basophils

	Low	Normal	High	
		■		Total RBCs
		■		Hemoglobin
		■		Hematocrit (PCV)
		■		MCV
			■	Nucleated RBCs
		■		Reticulocytes
		■		Heinz bodies
		■		Platelets
			■	RDW
		■		MPV

Urinalysis

	Low	Normal / none	High	
		■		pH
	■			Specific gravity
			■	Albumin
		■		Glucose
		■		Ketones
		■		Occult blood
		■		Bilirubin
		■		WBCs
		■		RBCs
		■		Epithelial cells
			■	Casts
		■		Crystals
		■		Bacteria

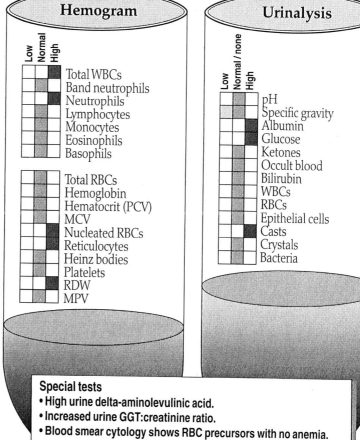

Special tests
- High urine delta-aminolevulinic acid.
- Increased urine GGT:creatinine ratio.
- Blood smear cytology shows RBC precursors with no anemia.
- Increased lead blood level >0.4 ppm.

Vitamin D Toxicity

excessive vitamin D increases serum calcium and phosphorus levels, leading to renal calcification

Excessive intake of vitamin D causes dystrophic calcification that eventually damages the kidneys enough to cause uremia. Increased absorption of calcium and phosphorus and increased release of material from the bone cause hypercalcemia. The most common cause is supplementation with excessive amounts of vitamin D, or ingestion of rodenticides containing cholecalciferol.

Interpretation
The high PCV and total plasma protein level indicate dehydration. Signs of kidney failure predominate, with increased BUN, creatinine, and phosphorus levels. The low serum bicarbonate level and acidic urine suggest acidosis. Normal serum Na and K levels help rule out hypoadrenocorticism.

Abnormal urine sediment, proteinuria, glycosuria, and low urine specific gravity suggest an active renal problem. A calcium $\times$ phosphorus product >60 suggests renal calcification.

Differential Diagnoses
- Hypoadrenocorticism: high serum urea nitrogen and calcium levels from hemoconcentration, low serum Na:K ratio (<23)
- Nephrotoxicosis: active urine sediment, renal calcification on radiographs
- Primary hyperparathyroidism: high serum calcium and chloride levels, low serum phosphorus level
- Chronic renal failure: anemia, low urine specific gravity

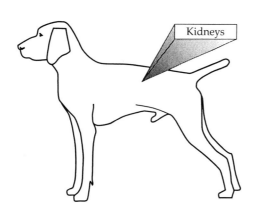

Kidneys

Signs
- Polyuria
- Polydipsia
- Listlessness
- Weakness
- Vomiting
- Anorexia
- Bradycardia

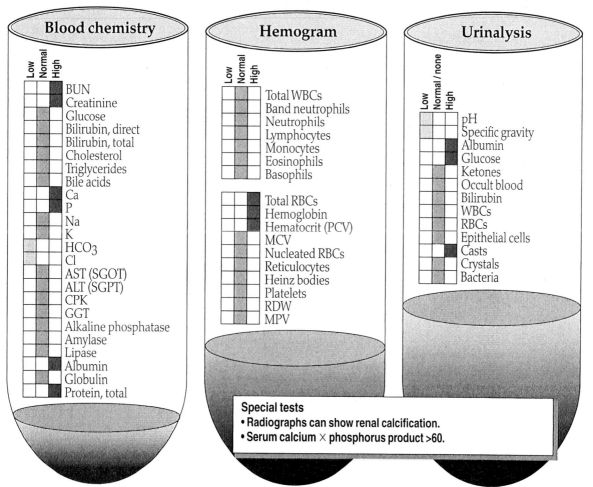

Blood chemistry

	Low	Normal	High	
			■	BUN
		■		Creatinine
		■		Glucose
		■		Bilirubin, direct
		■		Bilirubin, total
		■		Cholesterol
		■		Triglycerides
		■		Bile acids
			■	Ca
			■	P
		■		Na
		■		K
■				HCO3
		■		Cl
		■		AST (SGOT)
		■		ALT (SGPT)
		■		CPK
		■		GGT
		■		Alkaline phosphatase
		■		Amylase
		■		Lipase
		■		Albumin
		■		Globulin
		■		Protein, total

Hemogram

	Low	Normal	High	
		■		Total WBCs
		■		Band neutrophils
		■		Neutrophils
		■		Lymphocytes
		■		Monocytes
		■		Eosinophils
		■		Basophils

	Low	Normal	High	
			■	Total RBCs
			■	Hemoglobin
			■	Hematocrit (PCV)
	■			MCV
		■		Nucleated RBCs
		■		Reticulocytes
		■		Heinz bodies
		■		Platelets
		■		RDW
		■		MPV

Urinalysis

	Low	Normal / none	High	
■				pH
		■		Specific gravity
			■	Albumin
		■		Glucose
		■		Ketones
		■		Occult blood
		■		Bilirubin
		■		WBCs
		■		RBCs
		■		Epithelial cells
			■	Casts
		■		Crystals
		■		Bacteria

Special tests
- Radiographs can show renal calcification.
- Serum calcium × phosphorus product >60.

Zinc Toxicity

zinc toxicity
causes
intravascular
hemolytic
anemia

Ingestion of galvanized metal objects, pennies minted after 1993, and zinc-containing ointments may cause severe intravascular hemolysis and gastrointestinal irritation.

Interpretation
Intravascular hemolytic anemia with high nucleated RBC counts is the main laboratory sign of advanced zinc toxicity. This may be associated with increased ALT and AST, indicating acute liver necrosis and increased urine GGT:creatinine ratio, BUN, and creatinine, indicating kidney damage. Lethal cases may develop DIC.

Differential Diagnoses
- Immune hemolytic anemia: positive Coombs' test
- Parasitic anemia *(Babesia):* organisms seen, positive immune tests
- Heinz-body anemia: refractile bodies on RBC
- Lead toxicity: few reticulocytes, increased nucleated RBCs

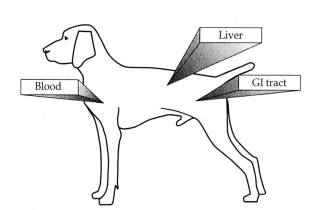

Signs
Early
- Depression
- Vomiting
- Diarrhea
- Anorexia

Advanced
- Icterus
- Hemoglobinuria
- Hematuria
- Anemia

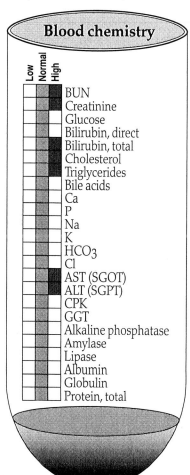

Blood chemistry

	Low	Normal	High
BUN			
Creatinine			
Glucose			
Bilirubin, direct			
Bilirubin, total			
Cholesterol			
Triglycerides			
Bile acids			
Ca			
P			
Na			
K			
HCO$_3$			
Cl			
AST (SGOT)			
ALT (SGPT)			
CPK			
GGT			
Alkaline phosphatase			
Amylase			
Lipase			
Albumin			
Globulin			
Protein, total			

Hemogram

	Low	Normal	High
Total WBCs			
Band neutrophils			
Neutrophils			
Lymphocytes			
Monocytes			
Eosinophils			
Basophils			
Total RBCs			
Hemoglobin			
Hematocrit (PCV)			
MCV			
Nucleated RBCs			
Reticulocytes			
Heinz bodies			
Platelets			
RDW			
MPV			

Urinalysis

	Low	Normal / none	High
pH			
Specific gravity			
Albumin			
Glucose			
Ketones			
Occult blood			
Bilirubin			
WBCs			
RBCs			
Epithelial cells			
Casts			
Crystals			
Bacteria			

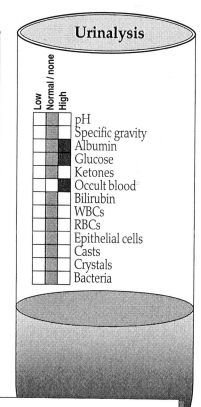

Special tests
- High serum zinc levels >2 µg/ml.
- Radiograph may show metal intestinal foreign body.
- ECG may show arrhythmias.
- Increased urine GGT:creatinine ratio indicates early kidney damage.
- Increased ACT, PT, PTT, and FDP indicate DIC.

Primary Hyperparathyroidism

primary hyper-
parathyroidism is
a rare cause of
hypercalcemia

Primary hyperparathyroidism is a rare cause of hypercalcemia. Elevated serum calcium levels normally inhibit release of parathormone (PTH) from the parathyroid gland. High serum calcium levels do not inhibit PTH secretion by parathyroid tumors or hyperplastic parathyroid tissue.

PTH acts on the bones and kidneys. High serum PTH levels raise blood calcium levels by decalcifying the bones, increasing renal calcium resorption, and increasing renal phosphorus excretion.

Interpretation
Renal failure can cause or result from hypercalcemia. Hypercalcemia and hypophosphatemia are present with both primary hyperparathyroidism and hypercalcemia of malignancy.

A ratio of serum chloride to phosphorus >33 suggests primary hyperparathyroidism because of concurrent hyperchloremic acidosis. A ratio of <33 suggests hypercalcemia induced by malignancy. Definitive diagnosis of a parathyroid tumor requires exploratory surgery of the neck. Hypercalcemia with normal or high serum PTH levels in a nonuremic cat suggests hyperparathyroidism

Differential Diagnoses
- Hypercalcemia of malignancy: serum Cl:P ratio <33, usually resulting from lymphosarcoma
- Primary renal failure: hypocalcemia, hyperphosphatemia
- Hypoadrenocorticism: high eosinophil and lymphocyte counts, low serum cortisol level, serum Na:K ratio below 23
- Bone tumors: osteolytic lesion visible on radiographs

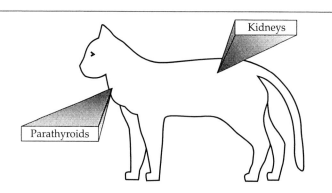

Signs
- Anorexia
- Lethargy
- Cervical mass
- Weakness

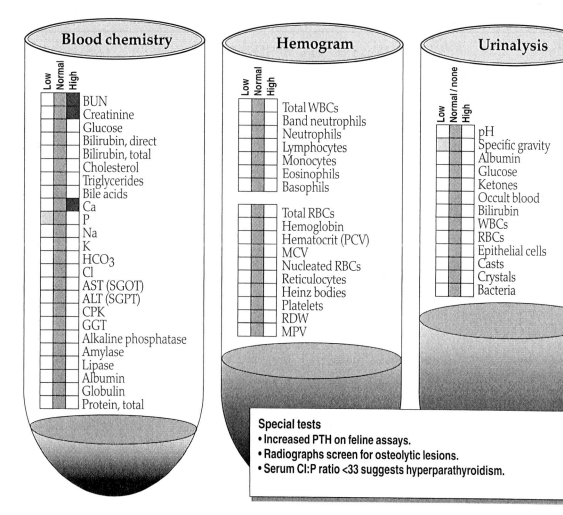

Blood chemistry

	Low	Normal	High	
				BUN
				Creatinine
				Glucose
				Bilirubin, direct
				Bilirubin, total
				Cholesterol
				Triglycerides
				Bile acids
				Ca
				P
				Na
				K
				HCO3
				Cl
				AST (SGOT)
				ALT (SGPT)
				CPK
				GGT
				Alkaline phosphatase
				Amylase
				Lipase
				Albumin
				Globulin
				Protein, total

Hemogram

	Low	Normal	High	
				Total WBCs
				Band neutrophils
				Neutrophils
				Lymphocytes
				Monocytes
				Eosinophils
				Basophils
				Total RBCs
				Hemoglobin
				Hematocrit (PCV)
				MCV
				Nucleated RBCs
				Reticulocytes
				Heinz bodies
				Platelets
				RDW
				MPV

Urinalysis

	Low	Normal / none	High	
				pH
				Specific gravity
				Albumin
				Glucose
				Ketones
				Occult blood
				Bilirubin
				WBCs
				RBCs
				Epithelial cells
				Casts
				Crystals
				Bacteria

Special tests
- Increased PTH on feline assays.
- Radiographs screen for osteolytic lesions.
- Serum Cl:P ratio <33 suggests hyperparathyroidism.

Dietary Secondary Hyperparathyroidism

high dietary phosphorus depresses serum calcium levels, stimulating PTH release

All-meat diets that are high in phosphorus and low in calcium cause release of parathormone (PTH). In kittens this produces major skeletal deformities because of deficient bone mineralization.

The bones of affected animals are not properly mineralized. High levels of serum phosphorus reduce levels of ionized calcium, causing PTH release and demineralization of bones. Affected animals show lameness, pathologic fractures, and faulty anatomic development of weight-bearing bones.

Interpretation
The serum chemistry profile is essentially normal but rules out several metabolic diseases. Diagnosis is based on a history of a low-calcium all-meat diet, lameness, bone deformity, and radiographs showing hypomineralization of bone.

Differential Diagnoses
• Trauma: normally calcified bones
• Renal hyperparathyroidism: high BUN level

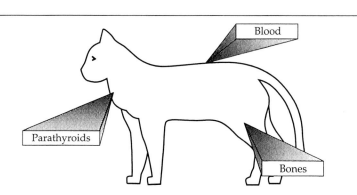

Signs
- Lameness
- Bone pain
- Constipation
- Neurologic dysfunction

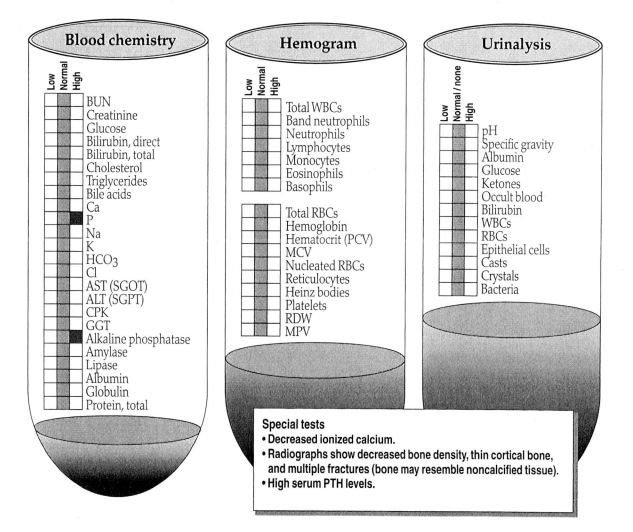

	Low	Normal	High	
				BUN
				Creatinine
				Glucose
				Bilirubin, direct
				Bilirubin, total
				Cholesterol
				Triglycerides
				Bile acids
				Ca
				P
				Na
				K
				HCO₃
				Cl
				AST (SGOT)
				ALT (SGPT)
				CPK
				GGT
				Alkaline phosphatase
				Amylase
				Lipase
				Albumin
				Globulin
				Protein, total

Blood chemistry

Hemogram

	Low	Normal	High	
				Total WBCs
				Band neutrophils
				Neutrophils
				Lymphocytes
				Monocytes
				Eosinophils
				Basophils
				Total RBCs
				Hemoglobin
				Hematocrit (PCV)
				MCV
				Nucleated RBCs
				Reticulocytes
				Heinz bodies
				Platelets
				RDW
				MPV

Urinalysis

	Low	Normal / none	High	
				pH
				Specific gravity
				Albumin
				Glucose
				Ketones
				Occult blood
				Bilirubin
				WBCs
				RBCs
				Epithelial cells
				Casts
				Crystals
				Bacteria

Special tests
- Decreased ionized calcium.
- Radiographs show decreased bone density, thin cortical bone, and multiple fractures (bone may resemble noncalcified tissue).
- High serum PTH levels.

Renal Secondary Hyperparathyroidism

phosphorus
retention
suppresses
serum calcium
levels,
stimulating PTH
release

In animals with chronic renal failure, secondary hyperparathyroidism occurs as a result of phosphorus retention and poor calcium absorption. Reaction with *phosphorus* reduces the serum level of ionized calcium. In addition, reduced activation of vitamin D in the diseased kidneys impairs intestinal absorption of calcium. The low serum calcium level stimulates parathormone release. This condition is both the result of and the cause of progressive kidney deterioration.

Interpretation
Signs of kidney failure predominate, with increased BUN, creatinine, and phosphorus levels. A low serum bicarbonate level and acidic urine indicate acidosis. Nonregenerative anemia is secondary to lack of erythropoietin.

Normal urine sediment and low urine specific gravity suggest chronic renal disease, rather than an acute problem. The danger of soft tissue mineralization is great because the serum calcium $\times$ phosphorus product is >60.

Differential Diagnoses
- Nutritional secondary hyperparathyroidism: hyperphosphatemia, hypocalcemia, no azotemia
- Hypoalbuminemia: normal corrected serum calcium value

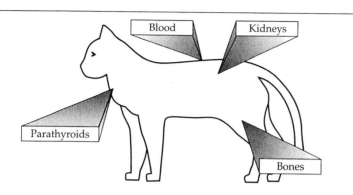

Blood

Kidneys

Parathyroids

Bones

Signs
- Polyuria
- Polydipsia
- Listlessness
- Weakness
- Vomiting
- Anorexia
- Pathologic fractures
- Loose teeth

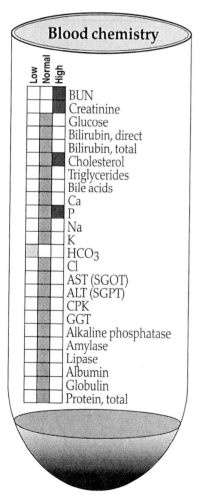

Blood chemistry

	Low	Normal	High
BUN			■
Creatinine		■	
Glucose		■	
Bilirubin, direct		■	
Bilirubin, total		■	
Cholesterol			■
Triglycerides		■	
Bile acids		■	
Ca		■	
P			■
Na		■	
K		■	
HCO₃	■		
Cl		■	
AST (SGOT)		■	
ALT (SGPT)		■	
CPK		■	
GGT		■	
Alkaline phosphatase		■	
Amylase		■	
Lipase		■	
Albumin		■	
Globulin		■	
Protein, total		■	

Hemogram

	Low	Normal	High
Total WBCs		■	
Band neutrophils		■	
Neutrophils		■	
Lymphocytes		■	
Monocytes		■	
Eosinophils		■	
Basophils		■	
Total RBCs	■		
Hemoglobin	■		
Hematocrit (PCV)	■		
MCV		■	
Nucleated RBCs		■	
Reticulocytes		■	
Heinz bodies		■	
Platelets		■	
RDW		■	
MPV		■	

Urinalysis

	Low	Normal / none	High
pH	■		
Specific gravity	■		
Albumin		■	
Glucose		■	
Ketones		■	
Occult blood		■	
Bilirubin		■	
WBCs		■	
RBCs		■	
Epithelial cells		■	
Casts		■	
Crystals		■	
Bacteria		■	

Special tests
- Low ionized calcium.
- Radiographs show renal calcification, shrunken kidneys, decreased bone density, or thin bone cortices.
- High serum PTH levels.
- Serum calcium × phosphorus product can be >60.
- Ultrasound may show renal calcification.

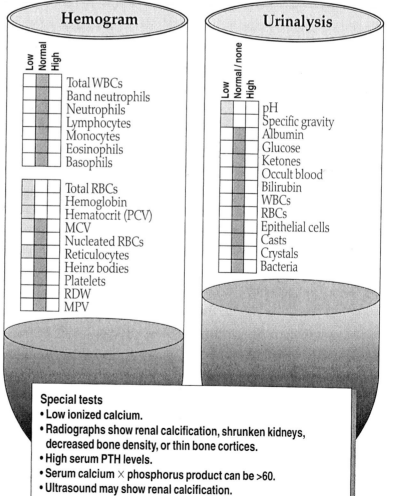

Acromegaly

insulin-resistant
diabetes mellitus
is the most
common
manifestation

Acromegaly is caused by oversecretion of growth hormone (GH). It usually occurs in mature animals more than 8 years old. In the cat the increase in GH is due to a pituitary tumor and not induced by drugs such as megestrol acetate. Insulin-resistant diabetes mellitus is the most common manifestation. Some cats show degenerative arthritis and cardiomegaly.

Growth hormone causes proliferation of connective tissue, increased weight, abdominal enlargement, and enlargement of the head. The most prominent clinical signs are polydipsia, polyuria, and glucosuria. Acromegaly should be suspected in cats that have severe insulin-resistant diabetes mellitus without ketosis.

Interpretation
The diabetes is characterized by severe insulin-resistant hyperglycemia and glucosuria without ketonuria. Mild increases in ALT, AST and alkaline phosphatase are due to hepatic lipidosis. Increased BUN, creatinine, and phosphorus are due to diabetic nephropathy and GH-induced increases in phosphorus resorption. Erythrocytosis may be due to the anabolic effects of GH excess. Because diabetic cats induce insulin-like growth factor without increased GH, this is not a confirmatory test for acromegaly.

Differential Diagnoses
- Simple diabetes mellitus: insulin responsive ±ketosis
- Hyperadrenocorticism: stress response, increased cortisol
- Hyperthyroidism: increased T_4
- Chronic renal failure: no hyperglycemia, dilute urine

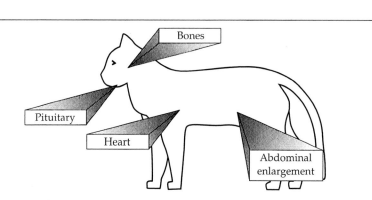

Bones

Pituitary

Heart

Abdominal enlargement

Signs
- Polydipsia
- Polyuria
- Altered appearance

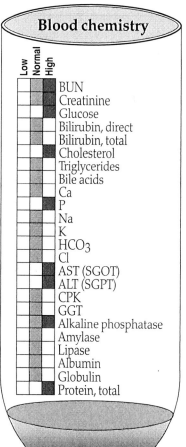

Blood chemistry

	Low	Normal	High
BUN			■
Creatinine			■
Glucose			■
Bilirubin, direct		■	
Bilirubin, total		■	
Cholesterol			■
Triglycerides		■	
Bile acids		■	
Ca		■	
P			■
Na		■	
K		■	
HCO3		■	
Cl		■	
AST (SGOT)		■	
ALT (SGPT)			■
CPK		■	
GGT		■	
Alkaline phosphatase			■
Amylase		■	
Lipase		■	
Albumin		■	
Globulin		■	
Protein, total			■

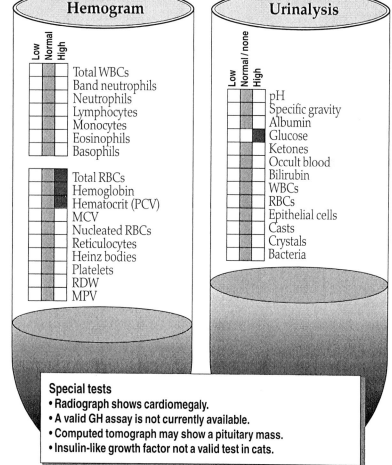

Hemogram

	Low	Normal	High
Total WBCs		■	
Band neutrophils		■	
Neutrophils		■	
Lymphocytes		■	
Monocytes		■	
Eosinophils		■	
Basophils		■	

	Low	Normal	High
Total RBCs			■
Hemoglobin			■
Hematocrit (PCV)			■
MCV		■	
Nucleated RBCs		■	
Reticulocytes		■	
Heinz bodies		■	
Platelets		■	
RDW		■	
MPV		■	

Urinalysis

	Low	Normal / none	High
pH		■	
Specific gravity		■	
Albumin		■	
Glucose			■
Ketones		■	
Occult blood		■	
Bilirubin		■	
WBCs		■	
RBCs		■	
Epithelial cells		■	
Casts		■	
Crystals		■	
Bacteria		■	

Special tests
- Radiograph shows cardiomegaly.
- A valid GH assay is not currently available.
- Computed tomograph may show a pituitary mass.
- Insulin-like growth factor not a valid test in cats.

Diabetes Insipidus, Central

insufficient ADH
is caused by
defective
secretion or
synthesis

persistent urine
SpGr <1.010
should be
investigated

Pituitary-dependent (central) diabetes insipidus, a deficiency of antidiuretic hormone (ADH), causes diuresis and hypotension. ADH is normally released in response to increased serum osmotic pressure, volume depletion, and drugs that increase blood pressure.

A lesion in the hypothalamus or the neurohypophysis of the pituitary causes permanent ADH deficiency. Chemicals (alcohol, xylazine, glucocorticoids) inhibit ADH secretion. Lack of ADH results in very dilute urine.

Interpretation
The blood panel can rule out common causes of polydipsia, such as kidney disease, liver disease, pyometra, and diabetes mellitus. Other causes of dilute urine must be distinguished with special tests. Increased BUN, creatinine, protein, and sodium are due to dehydration.

The vasopressin test can distinguish between central and nephrogenic diabetes insipidus. To be sure that prolonged polyuria has not washed out the osmotic gradient of the kidneys, a repository vasopressin test should be performed.

Water deprivation can rule out psychogenic water consumption but must not be done in a dehydrated animal.

Differential Diagnoses
- Diabetes mellitus: hyperglycemia, glycosuria
- Renal failure: anemia, high serum creatinine level, usually a urine specific gravity around 1.010 that does not respond to ADH
- Liver disease: increased serum bile acid levels, no response to ADH
- Hyperadrenocorticism: stress pattern on CBC, high serum cortisol level, high serum alkaline phosphatase activity
- Nephrogenic diabetes insipidus: no increase in urine specific gravity after ADH administration
- Hyperthyroidism: increased T_4

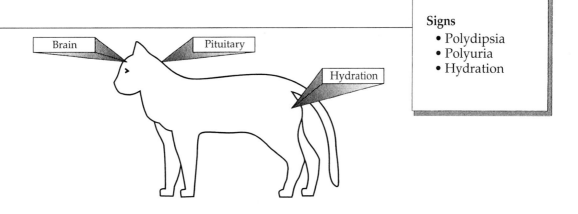

Signs
- Polydipsia
- Polyuria
- Hydration

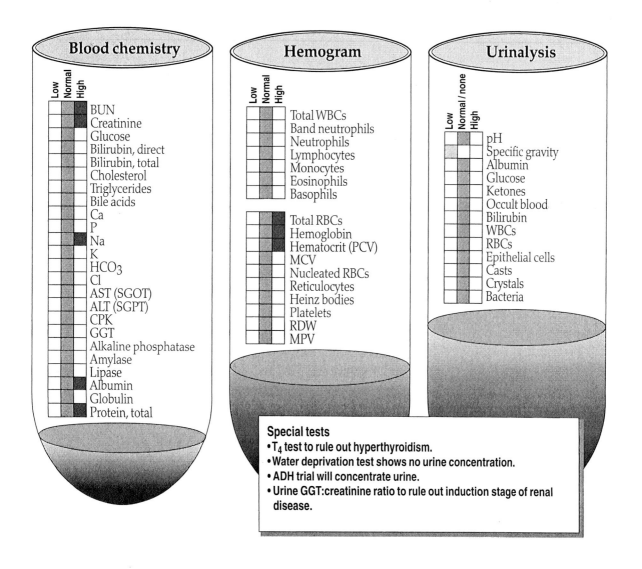

Blood chemistry

	Low	Normal	High	
				BUN
				Creatinine
				Glucose
				Bilirubin, direct
				Bilirubin, total
				Cholesterol
				Triglycerides
				Bile acids
				Ca
				P
				Na
				K
				HCO$_3$
				Cl
				AST (SGOT)
				ALT (SGPT)
				CPK
				GGT
				Alkaline phosphatase
				Amylase
				Lipase
				Albumin
				Globulin
				Protein, total

Hemogram

	Low	Normal	High	
				Total WBCs
				Band neutrophils
				Neutrophils
				Lymphocytes
				Monocytes
				Eosinophils
				Basophils
				Total RBCs
				Hemoglobin
				Hematocrit (PCV)
				MCV
				Nucleated RBCs
				Reticulocytes
				Heinz bodies
				Platelets
				RDW
				MPV

Urinalysis

	Low	Normal / none	High	
				pH
				Specific gravity
				Albumin
				Glucose
				Ketones
				Occult blood
				Bilirubin
				WBCs
				RBCs
				Epithelial cells
				Casts
				Crystals
				Bacteria

Special tests
- T$_4$ test to rule out hyperthyroidism.
- Water deprivation test shows no urine concentration.
- ADH trial will concentrate urine.
- Urine GGT:creatinine ratio to rule out induction stage of renal disease.

Hyperthyroidism

hyperthyroidism
is usually
diagnosed by an
elevated T_4

Hyperthyroidism is a common endocrinopathy of cats. Most cases are caused by a thyroid adenoma. Untreated cases result in hypertension and hypertrophic cardiomyopathy. Hyperthyroidism causes hypertension that induces renal pathology. Compensated cases of renal failure may worsen after treatment because decreased hypertension reduces glomerular filtration.

Interpretation
An elevated T_4 or an elevated fT_4d confirms hyperthyroidism because nonthyroidal disease may depress thyroxin levels.

Differential Diagnoses
- Diabetes mellitus: high blood sugar, high fructosamine
- Chronic renal failure: high BUN and creatinine
- Malabsorption syndromes: normal T_4, low cobalamin
- Primary heart failure: normal T_4, usually not a hypertrophic heart

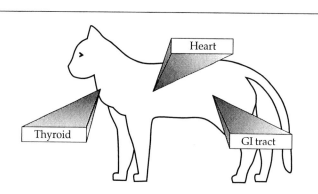

Signs
- Weight loss
- Tachycardia
- Polydipsia

Heart

Thyroid

GI tract

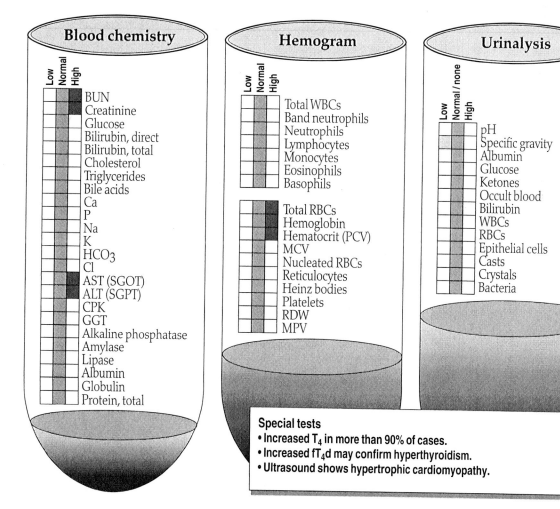

Blood chemistry

Low	Normal	High	
			BUN
			Creatinine
			Glucose
			Bilirubin, direct
			Bilirubin, total
			Cholesterol
			Triglycerides
			Bile acids
			Ca
			P
			Na
			K
			HCO₃
			Cl
			AST (SGOT)
			ALT (SGPT)
			CPK
			GGT
			Alkaline phosphatase
			Amylase
			Lipase
			Albumin
			Globulin
			Protein, total

Hemogram

Low	Normal	High	
			Total WBCs
			Band neutrophils
			Neutrophils
			Lymphocytes
			Monocytes
			Eosinophils
			Basophils

Low	Normal	High	
			Total RBCs
			Hemoglobin
			Hematocrit (PCV)
			MCV
			Nucleated RBCs
			Reticulocytes
			Heinz bodies
			Platelets
			RDW
			MPV

Urinalysis

Low	Normal / none	High	
			pH
			Specific gravity
			Albumin
			Glucose
			Ketones
			Occult blood
			Bilirubin
			WBCs
			RBCs
			Epithelial cells
			Casts
			Crystals
			Bacteria

Special tests
- Increased T₄ in more than 90% of cases.
- Increased fT₄d may confirm hyperthyroidism.
- Ultrasound shows hypertrophic cardiomyopathy.

Amyloidosis, Familial

signs are usually
due to liver
or renal
involvement

Pancreatic amyloidosis is a common finding in domestic cats and may be associated with diabetes mellitus. Less common is a familial form of systemic amyloidosis that occurs in Abyssinian, Siamese, and Oriental cats. The disease is inherited, but the mode of inheritance has not been fully determined. The characteristic of isolated amyloid protein indicates that this is reactive amyloid rather than immunoglobulin associated or the more common islet amyloid polypeptide.

In Abyssinians, myeloid deposits are found in the kidneys, adrenal glands, thyroid glands, spleen, stomach, small intestine, heart, liver, and tongue, but clinical signs are usually related to kidney failure. In other breeds, amyloid usually causes severe liver involvement.

Interpretation
Increased BUN, creatinine, and phosphorus are associated with renal failure secondary to tubular interstitial disease and sometimes proteinuria caused by glomerular deposits. Kidney failure also causes anemia, hypercholesterolemia, and acidosis. Hyperglycemia may be caused by insulin deficiency induced by pancreatic amyloid deposits. Hepatic amyloid deposits cause hyperbilirubinemia, liver failure, and occasionally hemorrhage from liver rupture.

Differential Diagnoses
- Glomerulonephritis: no amyloid in kidney biopsy
- Hepatic neoplasm: no amyloid on liver biopsy
- Primary coagulopathy: increased ACT, PT, PTT
- Abdominal trauma: usually normal-sized liver on x-ray and ultrasound, usually physical evidence of trauma

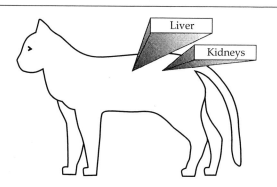

Signs
- Polydipsia
- Polyuria
- Unthriftiness
- Oral lesions

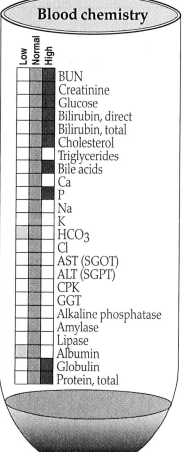

Blood chemistry

	Low	Normal	High	
				BUN
				Creatinine
				Glucose
				Bilirubin, direct
				Bilirubin, total
				Cholesterol
				Triglycerides
				Bile acids
				Ca
				P
				Na
				K
				HCO₃
				Cl
				AST (SGOT)
				ALT (SGPT)
				CPK
				GGT
				Alkaline phosphatase
				Amylase
				Lipase
				Albumin
				Globulin
				Protein, total

Hemogram

	Low	Normal	High	
				Total WBCs
				Band neutrophils
				Neutrophils
				Lymphocytes
				Monocytes
				Eosinophils
				Basophils

	Low	Normal	High	
				Total RBCs
				Hemoglobin
				Hematocrit (PCV)
				MCV
				Nucleated RBCs
				Reticulocytes
				Heinz bodies
				Platelets
				RDW
				MPV

Urinalysis

	Low	Normal / none	High	
				pH
				Specific gravity
				Albumin
				Glucose
				Ketones
				Occult blood
				Bilirubin
				WBCs
				RBCs
				Epithelial cells
				Casts
				Crystals
				Bacteria

Special tests
- Renal biopsy may show amyloid deposits in the glomeruli and interstitial medullary area.
- Serum protein electrophoresis reveals hyperglobulinemia with increased alpha-2 globulins.
- Radiographs may show hepatomegaly and splenomegaly.
- Increased protein:creatinine ratio.

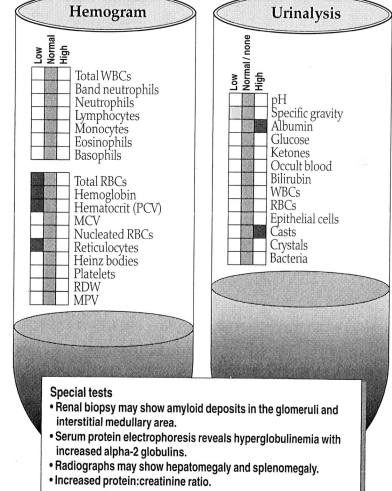

Diabetes Mellitus Ketoacidosis (DKA)

DKA is a severe complication of untreated diabetes mellitus

Diabetic ketoacidosis is a serious complication of diabetes mellitus that is characterized by hyperglycemia, hyperketonemia, and metabolic acidosis. It is a condition caused by insulin deficiency in combination with glucagon excess. This condition may occur in undiagnosed animals or may occur in treated animals in conjunction with an underlying disease. DKA is often a life-threatening emergency that requires prompt diagnosis and treatment. Because of the peripheral lipolysis, there is an influx of fatty acids into the liver and activation of liver enzymes that metabolize the fat to form ketones, acetoacetate, and β-hydroxybutyrate. These ketoacids cause metabolic acidosis.

Interpretation
Persistent hyperglycemia may be confirmed by increased fructose amine or glycosylated hemoglobin. These differentiate stress hyperglycemia from diabetes.

Shock causes increased formation of β-hydroxybutyrate a ketone that is not detected by the common nitroprusside test reaction but is demonstrated by adding hydrogen peroxide to the urine. Secondary liver damage is caused by hepatic lipidosis. The ketonemia induces acidosis, which causes an intracellular shift of potassium.

Differential Diagnoses
- Uncomplicated diabetes mellitus: normal ketone, normal potassium
- Common associated conditions: uremia, steroid administration, pancreatitis, hyperadrenocorticism, diestrus, and bacterial infections

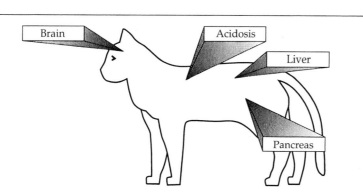

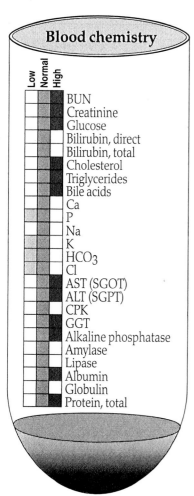

Blood chemistry

	Low	Normal	High	
				BUN
				Creatinine
				Glucose
				Bilirubin, direct
				Bilirubin, total
				Cholesterol
				Triglycerides
				Bile acids
				Ca
				P
				Na
				K
				HCO₃
				Cl
				AST (SGOT)
				ALT (SGPT)
				CPK
				GGT
				Alkaline phosphatase
				Amylase
				Lipase
				Albumin
				Globulin
				Protein, total

Hemogram

	Low	Normal	High	
				Total WBCs
				Band neutrophils
				Neutrophils
				Lymphocytes
				Monocytes
				Eosinophils
				Basophils
				Total RBCs
				Hemoglobin
				Hematocrit (PCV)
				MCV
				Nucleated RBCs
				Reticulocytes
				Heinz bodies
				Platelets
				RDW
				MPV

Urinalysis

	Low	Normal / none	High	
				pH
				Specific gravity
				Albumin
				Glucose
				Ketones
				Occult blood
				Bilirubin
				WBCs
				RBCs
				Epithelial cells
				Casts
				Crystals
				Bacteria

Special tests
- High anion gap >20.
- Decreased insulin: glucose ratio.
- Modified urine ketone test + for β-hydroxybutyrate.
- Increased glycerated hemoglobin, increased fructose amine.

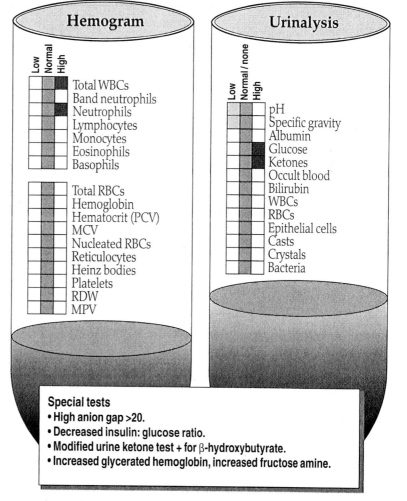

Diabetes Mellitus Hyperosmolar Syndrome

severe hyperglycemia in association with renal or heart disease may result in hyperosmolality and consequent CNS depression

Cats presented in a stupor or coma should be checked for diabetes, renal failure, and heart failure. Early in the disease classic signs of polydipsia, polyuria, and polyphagia are present. Usually renal excretion prevents blood glucose from exceeding 500 mg/dl, but when renal function fails either from renal or prerenal causes, blood glucose may rise above 600 mg/dl. This increases serum osmolality and impairs CNS function. Blood glucose >600 mg/dl causes osmolality >350 mOsm/kg.

Interpretation
The blood sugar is usually >600 mg/dl. High BUN, creatinine, and phosphorus suggest renal failure. Hepatic impairment is due to hepatic lipidosis. The modified urine ketone test is needed to rule out ketosis.

Differential Diagnoses
• Trauma: mild hyperglycemia
• Stroke: no hypoglycemia, no ketosis

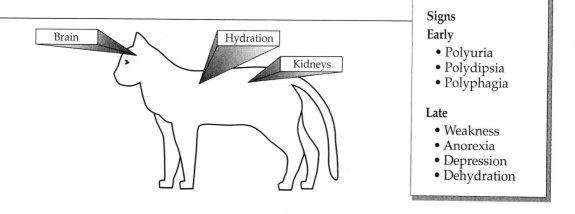

Signs
Early
- Polyuria
- Polydipsia
- Polyphagia

Late
- Weakness
- Anorexia
- Depression
- Dehydration

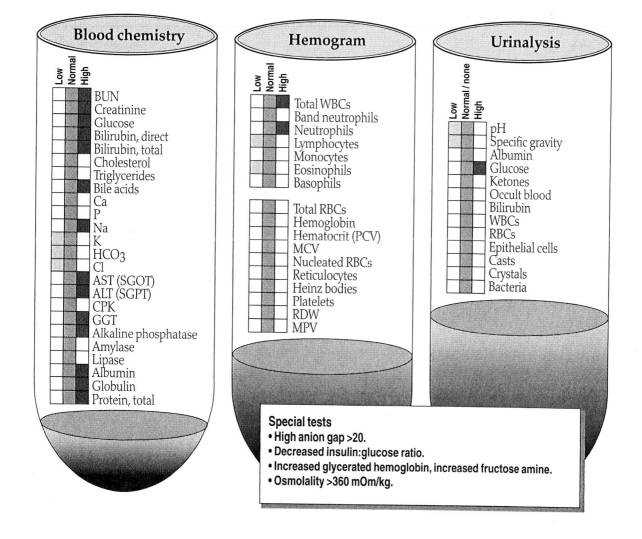

Blood chemistry

	Low	Normal	High	
				BUN
				Creatinine
				Glucose
				Bilirubin, direct
				Bilirubin, total
				Cholesterol
				Triglycerides
				Bile acids
				Ca
				P
				Na
				K
				HCO$_3$
				Cl
				AST (SGOT)
				ALT (SGPT)
				CPK
				GGT
				Alkaline phosphatase
				Amylase
				Lipase
				Albumin
				Globulin
				Protein, total

Hemogram

	Low	Normal	High	
				Total WBCs
				Band neutrophils
				Neutrophils
				Lymphocytes
				Monocytes
				Eosinophils
				Basophils
				Total RBCs
				Hemoglobin
				Hematocrit (PCV)
				MCV
				Nucleated RBCs
				Reticulocytes
				Heinz bodies
				Platelets
				RDW
				MPV

Urinalysis

	Low	Normal / none	High	
				pH
				Specific gravity
				Albumin
				Glucose
				Ketones
				Occult blood
				Bilirubin
				WBCs
				RBCs
				Epithelial cells
				Casts
				Crystals
				Bacteria

Special tests
- High anion gap >20.
- Decreased insulin:glucose ratio.
- Increased glycerated hemoglobin, increased fructose amine.
- Osmolality >360 mOm/kg.

Uncomplicated Diabetes Mellitus

uncomplicated diabetes mellitus may be transient, non-insulin-dependent, or insulin-dependent

Cats do not fit well into the human diabetes classification of insulin-dependent, non-insulin-dependent, and secondary diabetes mellitus because of overlapping mechanisms of disease progression. Impaired insulin secretion may occasionally be caused by destruction of islet cells from diseases such as pancreatitis or immune mechanisms. More often it is caused by abnormal amylin secretion that results in pancreatic amyloid deposits.

Amylin stabilizes glucose levels by facilitating storage as glucagon. A deficiency of amylin causes insulin resistance. Hormones or drugs such as cortisol or progestins also cause insulin resistance and may induce secondary diabetes. Both of these conditions, which at first may produce a non-insulin-dependent form of diabetes, eventually cause β-cells exhaustion or toxicity, resulting in absolute insulin deficiency.

Diabetes mellitus without stupor, marked ketosis, or hyperosmolarity is uncomplicated. In this stage, the cat can compensate for the osmotic diuresis and increased fat metabolism.

Interpretation
Persistent hyperglycemia is indicated by high fructosamine or high glycosylated hemoglobin. Low insulin levels are confirmed by the insulin/glucose tolerance test. No major complicating conditions such as marked ketosis and hyperosmolarity are present. The urine specific gravity may be normal or slightly decreased but is not isosthenuric.

Differential Diagnoses
- Complicated diabetes mellitus: ketosis, major diseases
- Stress hyperglycemia: no increase in fructose amine or glycerated hemoglobin
- Renal disease: increased BUN, creatinine, low urine specific gravity

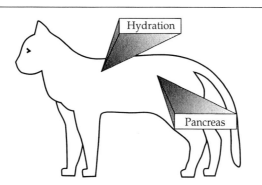

Signs
- Polydipsia
- Polyuria
- Weight loss
- Polyphagia

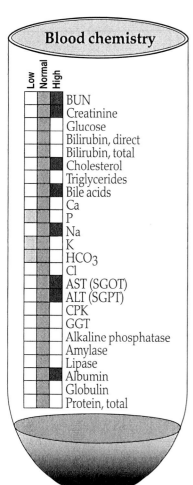

Blood chemistry

	Low	Normal	High	
				BUN
				Creatinine
				Glucose
				Bilirubin, direct
				Bilirubin, total
				Cholesterol
				Triglycerides
				Bile acids
				Ca
				P
				Na
				K
				HCO₃
				Cl
				AST (SGOT)
				ALT (SGPT)
				CPK
				GGT
				Alkaline phosphatase
				Amylase
				Lipase
				Albumin
				Globulin
				Protein, total

Hemogram

Total WBCs, Band neutrophils, Neutrophils, Lymphocytes, Monocytes, Eosinophils, Basophils

Total RBCs, Hemoglobin, Hematocrit (PCV), MCV, Nucleated RBCs, Reticulocytes, Heinz bodies, Platelets, RDW, MPV

Urinalysis

pH, Specific gravity, Albumin, Glucose, Ketones, Occult blood, Bilirubin, WBCs, RBCs, Epithelial cells, Casts, Crystals, Bacteria

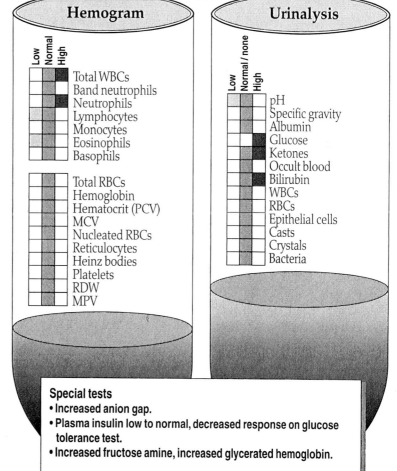

Special tests
- Increased anion gap.
- Plasma insulin low to normal, decreased response on glucose tolerance test.
- Increased fructose amine, increased glycerated hemoglobin.

Pancreatic Exocrine Insufficiency

pancreatic insufficiency is less common than inflammatory bowel disease and hyperthyroidism

Pancreatic exocrine insufficiency is uncommon but can be caused by chronic pancreatitis, neoplasms, and surgical resection. In some cases it is associated with diabetes mellitus. It results in deficiencies of digestive enzymes, resulting in impaired digestion and absorption of amino acids, sugars, and fats. The altered intestinal contents lead to small intestine bacterial overgrowth and steatorrhea. Malabsorption of fat-soluble vitamins and cobalamin lead to malnutrition and coagulopathy.

Interpretation
Most panel tests are normal. Occasionally the blood glucose will be elevated if the cat is also diabetic. Low levels of TLI confirm a diagnosis. Serum cobalamin levels are increased because of secondary bacterial overgrowth.

Differential Diagnoses
- Inflammatory bowel disease: normal TLI, confirmed with intestinal biopsy
- Hyperthyroidism: increased T_4

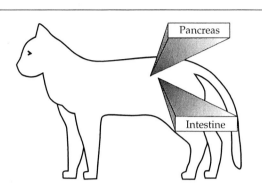

Signs
- Polyphagia
- Weight loss
- Diarrhea

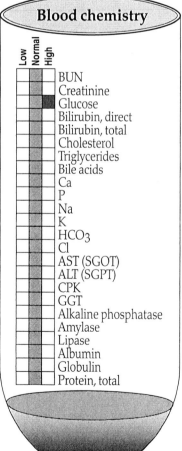

Blood chemistry

	Low	Normal	High	
		▓		BUN
		▓		Creatinine
			■	Glucose
		▓		Bilirubin, direct
		▓		Bilirubin, total
		▓		Cholesterol
		▓		Triglycerides
		▓		Bile acids
		▓		Ca
		▓		P
		▓		Na
		▓		K
		▓		HCO3
		▓		Cl
		▓		AST (SGOT)
		▓		ALT (SGPT)
		▓		CPK
		▓		GGT
		▓		Alkaline phosphatase
		▓		Amylase
		▓		Lipase
		▓		Albumin
		▓		Globulin
		▓		Protein, total

Hemogram

	Low	Normal	High	
		▓		Total WBCs
		▓		Band neutrophils
		▓		Neutrophils
		▓		Lymphocytes
		▓		Monocytes
		▓		Eosinophils
		▓		Basophils

	Low	Normal	High	
		▓		Total RBCs
		▓		Hemoglobin
		▓		Hematocrit (PCV)
		▓		MCV
		▓		Nucleated RBCs
		▓		Reticulocytes
		▓		Heinz bodies
		▓		Platelets
		▓		RDW
		▓		MPV

Urinalysis

	Low	Normal / none	High	
		▓		pH
		▓		Specific gravity
		▓		Albumin
		▓		Glucose
		▓		Ketones
		▓		Occult blood
		▓		Bilirubin
		▓		WBCs
		▓		RBCs
		▓		Epithelial cells
		▓		Casts
		▓		Crystals
		▓		Bacteria

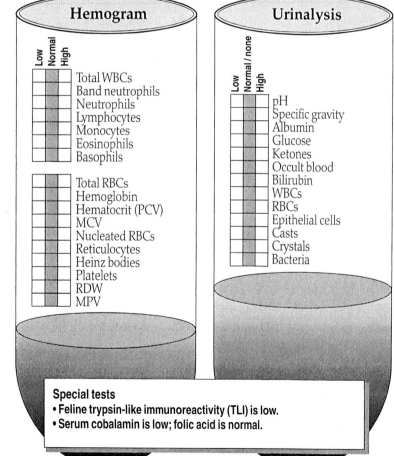

Special tests
- Feline trypsin-like immunoreactivity (TLI) is low.
- Serum cobalamin is low; folic acid is normal.

Acute Pancreatitis

feline pancreatitis is hard to diagnose because of the vague signs and the association of a variety of other common syndromes

Acute pancreatitis is difficult to diagnose in cats because the signs are vague and the usual tests inadequate. The pathogenesis is often less severe than in dogs. Although it rarely causes death, it may result in diabetes mellitus or cholangiohepatitis. The usual tests such as lipase and amylase are rarely helpful in making a diagnosis.

Interpretation

An elevation of feline trypsin-like immunoreactivity (TLI) is the best test to confirm acute pancreatitis. Other abnormalities on the blood panel are due to secondary disease such as cholangiohepatitis and diabetes mellitus. Azotemia is seen in some cases because of prerenal circulatory problems superimposed on preexisting renal disease.

Differential Diagnoses
- Diabetes mellitus: high blood glucose with increased fructosamine and glycosylated hemoglobin
- Cholangiohepatitis: increased bile acids, alkaline phosphatase, ALT
- Hepatic lipidosis: increased AST, large liver, hepatocytes filled with lipid

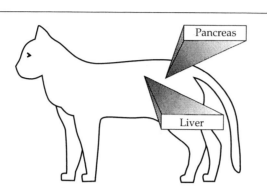

Signs
- Vague signs
- Lethargy
- Anorexia

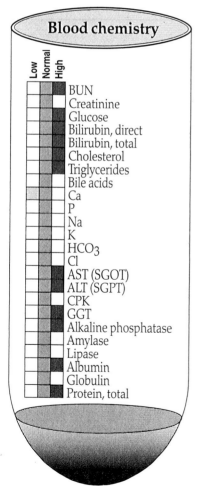

	Low	Normal	High
Blood chemistry			
BUN			
Creatinine			
Glucose			
Bilirubin, direct			
Bilirubin, total			
Cholesterol			
Triglycerides			
Bile acids			
Ca			
P			
Na			
K			
HCO$_3$			
Cl			
AST (SGOT)			
ALT (SGPT)			
CPK			
GGT			
Alkaline phosphatase			
Amylase			
Lipase			
Albumin			
Globulin			
Protein, total			

	Low	Normal	High
Hemogram			
Total WBCs			
Band neutrophils			
Neutrophils			
Lymphocytes			
Monocytes			
Eosinophils			
Basophils			
Total RBCs			
Hemoglobin			
Hematocrit (PCV)			
MCV			
Nucleated RBCs			
Reticulocytes			
Heinz bodies			
Platelets			
RDW			
MPV			

	Low	Normal / none	High
Urinalysis			
pH			
Specific gravity			
Albumin			
Glucose			
Ketones			
Occult blood			
Bilirubin			
WBCs			
RBCs			
Epithelial cells			
Casts			
Crystals			
Bacteria			

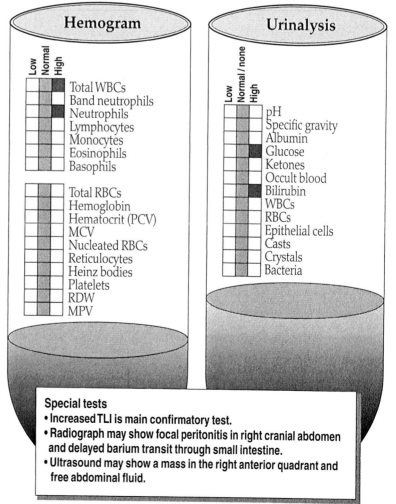

Special tests
- Increased TLI is main confirmatory test.
- Radiograph may show focal peritonitis in right cranial abdomen and delayed barium transit through small intestine.
- Ultrasound may show a mass in the right anterior quadrant and free abdominal fluid.

Aortic Thromboembolisms

thrombosis
is usually
secondary to
tissue injury,
blood stasis, and
altered blood
coagulation;
muscles and
kidneys are
damaged from
ischemia

Arterial emboli originate in the heart secondary to vascular pooling, cardiomyopathy, bacterial endocarditis, or advanced valvular heart disease. The thrombus breaks free from its point of origin, passes down the aorta, and usually lodges at the iliac artery bifurcation or in a femoral artery. Clinical signs depend on the site of obstruction. Thrombi can occlude the blood supply to the limbs or kidneys.

Interpretation
A high WBC count with mature neutrophilia, lymphopenia, and eosinopenia is caused by release of endogenous cortisol and epinephrine. Cortisol causes reduced numbers of lymphocytes and eosinophils, and epinephrine flushes the resting neutrophils from the marginated pool. A low platelet count and increased clotting time suggest consumption of clotting factors.

Elevated serum activity of muscle-derived enzymes (CPK, AST) indicates muscle necrosis. Eosinopenia rules out immune-mediated myositis. Hemoglobinuria or myoglobinuria suggests kidney damage and some breakdown of muscle cells.

Differential Diagnoses
• Localized myositis: eosinophilia, caudal paresis
• Peripheral neuropathy: no muscle necrosis
• Trauma: usually physical evidence of trauma

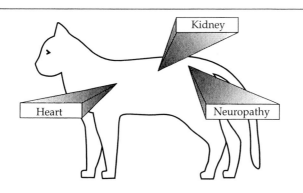

Signs
- Heart murmur
- Cardiac enlargement
- Paresis
- Paralysis
- Distress
- Pain

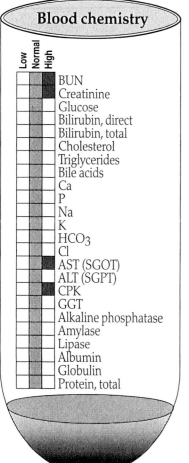

Blood chemistry	Low	Normal	High
BUN			High
Creatinine			High
Glucose		Normal	
Bilirubin, direct		Normal	
Bilirubin, total		Normal	
Cholesterol		Normal	
Triglycerides		Normal	
Bile acids		Normal	
Ca		Normal	
P		Normal	
Na		Normal	
K		Normal	
HCO3		Normal	
Cl		Normal	
AST (SGOT)			High
ALT (SGPT)		Normal	
CPK			High
GGT		Normal	
Alkaline phosphatase		Normal	
Amylase		Normal	
Lipase		Normal	
Albumin		Normal	
Globulin		Normal	
Protein, total		Normal	

Hemogram	Low	Normal	High
Total WBCs		Normal	
Band neutrophils			High
Neutrophils			High
Lymphocytes		Normal	
Monocytes		Normal	
Eosinophils		Normal	
Basophils		Normal	
Total RBCs		Normal	
Hemoglobin		Normal	
Hematocrit (PCV)		Normal	
MCV		Normal	
Nucleated RBCs		Normal	
Reticulocytes		Normal	
Heinz bodies		Normal	
Platelets	Low		
RDW		Normal	
MPV		Normal	

Urinalysis	Low	Normal / none	High
pH		Normal / none	
Specific gravity		Normal / none	
Albumin			High
Glucose		Normal / none	
Ketones		Normal / none	
Occult blood			High
Bilirubin		Normal / none	
WBCs		Normal / none	
RBCs			High
Epithelial cells		Normal / none	
Casts		Normal / none	
Crystals		Normal / none	
Bacteria		Normal / none	

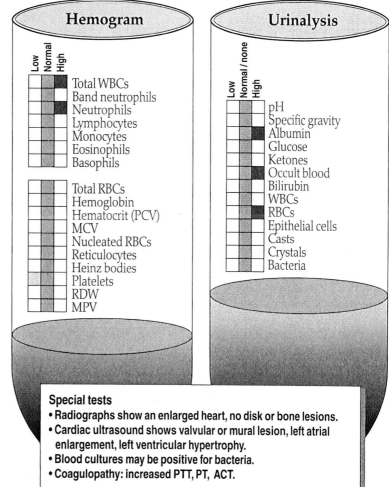

Special tests
- Radiographs show an enlarged heart, no disk or bone lesions.
- Cardiac ultrasound shows valvular or mural lesion, left atrial enlargement, left ventricular hypertrophy.
- Blood cultures may be positive for bacteria.
- Coagulopathy: increased PTT, PT, ACT.

Thoracic Lymphangiectasia (Chylothorax)

thoracic lymph-
angiectasia is
commonly
caused by heart
failure and
lymphosarcoma

Lymphangiectasia is a dilatation of lymph vessels caused by obstruction of the lymph drainage or by increased venous pressure. In intestinal lymphangiectasia the mesenteric lymph ducts obstructed by enlarged neoplastic or inflamed lymph nodes cause a protein-losing enteropathy.

In thoracic lymphangiectasia increased venous pressure obstructs the flow of the thoracic duct, resulting in lymphangiectasia and chylothorax. This is commonly seen in heart failure. Common causes of chylothorax are obstruction of the thoracic duct by lymphoma, rupture of the duct from trauma, hyperthyroidism, heartworm disease, and diaphragmatic hernia.

Interpretation
Most panel tests are normal. The fluid analysis shows a high triglyceride content (higher than serum) and large numbers of lymphocytes. Neutrophils may be present in chronic cases.

Differential Diagnoses
- Trauma: history or physical signs
- Lymphosarcoma: cytology shows immature and anaplastic lymphocytes
- Heart failure: abnormal findings on x-ray, ultrasound, or ECG
- Heartworm disease: +HW antibody test, heart failure
- T_4-induced cardiomyopathy: increased T_4

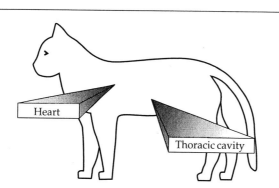

Signs
- Dyspnea
- Cough
- Muffled heart sounds

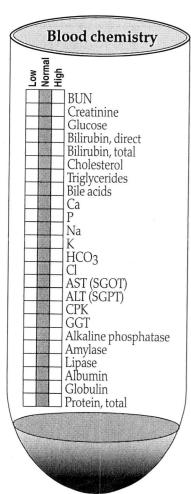

Blood chemistry

	Low	Normal	High	
		▓		BUN
		▓		Creatinine
		▓		Glucose
		▓		Bilirubin, direct
		▓		Bilirubin, total
		▓		Cholesterol
		▓		Triglycerides
		▓		Bile acids
		▓		Ca
		▓		P
		▓		Na
		▓		K
		▓		HCO3
		▓		Cl
		▓		AST (SGOT)
		▓		ALT (SGPT)
		▓		CPK
		▓		GGT
		▓		Alkaline phosphatase
		▓		Amylase
		▓		Lipase
		▓		Albumin
		▓		Globulin
		▓		Protein, total

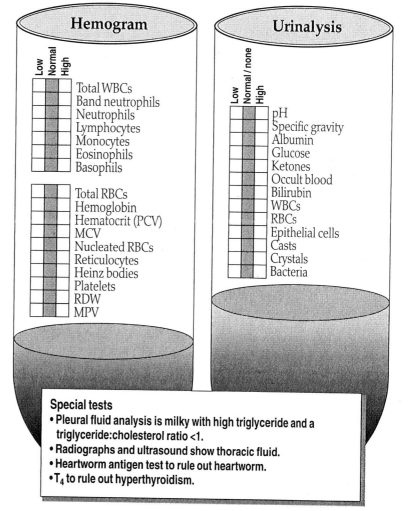

Hemogram

	Low	Normal	High	
		▓		Total WBCs
		▓		Band neutrophils
		▓		Neutrophils
		▓		Lymphocytes
		▓		Monocytes
		▓		Eosinophils
		▓		Basophils

	Low	Normal	High	
		▓		Total RBCs
		▓		Hemoglobin
		▓		Hematocrit (PCV)
		▓		MCV
		▓		Nucleated RBCs
		▓		Reticulocytes
		▓		Heinz bodies
		▓		Platelets
		▓		RDW
		▓		MPV

Urinalysis

	Low	Normal / none	High	
		▓		pH
		▓		Specific gravity
		▓		Albumin
		▓		Glucose
		▓		Ketones
		▓		Occult blood
		▓		Bilirubin
		▓		WBCs
		▓		RBCs
		▓		Epithelial cells
		▓		Casts
		▓		Crystals
		▓		Bacteria

Special tests
- Pleural fluid analysis is milky with high triglyceride and a triglyceride:cholesterol ratio <1.
- Radiographs and ultrasound show thoracic fluid.
- Heartworm antigen test to rule out heartworm.
- T_4 to rule out hyperthyroidism.

Heartworm

heartworm
antigen tests are
not diagnostic,
so only antibody
tests indicate
exposure

Adult feline heartworm causes obstructive pulmonary vascular problems, and larval migration causes problems in other organs. The cat is not a natural host for *Dirofilaria immitis,* and aberrant migration of the larvae to the brain and skin occurs more frequently in the cat than the dog. Clinical signs are usually related to lung and heart disease.

Interpretation
Vascular damage causes a consumptive thrombocytopenia with the compensatory release of large young platelets. The anemia when present is caused by the chronic inflammatory response to the heartworm. Eosinophilia occurs early in the infection as the larvae migrate. As the adults develop, eosinophilia decreases. Basophilia is less consistent than eosinophilia. Routine serum chemistries are normal unless heart failure causes prerenal azotemia and liver congestion.

Differential Diagnoses
- Feline asthma: radiograph shows bronchitis
- Lungworms: positive fecal examination using the Baermann apparatus

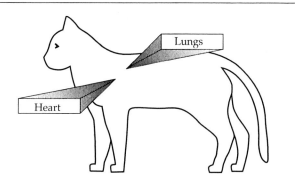

Signs
- Cough
- Dyspnea
- Vomiting
- CNS abnormalities
- ±Pleural effusion
- ±Ascites

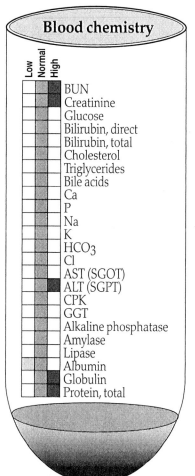

Blood chemistry

	Low	Normal	High
BUN			
Creatinine			
Glucose			
Bilirubin, direct			
Bilirubin, total			
Cholesterol			
Triglycerides			
Bile acids			
Ca			
P			
Na			
K			
HCO$_3$			
Cl			
AST (SGOT)			
ALT (SGPT)			
CPK			
GGT			
Alkaline phosphatase			
Amylase			
Lipase			
Albumin			
Globulin			
Protein, total			

Hemogram

	Low	Normal	High
Total WBCs			
Band neutrophils			
Neutrophils			
Lymphocytes			
Monocytes			
Eosinophils			
Basophils			
Total RBCs			
Hemoglobin			
Hematocrit (PCV)			
MCV			
Nucleated RBCs			
Reticulocytes			
Heinz bodies			
Platelets			
RDW			
MPV			

Urinalysis

	Low	Normal / none	High
pH			
Specific gravity			
Albumin			
Glucose			
Ketones			
Occult blood			
Bilirubin			
WBCs			
RBCs			
Epithelial cells			
Casts			
Crystals			
Bacteria			

Special tests
- Heartworm antigen tests are specific but give false negative results if only male worms, immature worms, or few worms are present.
- Heartworm antibody tests indicate exposure but do not determine if living worms are present.
- Radiographs show infiltrative lung disease, enlargement of caudal pulmonary arteries, and an enlarged heart.

Inflammatory Bowel Disease

inflammatory
bowel disease
has many causes

Lymphocytic-plasmacytic enteritis (LPE) is the most common histopathologic form of inflammatory bowel disease. It represents a spectrum of disease from mild to severe infiltration to lymphosarcoma (LSA). LPE can be difficult to differentiate histologically from LSA, and both have been found in adjacent tissues. The lamina propria infiltrate that is found in LPE may be associated with parasitism, giardiasis, lymphangiectasia, regional enteritis, and LSA, or may be an abnormal response to bacterial, dietary, or self-antigens. These lymphocyte infiltrations are often T suppressor cells.

Although endoscopic biopsy of the small intestine is the common method of confirming a diagnosis, it has limitations. Lack of histologic changes in biopsy specimens is frequent because often only the proximal small intestine or large intestine is examined and the involved area may be missed. Nonbiopsy methods such as fecal examination, serum folate, and cobalamin levels, and trypsin-like immunoreactivity can be used to assess digestion, absorption, and some etiologic agents.

Interpretation
Most tests are normal except those associated with digestion. Low proteins are due to protein-losing enteropathy and malnutrition. Raised liver enzymes are secondary to the enteritis. The low potassium is caused by the diarrhea. Hair ball type densities on radiographs may be a sign of impaired bowel motility.

Differential Diagnoses
• Parasitic enteritis *(Giardia):* positive fecal tests
• Hair ball obstruction: foreign body on radiograph
• Intestinal lymphosarcoma: intestinal biopsy

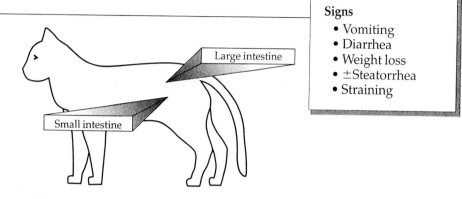

Signs
- Vomiting
- Diarrhea
- Weight loss
- ±Steatorrhea
- Straining

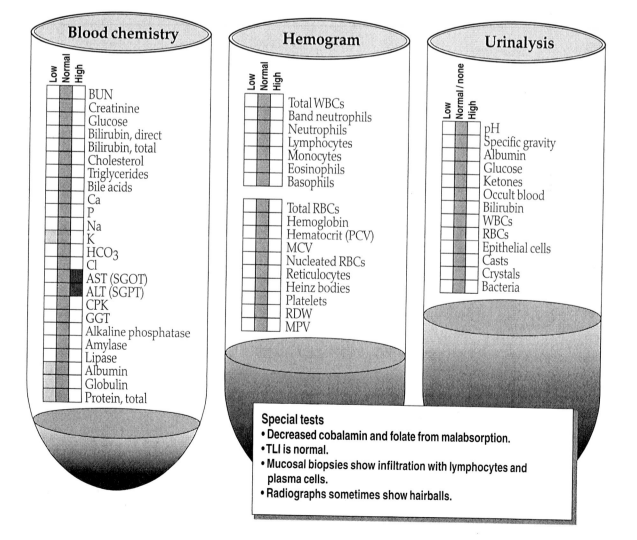

Blood chemistry	Low	Normal	High
BUN		■	
Creatinine		■	
Glucose		■	
Bilirubin, direct		■	
Bilirubin, total		■	
Cholesterol		■	
Triglycerides		■	
Bile acids		■	
Ca		■	
P		■	
Na		■	
K	■		
HCO3		■	
Cl		■	
AST (SGOT)			■
ALT (SGPT)			■
CPK		■	
GGT		■	
Alkaline phosphatase		■	
Amylase		■	
Lipase		■	
Albumin	■		
Globulin		■	
Protein, total	■		

Hemogram	Low	Normal	High
Total WBCs		■	
Band neutrophils		■	
Neutrophils		■	
Lymphocytes		■	
Monocytes		■	
Eosinophils		■	
Basophils		■	
Total RBCs		■	
Hemoglobin		■	
Hematocrit (PCV)		■	
MCV		■	
Nucleated RBCs		■	
Reticulocytes		■	
Heinz bodies		■	
Platelets		■	
RDW		■	
MPV		■	

Urinalysis	Low	Normal / none	High
pH		■	
Specific gravity		■	
Albumin		■	
Glucose		■	
Ketones		■	
Occult blood		■	
Bilirubin		■	
WBCs		■	
RBCs		■	
Epithelial cells		■	
Casts		■	
Crystals		■	
Bacteria		■	

Special tests
- Decreased cobalamin and folate from malabsorption.
- TLI is normal.
- Mucosal biopsies show infiltration with lymphocytes and plasma cells.
- Radiographs sometimes show hairballs.

Hypereosinophilic Syndrome

mature eosino-
phils distinguish
hypereosinophilic
syndrome from
myeloprolifera-
tive diseases

Hypereosinophilic syndrome is a disorder associated with a persistent marked increased eosinophil count of unknown etiology, bone marrow hyperplasia of eosinophilic precursors, and multiple organ infiltration by mature eosinophils. Clinical signs are nonspecific and vary with the organ(s) involved, but they most commonly reflect gastrointestinal disease. Affected cats minimally respond to recommended treatment, and prognosis for long-term survival is poor.

This condition is distinguished from eosinophilic leukemia and myeloproliferative disease by a lack of immaturity of the infiltrate. Clinical signs are similar, and both have poor long-term prognosis. There is some speculation as to whether the two syndromes are variants of the same disorder.

The intestine, liver, spleen, lymph nodes, bone marrow, lung, pancreas, adrenal glands, and skin can be affected. A lack of steroid responsiveness distinguishes this disease from inflammatory diseases.

Interpretation
The lack of steroid depression of the eosinophils is characteristic for this syndrome

Differential Diagnoses
- Asthma: eosinophilia limited to lungs
- Eosinophilic inflammatory bowel disease: eosinophils mainly in intestine
- Eosinophilic myeloproliferative disease: immature eosinophilic infiltration
- Addison's disease: high lymphocyte counts, low Na/K ratio, low serum cortisol

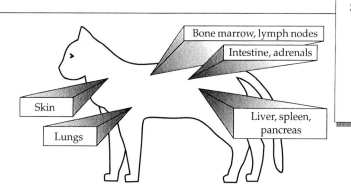

Bone marrow, lymph nodes

Intestine, adrenals

Skin

Lungs

Liver, spleen, pancreas

Signs
- Marked eosinophilia
- Lethargy
- Anorexia
- Vomiting
- Weight loss
- Fever

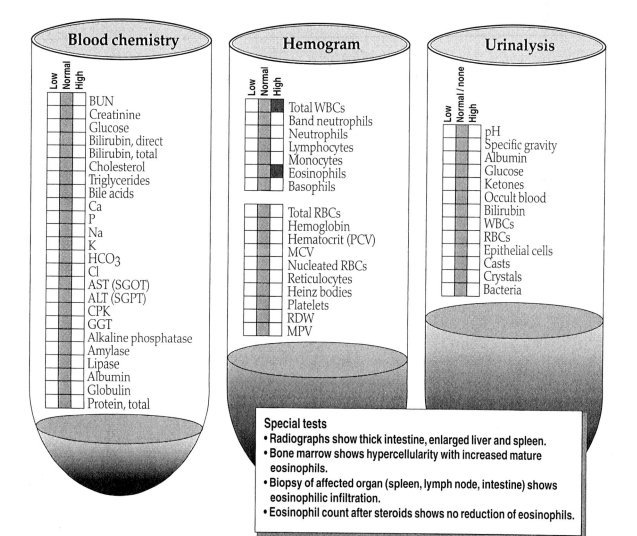

Blood chemistry

	Low	Normal	High
BUN		■	
Creatinine		■	
Glucose		■	
Bilirubin, direct		■	
Bilirubin, total		■	
Cholesterol		■	
Triglycerides		■	
Bile acids		■	
Ca		■	
P		■	
Na		■	
K		■	
HCO₃		■	
Cl		■	
AST (SGOT)		■	
ALT (SGPT)		■	
CPK		■	
GGT		■	
Alkaline phosphatase		■	
Amylase		■	
Lipase		■	
Albumin		■	
Globulin		■	
Protein, total		■	

Hemogram

	Low	Normal	High
Total WBCs			■
Band neutrophils		■	
Neutrophils		■	
Lymphocytes		■	
Monocytes			■
Eosinophils			■
Basophils		■	

	Low	Normal	High
Total RBCs	■		
Hemoglobin	■		
Hematocrit (PCV)	■		
MCV		■	
Nucleated RBCs		■	
Reticulocytes		■	
Heinz bodies		■	
Platelets		■	
RDW		■	
MPV		■	

Urinalysis

	Low	Normal / none	High
pH		■	
Specific gravity		■	
Albumin		■	
Glucose		■	
Ketones		■	
Occult blood		■	
Bilirubin		■	
WBCs		■	
RBCs		■	
Epithelial cells		■	
Casts		■	
Crystals		■	
Bacteria		■	

Special tests
- Radiographs show thick intestine, enlarged liver and spleen.
- Bone marrow shows hypercellularity with increased mature eosinophils.
- Biopsy of affected organ (spleen, lymph node, intestine) shows eosinophilic infiltration.
- Eosinophil count after steroids shows no reduction of eosinophils.

Coagulopathy of Liver Disease

severe liver disease may cause bleeding problems

Cats with liver disease usually have hemostatic defects but do not clinically bleed unless marked liver cirrhosis is present. Since hepatocytes produce most clotting factors and the mononuclear phagocyte system removes FDPs from circulation, severe liver disease can produce hemostatic abnormalities. Usually this liver dysfunction does not produce spontaneous bleeding, but excess bleeding may occur during surgery. Increase in alkaline phosphatase activity correlates with coagulation abnormalities. Cats with marked increases in alkaline phosphatase activity are more likely to have coagulation abnormalities than those with only mild increases in ALP activity

Interpretation
Increased AST and ALT indicate active liver necrosis. These enzymes may decrease as normal liver tissue is replaced by fibrous tissue. Prolonged PT, PTT, ACT, and PIVKA tests indicate decreased clotting factors. High FDPs occur because of decreased hepatic clearance.

Differential Diagnoses
- Vitamin K deficiency resulting from rodenticides: normal liver function, history of exposure.
- Disseminated intravascular coagulation: normal alkaline phosphatase
- Trauma: normal ACT, PT, PTT

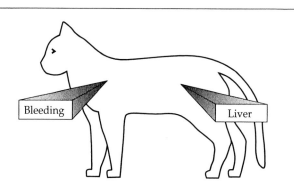

Signs
- Melena
- Prolonged bleeding
- Petechia
- Ecchymosis

Bleeding

Liver

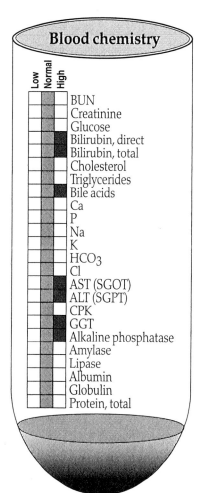

Blood chemistry

	Low	Normal	High	
				BUN
				Creatinine
				Glucose
				Bilirubin, direct
				Bilirubin, total
				Cholesterol
				Triglycerides
				Bile acids
				Ca
				P
				Na
				K
				HCO3
				Cl
				AST (SGOT)
				ALT (SGPT)
				CPK
				GGT
				Alkaline phosphatase
				Amylase
				Lipase
				Albumin
				Globulin
				Protein, total

Hemogram

	Low	Normal	High	
				Total WBCs
				Band neutrophils
				Neutrophils
				Lymphocytes
				Monocytes
				Eosinophils
				Basophils
				Total RBCs
				Hemoglobin
				Hematocrit (PCV)
				MCV
				Nucleated RBCs
				Reticulocytes
				Heinz bodies
				Platelets
				RDW
				MPV

Urinalysis

	Low	Normal / none	High	
				pH
				Specific gravity
				Albumin
				Glucose
				Ketones
				Occult blood
				Bilirubin
				WBCs
				RBCs
				Epithelial cells
				Casts
				Crystals
				Bacteria

Special tests
- Coagulation tests may show increased values for ACT, PT, PTT, FDP and decreased fibrinogen; PIVKA values may be increased.
- Increased BSP retention shows marked parenchymal loss secondary to fibrosis.

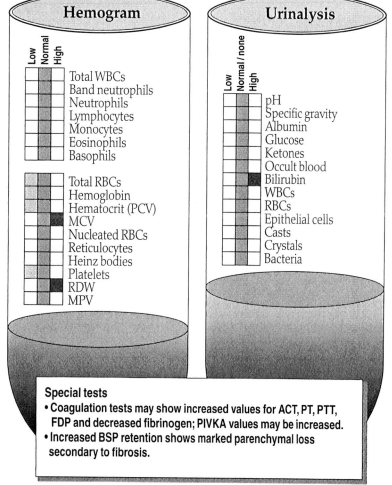

Lymphocytic Cholangitis

cholangitis starts
as an immune
reaction to viral
or chemical
agents

Cholangitis (inflammation of the bile ducts) or cholangiohepatitis (inflammation of the bile ducts and liver parenchyma) is more common in cats than in dogs. Inflammation can start as an immune-mediated reaction to viral or chemical agents but later becomes secondarily infected with bacteria.

The disease progresses from lymphocytic infiltration of the portal areas to bile duct proliferation and fibrosis. Some cases develop after an episode of acute pancreatitis. Inflammation causes biliary stasis, hyperplasia, and eventual hepatic portal fibrosis. The disease is chronic, with periods of clinical remission.

Interpretation
High serum ALT and AST activities indicate acute liver necrosis. High serum alkaline phosphatase, GGT, and bilirubin values indicate cholestasis and portal damage. Decreased serum albumin and increased serum globulin suggest chronicity. High ammonia and bile acid levels indicate liver failure and shunting. The WBC count is variable. The earliest change is usually bilirubinuria.

Differential Diagnoses
- Hepatic lipidosis: lipid droplets within hepatocytes on cytologic examination of biopsies
- FeLV-related liver disease: can have positive FeLV test, abnormal lymphocytes on liver biopsy
- FIP-related liver disease: high serum globulin level, low serum albumin level, rising titer on FIP test
- Toxin-induced liver failure: marked liver fibrosis
- Suppurative cholangitis: high WBC count, many neutrophils on cytologic examination of liver biopsies

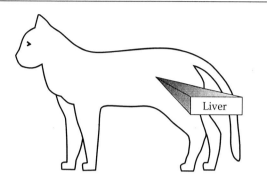

Signs
- Intermittent fever
- Hepatomegaly
- Vomiting
- Weight loss
- Depression
- Icterus
- ±Ascites

Liver

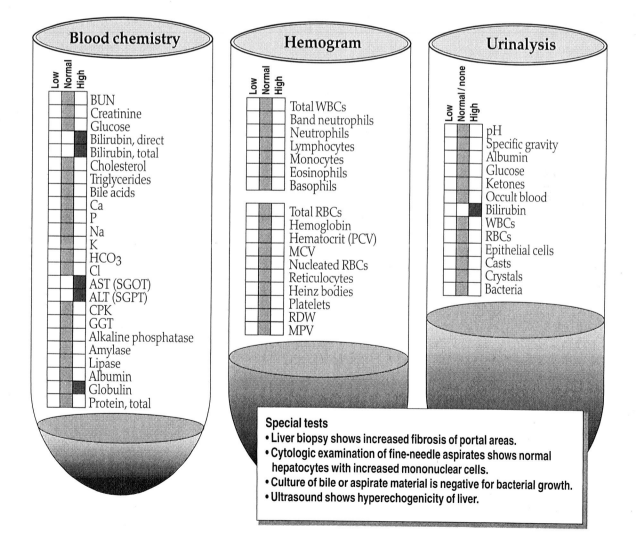

Blood chemistry

	Low	Normal	High	
		▨		BUN
		▨		Creatinine
		▨		Glucose
			■	Bilirubin, direct
			▨	Bilirubin, total
		▨		Cholesterol
		▨		Triglycerides
		▨		Bile acids
		▨		Ca
		▨		P
		▨		Na
		▨		K
		▨		HCO$_3$
		▨		Cl
			■	AST (SGOT)
			■	ALT (SGPT)
		▨		CPK
		▨		GGT
		▨		Alkaline phosphatase
		▨		Amylase
		▨		Lipase
		▨		Albumin
			■	Globulin
		▨		Protein, total

Hemogram

	Low	Normal	High	
		▨		Total WBCs
		▨		Band neutrophils
		▨		Neutrophils
		▨		Lymphocytes
		▨		Monocytes
		▨		Eosinophils
		▨		Basophils

	Low	Normal	High	
		▨		Total RBCs
		▨		Hemoglobin
		▨		Hematocrit (PCV)
		▨		MCV
		▨		Nucleated RBCs
		▨		Reticulocytes
		▨		Heinz bodies
		▨		Platelets
		▨		RDW
		▨		MPV

Urinalysis

	Low	Normal / none	High	
		▨		pH
		▨		Specific gravity
		▨		Albumin
		▨		Glucose
		▨		Ketones
		▨		Occult blood
			■	Bilirubin
		▨		WBCs
		▨		RBCs
		▨		Epithelial cells
		▨		Casts
		▨		Crystals
		▨		Bacteria

Special tests
- Liver biopsy shows increased fibrosis of portal areas.
- Cytologic examination of fine-needle aspirates shows normal hepatocytes with increased mononuclear cells.
- Culture of bile or aspirate material is negative for bacterial growth.
- Ultrasound shows hyperechogenicity of liver.

Suppurative Cholangitis

enteric bacteria infect bile ducts damaged by chemical, viruses, or immune reactions to cause suppurative cholangitis

Suppurative cholangitis (inflammation of the bile ducts) or cholangiohepatitis (inflammation of the bile ducts and liver parenchyma) is usually caused by invasion of the bile ducts by enteric bacteria. Many cases are associated with acute pancreatitis or occur secondary to immune-mediated or viral cholangitis. Inflammation causes biliary stasis, bile duct hyperplasia, and eventual hepatic portal fibrosis.

Interpretation
Increased serum ALT and AST activities indicate acute liver necrosis. Increased serum alkaline phosphatase and GGT activities and increased bilirubin levels in the blood and urine indicate cholestasis and portal damage. Low serum albumin and high serum globulin, bile acid, and ammonia levels indicate liver failure and vascular shunts. The WBC count is variable. Neutrophilic leukocytosis with a left shift is usual, but infection with some gram-negative bacteria causes leukopenia.

Differential Diagnoses
- Hepatic lipidosis: normal WBC count, liver biopsy shows lipid vacuoles
- Lymphocytic cholangiohepatitis: normal WBC count, liver biopsy shows no lipid vacuoles
- FeLV-related liver disease: may have positive FeLV test, liver biopsy can show immature lymphocytes
- FIP-related liver disease: high serum globulin levels and normal serum albumin levels, rising titer on FIP test
- Toxin-induced liver failure: Heinz-body anemia is common
- Hepatic biliary neoplasm: neoplastic cells on liver biopsy

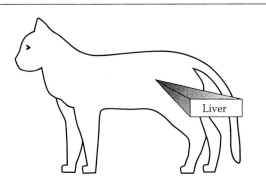

Signs
- Intermittent fever
- Anorexia
- Vomiting
- Weight loss
- Depression
- Icterus
- ± Ascites

Blood chemistry

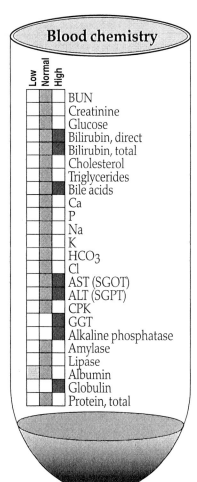

	Low	Normal	High
BUN		■	
Creatinine		■	
Glucose		■	
Bilirubin, direct			■
Bilirubin, total			■
Cholesterol		■	
Triglycerides		■	
Bile acids			■
Ca		■	
P		■	
Na		■	
K		■	
HCO₃		■	
Cl		■	
AST (SGOT)			■
ALT (SGPT)			■
CPK		■	
GGT			■
Alkaline phosphatase			■
Amylase		■	
Lipase		■	
Albumin	■		
Globulin			■
Protein, total		■	

Hemogram

	Low	Normal	High
Total WBCs			■
Band neutrophils			■
Neutrophils			■
Lymphocytes		■	
Monocytes		■	
Eosinophils		■	
Basophils		■	
Total RBCs		■	
Hemoglobin		■	
Hematocrit (PCV)		■	
MCV		■	
Nucleated RBCs		■	
Reticulocytes		■	
Heinz bodies		■	
Platelets		■	
RDW		■	
MPV		■	

Urinalysis

	Low	Normal / none	High
pH		■	
Specific gravity		■	
Albumin		■	
Glucose		■	
Ketones		■	
Occult blood		■	
Bilirubin			■
WBCs		■	
RBCs		■	
Epithelial cells		■	
Casts		■	
Crystals		■	
Bacteria		■	

Special tests
- Liver biopsy shows hepatic portal fibrosis, bile duct hyperplasia, suppurative exudate within dilated bile ducts, neutrophilic infiltration of portal areas.
- Ultrasound sometimes shows dilated bile ducts and a thick-walled gallbladder.
- Bile samples should be cultured anaerobically and aerobically.

Biliary Cirrhosis

chronic
cholangitis and
biliary
obstruction
cause biliary
cirrhosis

Chronic cholangitis or biliary obstruction can produce portal fibrosis. The liver is firm, nodular, and large. Histologically there is increased fibrous tissue, bile duct hyperplasia, and variable amounts of mixed inflammatory cells. Diagnosis is confirmed by biopsy, but there is some danger of bleeding from coagulopathies.

Interpretation
Liver enzymes such as ALT and AST may be normal or increased, depending on involvement of the liver parenchyma. The alkaline phosphatase and GGT is increased if there is biliary obstruction. Hyperbilirubinemia may mask rises in bile acids. The low BUN, albumin, and clotting factors are poor prognostic signs, indicating defective liver metabolism. Hepatic biopsy will confirm a diagnosis.

Differential Diagnoses
• Hepatic lipidosis: large liver, hepatocytes filled with fat
• Heart failure: enlarged heart
• Cholangiohepatitis: normal-sized liver, no increase in fibrous tissue

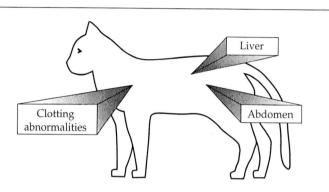

Signs
- Lethargy
- Weakness
- CNS abnormalities
- Vomiting
- Abdominal distention
- Diarrhea
- Icterus

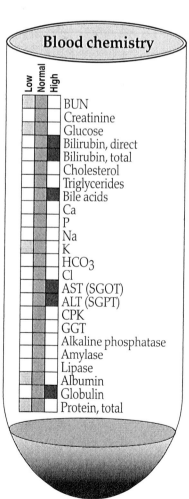

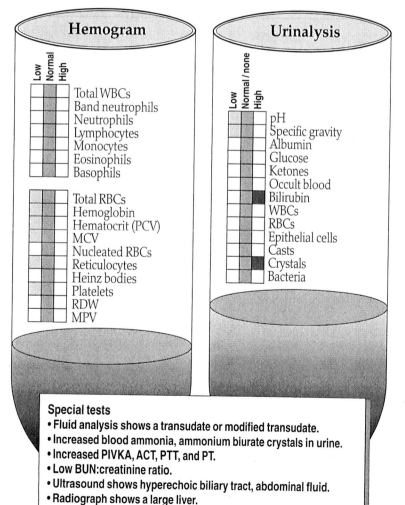

Special tests
- Fluid analysis shows a transudate or modified transudate.
- Increased blood ammonia, ammonium biurate crystals in urine.
- Increased PIVKA, ACT, PTT, and PT.
- Low BUN:creatinine ratio.
- Ultrasound shows hyperechoic biliary tract, abdominal fluid.
- Radiograph shows a large liver.

Hepatic Lipidosis

fat-filled hepato-
cytes distend the
parenchyma and
occlude bile flow
through the
portal area

Lipid infiltration of the liver occurs in obese cats that rapidly lose weight. Usually these animals are healthy before the weight loss. Other causes of hepatic lipidosis are starvation, diabetes mellitus, cortisol excess, and conditions that decrease serum levels of very-low-density lipids, which normally transport triglycerides from the liver. Fat accumulation in the liver leads to hepatomegaly.

Interpretation
Slightly increased serum ALT and AST activities indicate enzyme leakage from damaged liver cells. Increased serum alkaline phosphatase, GGT, and bilirubin values indicate biliary stasis from intrahepatic obstruction of the bile ducts. Although serum bile acid levels are increased, it is usually unnecessary to perform this assay because bilirubinemia is apparent.

The WBC count is usually normal or shows a stress response. A normal blood glucose level rules out diabetes mellitus as a cause of hepatic lipidosis.

Differential Diagnoses
- Cholangitis: usually occurs in a thin cat, no lipid droplets in hepatocytes on liver biopsies
- FeLV-related liver disease: may have positive FeLV test, liver biopsy can show many immature lymphocytes
- Diabetes mellitus: high blood glucose level
- Primary hepatic tumors: liver biopsy shows fibrosis and neoplastic cells; ultrasonographic examination shows hypoechoic areas with abnormal architecture

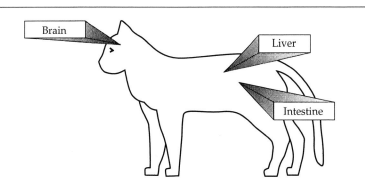

Signs
- Depression
- Ataxia
- Paresis
- Seizure
- Salivation
- Vomiting
- Icterus
- Melena

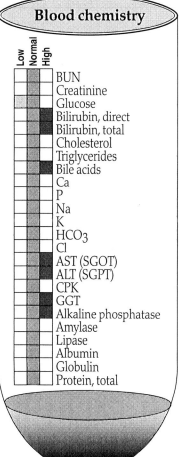

Blood chemistry

	Low	Normal	High	
		▨		BUN
	▨			Creatinine
	▨	▨		Glucose
		▨	■	Bilirubin, direct
		▨	■	Bilirubin, total
		▨		Cholesterol
		▨		Triglycerides
		▨	■	Bile acids
		▨		Ca
		▨		P
		▨		Na
		▨		K
		▨		HCO₃
		▨		Cl
		▨	■	AST (SGOT)
		▨	■	ALT (SGPT)
			▨	CPK
		▨	■	GGT
		▨		Alkaline phosphatase
		▨		Amylase
		▨		Lipase
		▨		Albumin
		▨		Globulin
		▨		Protein, total

Hemogram

	Low	Normal	High	
		▨		Total WBCs
		▨		Band neutrophils
		▨		Neutrophils
		▨		Lymphocytes
		▨		Monocytes
		▨		Eosinophils
		▨		Basophils
		▨		Total RBCs
		▨		Hemoglobin
		▨		Hematocrit (PCV)
		▨		MCV
		▨		Nucleated RBCs
		▨		Reticulocytes
		▨		Heinz bodies
		▨		Platelets
		▨		RDW
		▨		MPV

Urinalysis

	Low	Normal / none	High	
		▨		pH
	▨	▨		Specific gravity
		▨		Albumin
		▨		Glucose
		▨		Ketones
		▨		Occult blood
		▨	■	Bilirubin
		▨		WBCs
		▨		RBCs
		▨		Epithelial cells
		▨		Casts
		▨		Crystals
		▨		Bacteria

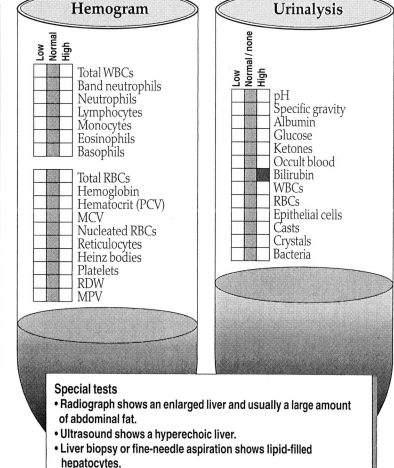

Special tests
- Radiograph shows an enlarged liver and usually a large amount of abdominal fat.
- Ultrasound shows a hyperechoic liver.
- Liver biopsy or fine-needle aspiration shows lipid-filled hepatocytes.

Hepatic Tumors

lymphosarcoma is the most common hepatic neoplasm

Lymphosarcoma is the most common hepatic neoplasm in the cat. Other neoplasms may either arise from the ductal or parenchymal tissue of the liver or more commonly be metastatic. Primary neoplasms may be solitary or multiple discrete nodules in several lobes of the liver. In aged cats a benign cystic condition (cystadenoma) may be incidentally found during ultra sound examination.

Interpretation
Laboratory findings are variable but may include nonregenerative anemia. The RDW may increase without reticulocytosis because of the small fragmented cells. ALT, alkaline phosphatase, bilirubin, and bile acids increase from liver necrosis and impingement on the bile canaliculi. Bilirubin may appear in the urine before icterus is apparent. Normal findings, however, do not rule out liver tumors. A definitive diagnosis is based on biopsy or fine-needle aspiration of the suspected mass.

Differential Diagnoses
- Hepatic cysts: cystic mass on ultrasound
- Amyloidosis: confirmed with liver biopsy

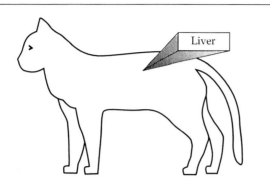

Signs
- Abdominal mass
- ±Sudden collapse

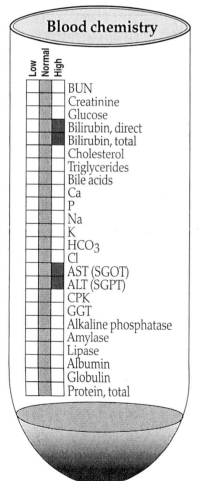

Blood chemistry

	Low	Normal	High	
BUN				
Creatinine				
Glucose				
Bilirubin, direct				
Bilirubin, total				
Cholesterol				
Triglycerides				
Bile acids				
Ca				
P				
Na				
K				
HCO3				
Cl				
AST (SGOT)				
ALT (SGPT)				
CPK				
GGT				
Alkaline phosphatase				
Amylase				
Lipase				
Albumin				
Globulin				
Protein, total				

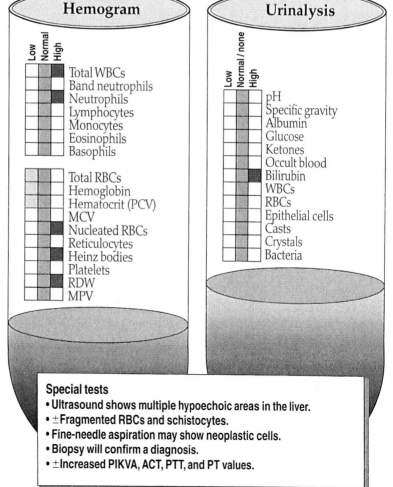

Hemogram

	Low	Normal	High
Total WBCs			
Band neutrophils			
Neutrophils			
Lymphocytes			
Monocytes			
Eosinophils			
Basophils			
Total RBCs			
Hemoglobin			
Hematocrit (PCV)			
MCV			
Nucleated RBCs			
Reticulocytes			
Heinz bodies			
Platelets			
RDW			
MPV			

Urinalysis

	Low	Normal / none	High
pH			
Specific gravity			
Albumin			
Glucose			
Ketones			
Occult blood			
Bilirubin			
WBCs			
RBCs			
Epithelial cells			
Casts			
Crystals			
Bacteria			

Special tests
- Ultrasound shows multiple hypoechoic areas in the liver.
- ±Fragmented RBCs and schistocytes.
- Fine-needle aspiration may show neoplastic cells.
- Biopsy will confirm a diagnosis.
- ±Increased PIKVA, ACT, PTT, and PT values.

Hepatic Amyloidosis

amyloidosis is most common in Abyssinian, Oriental, Siamese, and Burmese cats

The pathogenesis of amyloidosis is unknown. Current evidence suggests that amyloid proteins are derived by partial protein degradation of acute phase proteins (secondary amyloidosis) or by a genetic abnormality that results in the production of a chemically abnormal precursor protein (primary amyloidosis). All reported cases of hepatic amyloidosis in cats are secondary amyloidosis.

Certain breeds (Abyssinian, Oriental, Siamese, and Burmese) show a higher incidence of amyloidosis than other breeds, but no primary site of inflammation has been found. It is possible that these animals have a deficiency in degrading serum amyloid to a soluble polypeptide that can be secreted.

Interpretation
In early cases the primary laboratory abnormalities are related to the liver. If the liver ruptures, the acute hemorrhage causes anemia. Chronic cases may present in renal failure. The only definitive test is histopathologic examination of biopsy material stained with Congo red.

Differential Diagnoses
- Hepatic neoplasm: confirmed with liver biopsy
- Coagulopathy: altered clotting tests without liver enlargement
- Abdominal trauma: usually history is not suggestive, liver is usually not enlarged

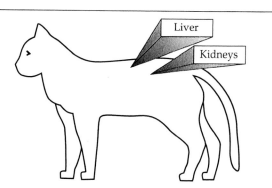

Signs
- Sudden death
- Liver rupture
- Hepatomegaly
- Abdominal distention

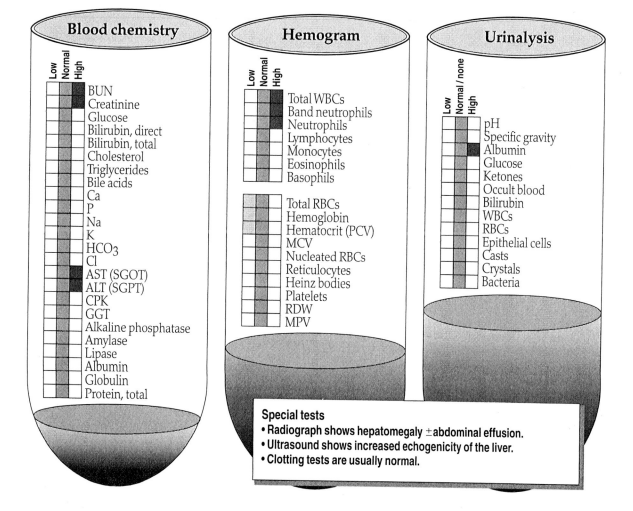

Blood chemistry

	Low	Normal	High	
		▓	▓	BUN
		▓	▓	Creatinine
		▓		Glucose
		▓		Bilirubin, direct
		▓		Bilirubin, total
		▓		Cholesterol
		▓		Triglycerides
		▓		Bile acids
		▓		Ca
		▓		P
		▓		Na
		▓		K
		▓		HCO₃
		▓		Cl
			█	AST (SGOT)
			█	ALT (SGPT)
		▓		CPK
		▓		GGT
		▓		Alkaline phosphatase
		▓		Amylase
		▓		Lipase
		▓		Albumin
		▓		Globulin
		▓		Protein, total

Hemogram

	Low	Normal	High	
		▓	▓	Total WBCs
			█	Band neutrophils
		▓	▓	Neutrophils
	▓			Lymphocytes
		▓		Monocytes
		▓		Eosinophils
		▓		Basophils

▓				Total RBCs
▓				Hemoglobin
▓				Hematocrit (PCV)
	▓			MCV
	▓			Nucleated RBCs
	▓			Reticulocytes
	▓			Heinz bodies
	▓			Platelets
	▓			RDW
	▓			MPV

Urinalysis

	Low	Normal / none	High	
		▓	▓	pH
		▓		Specific gravity
			█	Albumin
		▓		Glucose
		▓		Ketones
		▓		Occult blood
		▓		Bilirubin
		▓		WBCs
		▓		RBCs
		▓		Epithelial cells
		▓		Casts
		▓		Crystals
		▓		Bacteria

Special tests
- Radiograph shows hepatomegaly ±abdominal effusion.
- Ultrasound shows increased echogenicity of the liver.
- Clotting tests are usually normal.

Renal Diabetes Insipidus

decreased renal responsiveness to ADH may be caused by renal disease that affects the tubules and collecting ducts; hypercalcemia, hypokalemia, liver failure, and adrenal or hyperthyroidism are common causes

Renal diabetes insipidus is a tubular insensitivity to antidiuretic hormone (ADH, vasopressin). A number of systemic diseases can damage the ADH receptor sites in the distal convoluted tubules and collecting ducts of the kidney. Chronic renal failure, pyelonephritis, obstructive nephropathy, hypercalcemia, hepatic failure, pyometra, hypokalemia, and hyperadrenocorticism are common conditions causing this problem. Congenital dysfunction is rare.

Interpretation
The blood panel and hemogram can be used to rule out common causes of polydipsia, such as uremia, liver disease, pyometra, and diabetes mellitus.

Special tests distinguish other causes of the very dilute urine. An exogenous vasopressin test distinguishes between central and nephrogenic diabetes insipidus. Negative results of vasopressin and repository vasopressin tests confirm nephrogenic diabetes insipidus.

Differential Diagnoses
- Diabetes mellitus: high blood glucose level, glycosuria
- Subclinical renal failure: slightly increased serum creatinine level
- Liver disease: usually low serum albumin level, high serum bile acid levels
- Hyperadrenocorticism: stress response on the hemogram
- Central diabetes insipidus: polydipsia and polyuria controlled by vasopressin
- Hyperthyroidism: increased T_4

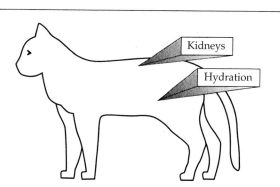

Kidneys

Hydration

Signs
- Polydipsia
- Polyuria
- Incontinence

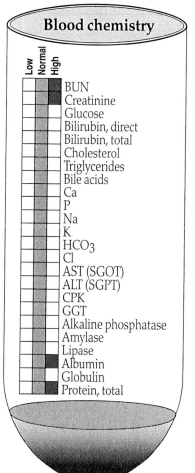

Blood chemistry

	Low	Normal	High	
			▓	BUN
			▓	Creatinine
		▓		Glucose
		▓		Bilirubin, direct
		▓		Bilirubin, total
		▓		Cholesterol
		▓		Triglycerides
		▓		Bile acids
		▓		Ca
		▓		P
		▓		Na
		▓		K
		▓		HCO₃
		▓		Cl
		▓		AST (SGOT)
		▓		ALT (SGPT)
		▓		CPK
		▓		GGT
		▓		Alkaline phosphatase
		▓		Amylase
		▓		Lipase
	▓			Albumin
		▓		Globulin
			▓	Protein, total

Hemogram

	Low	Normal	High	
		▓		Total WBCs
		▓		Band neutrophils
		▓		Neutrophils
		▓		Lymphocytes
		▓		Monocytes
		▓		Eosinophils
		▓		Basophils
		▓		Total RBCs
		▓		Hemoglobin
		▓		Hematocrit (PCV)
		▓		MCV
		▓		Nucleated RBCs
		▓		Reticulocytes
		▓		Heinz bodies
		▓		Platelets
		▓		RDW
		▓		MPV

Urinalysis

	Low	Normal / none	High	
		▓		pH
▓				Specific gravity
			▓	Albumin
		▓		Glucose
		▓		Ketones
		▓		Occult blood
		▓		Bilirubin
		▓		WBCs
		▓		RBCs
		▓		Epithelial cells
			▓	Casts
		▓		Crystals
		▓		Bacteria

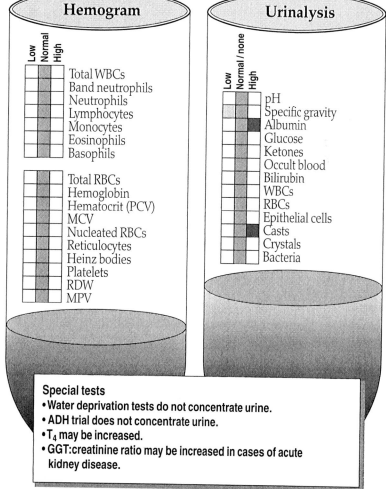

Special tests
- Water deprivation tests do not concentrate urine.
- ADH trial does not concentrate urine.
- T₄ may be increased.
- GGT:creatinine ratio may be increased in cases of acute kidney disease.

Urinary Tract Obstruction

urethral
obstruction
causes reflux of
urine into the
renal pelvis,
leading to
pyelonephritis

Lower urinary tract disease (feline urologic syndrome) often causes urethral obstruction that results initially in postrenal uremia and eventually in kidney failure. With obstruction, the kidneys are initially normal, but increased renal tubular pressure leads to renal failure. The obstruction can occur anywhere from the renal pelvis to the urethra, but both kidneys must be affected by the obstruction before uremia becomes evident.

Interpretation
Dehydration and poor renal perfusion cause high blood urea nitrogen, creatinine, and phosphorus levels. An elevated PCV and high total plasma protein and albumin levels suggest dehydration. Low blood bicarbonate with an anion gap indicates acidosis. Platelet dysfunction causes increased bleeding time and lack of clot retraction.

Reduced renal clearance causes high serum lipase and amylase activities. Urinary obstruction can be distinguished from the anuric phase of acute renal failure by the lack of casts and the enlarged bladder.

Differential Diagnoses
- Anuric renal failure: casts and protein in the urine sediment, normal urine protein/creatinine ratio
- Uroabdomen: normal urine, abdominocentesis yields urine
- Urinary calculi: visible on radiographs or ultrasonograms

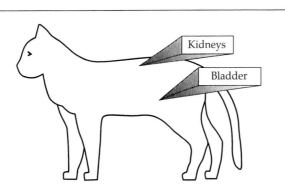

Signs
- Anuria
- Dysuria
- Painful abdomen
- Straining
- Vomiting

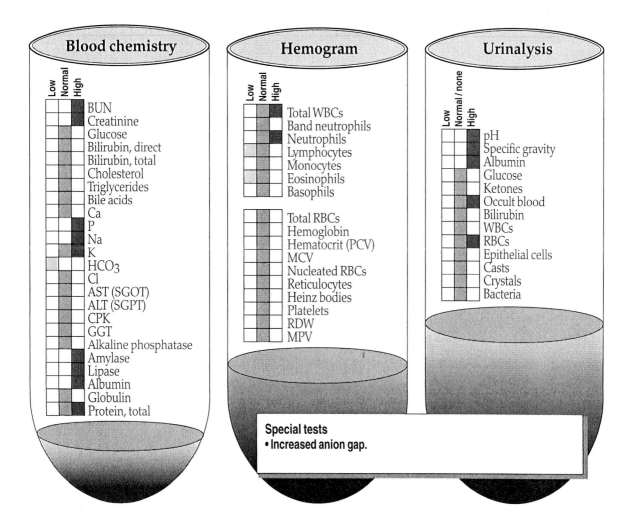

Blood chemistry

	Low	Normal	High	
			■	BUN
		■		Creatinine
		■		Glucose
		■		Bilirubin, direct
		■		Bilirubin, total
		■		Cholesterol
		■		Triglycerides
		■		Bile acids
				Ca
			■	P
		■		Na
			■	K
	░			HCO₃
		■		Cl
		■		AST (SGOT)
		■		ALT (SGPT)
		■		CPK
		■		GGT
				Alkaline phosphatase
			■	Amylase
			■	Lipase
		■		Albumin
		■		Globulin
			■	Protein, total

Hemogram

	Low	Normal	High	
		░	■	Total WBCs
			■	Band neutrophils
			■	Neutrophils
	░			Lymphocytes
		■		Monocytes
	░			Eosinophils
		■		Basophils

	Low	Normal	High	
		░		Total RBCs
		░		Hemoglobin
		░		Hematocrit (PCV)
		■		MCV
		■		Nucleated RBCs
		■		Reticulocytes
		■		Heinz bodies
		■		Platelets
		■		RDW
		■		MPV

Urinalysis

	Low	Normal / none	High	
			■	pH
			■	Specific gravity
		■		Albumin
		■		Glucose
		░		Ketones
		░	■	Occult blood
		■		Bilirubin
		░		WBCs
			■	RBCs
		■		Epithelial cells
		■		Casts
		░		Crystals
		░		Bacteria

Special tests
- Increased anion gap.

Acute Renal Failure, Maintenance Stage

during the maintenance stage, repair and adaptation occur; the patient may be anuric, oliguric, or polyuric

In the maintenance phase of acute renal failure, renal function deteriorates because of reduced glomerular filtration. This is caused by tubular obstruction, tubular backleak, afferent arteriolar vasoconstriction, efferent arteriolar vasodilatation, and decreased glomerular permeability. Azotemia progresses because of irreversible damage to the nephron despite correction of the inciting causes. The final level depends on the number of surviving nephrons.

Interpretation

Blood urea nitrogen, creatinine, and phosphorus levels continue to rise. Cholesterol and triglycerides are high because of defective lipoprotein lipase activity in the blood vessels. A high serum phosphorus level is usually associated with a decreased serum calcium level. If the serum phosphorus level remains high and the serum calcium level also is high, the kidneys could be further damaged by dystrophic calcification.

Low blood HCO_3 and an anion gap indicate acidosis. Increased bleeding time and lack of clot retraction indicate platelet dysfunction. High serum lipase and amylase activities are caused by decreased kidney clearance, not by acute pancreatitis. Urinary sodium loss and phosphorus retention produce low serum sodium and high potassium levels. High urine flow, low specific gravity, and casts in the urinary sediment indicate active kidney damage. Increased levels of urinary GGT indicate continued renal tubule damage.

Differential Diagnoses

- Chronic renal failure: usually produces nonregenerative anemia and inactive urine sediment
- Diabetes mellitus: high blood glucose level with glycosuria
- Pyelonephritis: usually no marked sodium loss; protein, RBCs, and WBCs in urine sediment

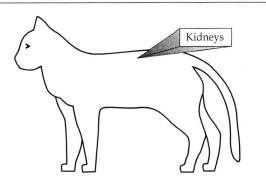

Signs
- $\pm$ Anuria
- $\pm$ Polyuria
- Depression
- Anorexia
- Vomiting

Kidneys

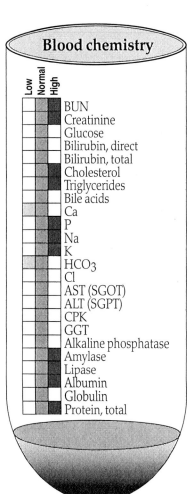

Blood chemistry

	Low	Normal	High	
				BUN
				Creatinine
				Glucose
				Bilirubin, direct
				Bilirubin, total
				Cholesterol
				Triglycerides
				Bile acids
				Ca
				P
				Na
				K
				HCO3
				Cl
				AST (SGOT)
				ALT (SGPT)
				CPK
				GGT
				Alkaline phosphatase
				Amylase
				Lipase
				Albumin
				Globulin
				Protein, total

Hemogram

	Low	Normal	High	
				Total WBCs
				Band neutrophils
				Neutrophils
				Lymphocytes
				Monocytes
				Eosinophils
				Basophils

	Low	Normal	High	
				Total RBCs
				Hemoglobin
				Hematocrit (PCV)
				MCV
				Nucleated RBCs
				Reticulocytes
				Heinz bodies
				Platelets
				RDW
				MPV

Urinalysis

	Low	Normal / none	High	
				pH
				Specific gravity
				Albumin
				Glucose
				Ketones
				Occult blood
				Bilirubin
				WBCs
				RBCs
				Epithelial cells
				Casts
				Crystals
				Bacteria

Special tests
- Normal BUN:Cr ratio indicates a renal cause rather than a prerenal cause of the uremia.
- Increased GGT:Cr ratio indicates continued nephron damage.
- Increased fractional excretion of Na indicates continued nephron damage.

Acute Renal Failure, Induction Stage

polyuria with high serum cholesterol is a sign of the induction stage of acute renal failure

The induction stage of acute renal failure is hard to diagnose. Often the signs consist only of listlessness, polyuria, and high serum cholesterol. By the time casts are seen in the urine and azotemia occurs, the patient is already in the maintenance state of renal failure and the renal tubular epithelium cannot be regenerated. If treatment can be initiated during the induction stage, many of the tubular cells may be saved and limited numbers of nephrons lost.

The key tests for diagnosis in this stage are the GGT:Cr ratio and the fractional excretion of sodium. If these are high, the tubules of the epithelium are damaged. Treatment currently consists of a protective diet (acute stage renal diet) that provides high protein and high omega-3 oils.

Interpretation
The panel often shows only a rise in cholesterol, which may be masked by lipemia. This is due to inhibition of lipoprotein lipase. There are no azotemia or other indications of kidney failure. The urine also shows minimal changes such as a low specific gravity. The usual signs of kidney damage such as casts, protein, and glucose are not present. The GGT:Cr ratio is high, indicating renal tubular epithelial damage, and the fractional excretion of sodium is high, indicating leakage through the tight junctions.

Differential Diagnoses
- Diabetes mellitus: high blood sugar, high fructosamine
- Diabetes insipidus: usually no alterations in serum lipids
- Chronic renal failure: high BUN and creatinine
- Maintenance stage of acute renal failure: high BUN creatinine and active urine sediment

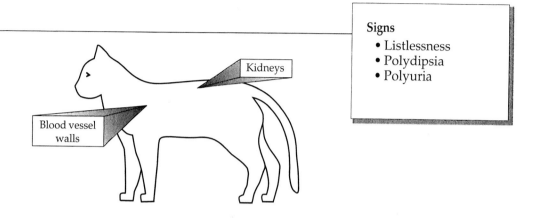

Signs
- Listlessness
- Polydipsia
- Polyuria

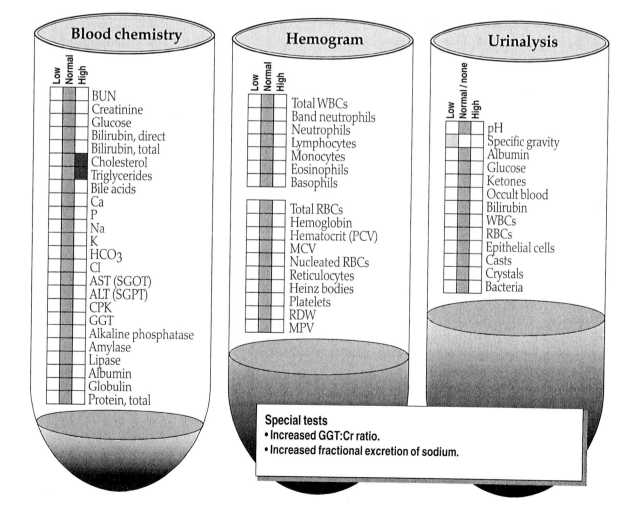

Blood chemistry

	Low	Normal	High	
				BUN
				Creatinine
				Glucose
				Bilirubin, direct
				Bilirubin, total
				Cholesterol
				Triglycerides
				Bile acids
				Ca
				P
				Na
				K
				HCO3
				Cl
				AST (SGOT)
				ALT (SGPT)
				CPK
				GGT
				Alkaline phosphatase
				Amylase
				Lipase
				Albumin
				Globulin
				Protein, total

Hemogram

	Low	Normal	High	
				Total WBCs
				Band neutrophils
				Neutrophils
				Lymphocytes
				Monocytes
				Eosinophils
				Basophils

	Low	Normal	High	
				Total RBCs
				Hemoglobin
				Hematocrit (PCV)
				MCV
				Nucleated RBCs
				Reticulocytes
				Heinz bodies
				Platelets
				RDW
				MPV

Urinalysis

	Low	Normal / none	High	
				pH
				Specific gravity
				Albumin
				Glucose
				Ketones
				Occult blood
				Bilirubin
				WBCs
				RBCs
				Epithelial cells
				Casts
				Crystals
				Bacteria

Special tests
- Increased GGT:Cr ratio.
- Increased fractional excretion of sodium.

Glomerulonephritis

glomerulonephritis is usually caused by deposition of immune complexes secondary to an antigen-antibody reaction

Glomerulonephritis is a protein-losing nephropathy usually caused by reactions to immune complexes in the blood, which indirectly damage the kidney. These antigen-antibody complexes are deposited in the small blood vessels of the renal glomeruli. The antigen often consists of virus particles (FeLV, FIP), microfilariae, or debris from inflammation of any organ. Occasionally antibodies to medicines such as insulin are the antigens. Clinical signs are related to loss of serum albumin and rarely uremia.

Interpretation
Glomerular leakage is the usual cause of proteinuria without hemorrhage or pyuria. The amount of protein loss can be estimated by the urine protein:creatinine ratio. Normal serum globulin levels suggest renal loss rather than intestinal or exudative loss. As the condition worsens and edema develops, the serum cholesterol level rises and the animal becomes hypertensive. Kidney biopsy confirms the diagnosis. Later the patient may have renal failure.

Differential Diagnoses
- Amyloidosis: demonstrated with special staining of kidney biopsies
- Urinary tract infection: positive urine cultures, WBCs in urine
- Hepatic insufficiency: no significant urine protein, high serum bile acid levels, low BUN level
- Malnutrition: very thin animal, anorexia, no urine protein loss
- Protein-losing enteropathy: no urine protein loss, low serum globulin level
- Chronic hemorrhage: anemia, low serum globulin level, proteinuria from hemorrhage

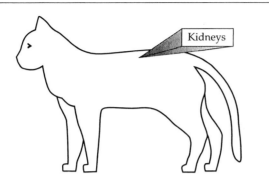

Signs
- Primary disease signs may predominate
- ±Ascites
- ±Edema

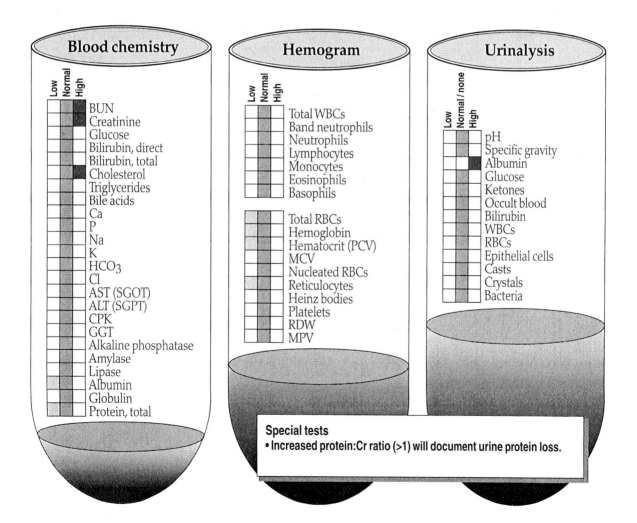

Blood chemistry

	Low	Normal	High	
				BUN
				Creatinine
				Glucose
				Bilirubin, direct
				Bilirubin, total
				Cholesterol
				Triglycerides
				Bile acids
				Ca
				P
				Na
				K
				HCO3
				Cl
				AST (SGOT)
				ALT (SGPT)
				CPK
				GGT
				Alkaline phosphatase
				Amylase
				Lipase
				Albumin
				Globulin
				Protein, total

Hemogram

	Low	Normal	High	
				Total WBCs
				Band neutrophils
				Neutrophils
				Lymphocytes
				Monocytes
				Eosinophils
				Basophils
				Total RBCs
				Hemoglobin
				Hematocrit (PCV)
				MCV
				Nucleated RBCs
				Reticulocytes
				Heinz bodies
				Platelets
				RDW
				MPV

Urinalysis

	Low	Normal / none	High	
				pH
				Specific gravity
				Albumin
				Glucose
				Ketones
				Occult blood
				Bilirubin
				WBCs
				RBCs
				Epithelial cells
				Casts
				Crystals
				Bacteria

Special tests
- Increased protein:Cr ratio (>1) will document urine protein loss.

Pyelonephritis

renal infections
are usually
caused by
bacteria
ascending from
the lower urinary
tract

Pyelonephritis is a bacterial infection of the kidney. Bacteria ascending from the lower urinary tract are the usual source of infection. The chance of infection increases with urine stasis and cystitis. Infections elsewhere in the body may occasionally cause septicemia and kidney infection. Trauma, nephroliths, diabetes mellitus, and immunosuppression increase the risk of kidney infection. Pyelonephritis causes bacteriuria, bacteremia, nephrolithiasis, and renal failure.

Interpretation
Not all affected animals are azotemic, but when 75% or more of the kidney is damaged, BUN, creatinine, and phosphorus levels increase. Serum globulin levels increase in chronic infections. The WBCs, RBCs, casts, and bacteria in urine samples suggest kidney infection. The presence of casts distinguishes a kidney lesion from a lower urinary tract lesion.

Differential Diagnoses
- Nephrolithiasis: nephroliths visible on radiographs, pyelograms, or sonograms
- Lower urinary tract infection: usually no casts in urine sediment

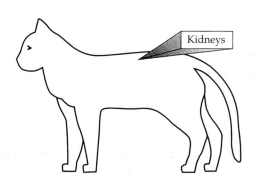

Signs
Acute
- Fever
- Depression
- Anorexia
- Lumbar pain

Chronic
- Polydipsia
- Asymptomatic
- Incidental finding

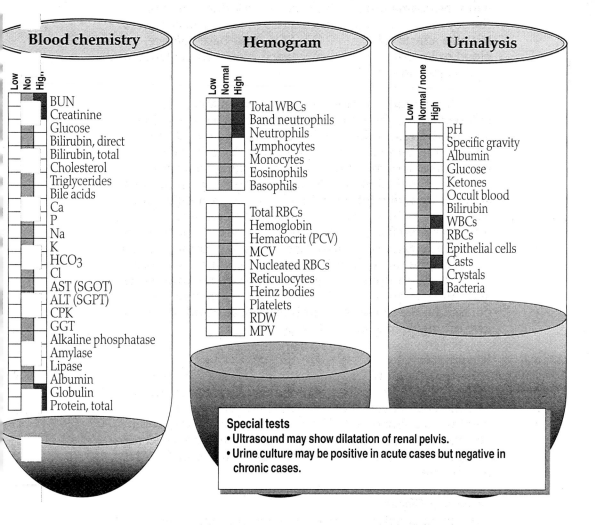

Blood chemistry

	Low	Normal	High
BUN			
Creatinine			
Glucose			
Bilirubin, direct			
Bilirubin, total			
Cholesterol			
Triglycerides			
Bile acids			
Ca			
P			
Na			
K			
HCO₃			
Cl			
AST (SGOT)			
ALT (SGPT)			
CPK			
GGT			
Alkaline phosphatase			
Amylase			
Lipase			
Albumin			
Globulin			
Protein, total			

Hemogram

	Low	Normal	High
Total WBCs			
Band neutrophils			
Neutrophils			
Lymphocytes			
Monocytes			
Eosinophils			
Basophils			
Total RBCs			
Hemoglobin			
Hematocrit (PCV)			
MCV			
Nucleated RBCs			
Reticulocytes			
Heinz bodies			
Platelets			
RDW			
MPV			

Urinalysis

	Low	Normal / none	High
pH			
Specific gravity			
Albumin			
Glucose			
Ketones			
Occult blood			
Bilirubin			
WBCs			
RBCs			
Epithelial cells			
Casts			
Crystals			
Bacteria			

Special tests
- Ultrasound may show dilatation of renal pelvis.
- Urine culture may be positive in acute cases but negative in chronic cases.

Chronic Renal Failure

correcting >PTH levels may slow the deterioration of renal failure

Chronic renal failure is a state of progressive and irreversible deterioration of renal function that results from continued exposure to agents that cause acute renal failure. In addition, polycystic kidneys, hypertension, hyperparathyroidism, and lymphosarcoma progressively decrease kidney function. Kidney failure not only causes a rise in BUN and creatinine but also affects calcium metabolism, acid-base balance, red blood cell production, water balance, electrolyte balance, and neurologic function.

The clinical manifestations of chronic renal failure are independent of the initial insult that damaged the kidneys and instead reflect the inability of the kidney to excrete nitrogenous wastes, regulate fluid and electrolyte balances, and secrete or excrete hormones. Managing patients with advanced renal failure partly depends on the presence of an active urine sediment (proteinuria, casts, enzymuria, and alterations in the fractional excretion of electrolytes) or the results of a renal biopsy for tumor or amyloid. The exogenous creatinine clearance or plotting the serum creatinine (1/Cr) estimates the rate of kidney deterioration. Increased fraction excretion of phosphorus suggests increased parathormone and can be confirmed with a PTH assay. Sequential assays for potassium, red blood cells, and reticulocytes and bicarbonate give estimates of effective therapy.

Interpretation
Persistently high BUN and creatinine levels indicate the loss of more than 80% of the functional kidneys. Phosphorus retention decreases serum calcium and activates the parathyroids. Increased PTH and high serum phosphorus may be nephrotoxic. To estimate the need for therapy to decrease PTH, a screening test (Fe phosphorus) or an assay for PTH may be run.

Differential Diagnoses
• Acute renal failure: recovery of concentrating ability

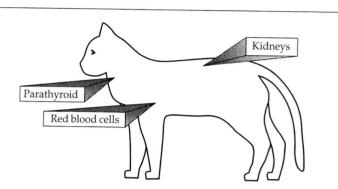

Signs
- Chronic polyuria
- Chronic polydipsia
- Anorexia
- Weight loss
- ±Seizures
- ±Osteodystrophy

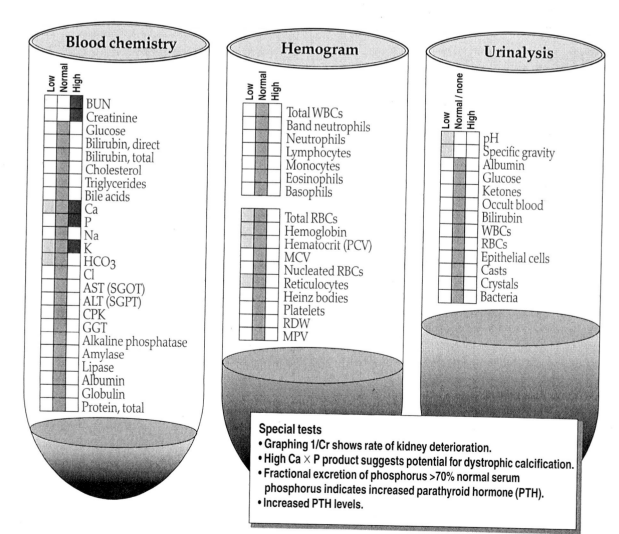

Blood chemistry

	Low	Normal	High	
				BUN
				Creatinine
				Glucose
				Bilirubin, direct
				Bilirubin, total
				Cholesterol
				Triglycerides
				Bile acids
				Ca
				P
				Na
				K
				HCO3
				Cl
				AST (SGOT)
				ALT (SGPT)
				CPK
				GGT
				Alkaline phosphatase
				Amylase
				Lipase
				Albumin
				Globulin
				Protein, total

Hemogram

	Low	Normal	High	
				Total WBCs
				Band neutrophils
				Neutrophils
				Lymphocytes
				Monocytes
				Eosinophils
				Basophils
				Total RBCs
				Hemoglobin
				Hematocrit (PCV)
				MCV
				Nucleated RBCs
				Reticulocytes
				Heinz bodies
				Platelets
				RDW
				MPV

Urinalysis

	Low	Normal / none	High	
				pH
				Specific gravity
				Albumin
				Glucose
				Ketones
				Occult blood
				Bilirubin
				WBCs
				RBCs
				Epithelial cells
				Casts
				Crystals
				Bacteria

Special tests
- Graphing 1/Cr shows rate of kidney deterioration.
- High Ca × P product suggests potential for dystrophic calcification.
- Fractional excretion of phosphorus >70% normal serum phosphorus indicates increased parathyroid hormone (PTH).
- Increased PTH levels.

Effusive Feline Infectious Peritonitis (Wet FIP)

FIP may be tentatively diagnosed by hyperglobulinemia, a serologic test or typical fluid exudation

Effusive ("wet") FIP is a chronic debilitating coronavirus infection that produces a peritoneal and/or pleural effusion. The basic lesion is an Arthus type immune-complex vasculitis. Most cats with the effusive form of FIP die.

Interpretation
High total plasma protein and globulin levels with a persistent fever suggest FIP. This diagnosis is supported by a high-protein, noncellular effusion. A positive polymerase chain reaction test supports a diagnosis of FIP. Increased serum titers for either feline corona virus or the modified FIP virus confirm exposure and can be used to support a diagnosis, not confirm one.

High serum activity of liver-derived enzymes reflects concurrent liver damage. The high protein content of the effusion indicates an exudate. Some affected cats have many WBCs in the exudate. Proteinuria is due to immune complex glomerulonephritis.

Differential Diagnoses
- Congestive heart failure: peritoneal effusion is a transudate with a low protein count
- Bacterial peritonitis or pleuritis: effusion is an exudate containing many degenerate WBCs
- Ascites: low total plasma protein and globulin levels

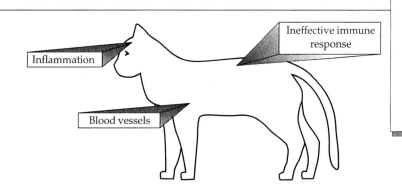

Signs
- Fever
- Weight loss
- Swollen abdomen
- Pleural effusion
- Abdominal effusion
- Uveitis
- Neurologic signs

Inflammation

Ineffective immune response

Blood vessels

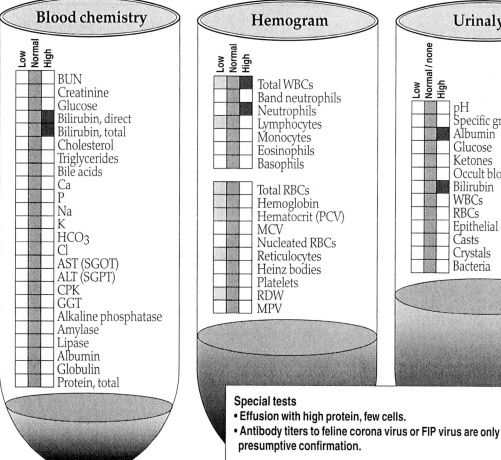

Blood chemistry

	Low	Normal	High	
		■		BUN
		■		Creatinine
		■		Glucose
			■	Bilirubin, direct
			■	Bilirubin, total
		■		Cholesterol
		■		Triglycerides
		■		Bile acids
		■		Ca
		■		P
		■		Na
		■		K
		■		HCO₃
		■		Cl
		■		AST (SGOT)
		■		ALT (SGPT)
		■		CPK
		■		GGT
		■		Alkaline phosphatase
		■		Amylase
		■		Lipase
		■		Albumin
			■	Globulin
		■		Protein, total

Hemogram

	Low	Normal	High	
			■	Total WBCs
		■		Band neutrophils
			■	Neutrophils
		■		Lymphocytes
		■		Monocytes
		■		Eosinophils
		■		Basophils

	Low	Normal	High	
		■		Total RBCs
		■		Hemoglobin
		■		Hematocrit (PCV)
		■		MCV
		■		Nucleated RBCs
		■		Reticulocytes
		■		Heinz bodies
		■		Platelets
		■		RDW
		■		MPV

Urinalysis

	Low	Normal / none	High	
		■		pH
		■		Specific gravity
			■	Albumin
		■		Glucose
		■		Ketones
		■		Occult blood
			■	Bilirubin
		■		WBCs
		■		RBCs
		■		Epithelial cells
		■		Casts
		■		Crystals
		■		Bacteria

Special tests
- Effusion with high protein, few cells.
- Antibody titers to feline corona virus or FIP virus are only presumptive confirmation.

Noneffusive Feline Infectious Peritonitis (Dry FIP)

dry FIP is
confirmed by
biopsy

Noneffusive ("dry") FIP is a coronavirus infection characterized by pyogranulomatous vasculitis. These perivascular infiltrates may damage the kidneys, liver, pancreas, lungs, brain, or eye. Clinical signs vary with the organs affected. Most infected cats have a fever and hyperproteinemia.

Interpretation
High total plasma protein and globulin levels with persistent fever suggest FIP. Biopsy of affected tissue may confirm corona viral particles. Increased serum titers for either feline corona virus or the modified FIP virus confirm exposure and can be used only to support a diagnosis, not confirm one.

High serum activity of liver-derived enzymes indicates liver necrosis. A low platelet count and impaired clotting indicate impending disseminated intravascular coagulation induced by the many vascular lesions. A definitive diagnosis often depends on special stains on biopsy specimens.

Concurrent Disease
FeLV infection: The FeLV test is often positive in free-roaming animals, but is usually negative in closed colonies of cats.

Differential Diagnosis
• Bacterial infection: response to antibiotics
• Viral infection: low WBC, clinical signs
• Tumor: increased WBC, ultrasound or x-rays
• Toxoplasmosis: rising titer

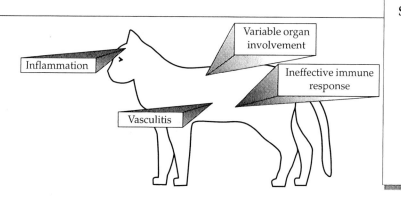

Signs
- Anorexia
- Depression
- Wasting
- Dehydration
- Fever
- Paresis
- Ataxia
- Anterior uveitis
- Abortion
- Infertility

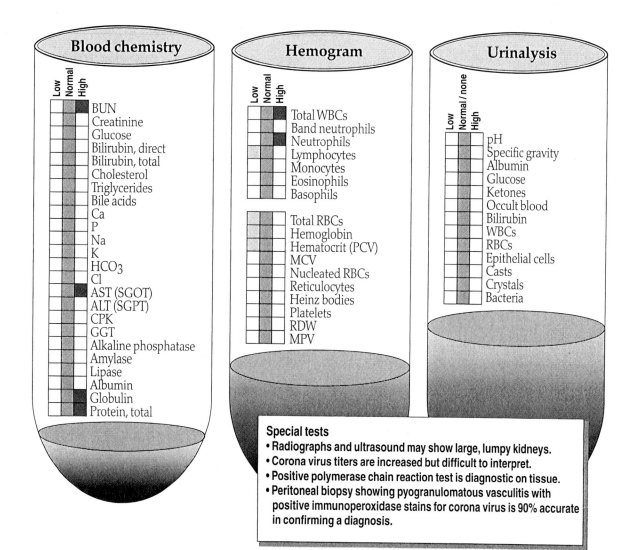

Special tests
- Radiographs and ultrasound may show large, lumpy kidneys.
- Corona virus titers are increased but difficult to interpret.
- Positive polymerase chain reaction test is diagnostic on tissue.
- Peritoneal biopsy showing pyogranulomatous vasculitis with positive immunoperoxidase stains for corona virus is 90% accurate in confirming a diagnosis.

Toxoplasmosis

cats showing
clinical disease
are not infectious
to humans

Infection of the cat with *Toxoplasma gondii* usually occurs after ingestion of an infected animal. In many cats the organism goes through an active life cycle in the intestine, and oocysts are shed in the feces. Exposure to infected feces can result in toxoplasma infection in many animals including humans. Cats usually shed large numbers of cysts only once in their life. This shedding occurs for less than 2 weeks and then the cat becomes immune.

A few cats may become clinically infected when the organisms penetrate the small intestinal and spread to other organs via the lymph or blood. The lungs and liver are the most common organs involved, but the muscles, heart, eye, pancreas, and CNS are sometimes affected. These animals are usually not infective to others.

Interpretation
Abnormal laboratory tests vary with the organs affected. A high antibody titer is not diagnostic in itself, but it does indicate exposure. A rising titer is more diagnostic of active infection.

Differential Diagnoses
- FIP: no rising *Toxoplasma* titers, high serum globulin, positive antibody test or biopsy results
- FeLV: positive FeLV test
- Immune-mediated disease: no rising titer to *Toxoplasma*
- Lymphosarcoma: lymphoblasts seen on cytology
- Other neoplasms: no rising tier to *Toxoplasma*, positive cytologic tests

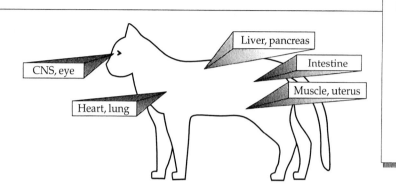

Signs
- Depend on organs involved
- Fever
- Anorexia
- ±Dyspnea
- ±Seizure
- ±Icterus
- ±Uveitis
- ±Abortion

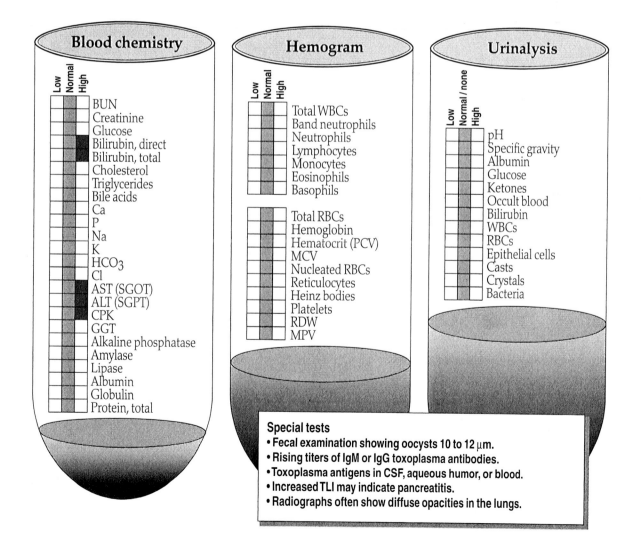

Blood chemistry

	Low	Normal	High	
				BUN
				Creatinine
				Glucose
				Bilirubin, direct
				Bilirubin, total
				Cholesterol
				Triglycerides
				Bile acids
				Ca
				P
				Na
				K
				HCO3
				Cl
				AST (SGOT)
				ALT (SGPT)
				CPK
				GGT
				Alkaline phosphatase
				Amylase
				Lipase
				Albumin
				Globulin
				Protein, total

Hemogram

	Low	Normal	High	
				Total WBCs
				Band neutrophils
				Neutrophils
				Lymphocytes
				Monocytes
				Eosinophils
				Basophils
				Total RBCs
				Hemoglobin
				Hematocrit (PCV)
				MCV
				Nucleated RBCs
				Reticulocytes
				Heinz bodies
				Platelets
				RDW
				MPV

Urinalysis

	Low	Normal / none	High	
				pH
				Specific gravity
				Albumin
				Glucose
				Ketones
				Occult blood
				Bilirubin
				WBCs
				RBCs
				Epithelial cells
				Casts
				Crystals
				Bacteria

Special tests
- Fecal examination showing oocysts 10 to 12 μm.
- Rising titers of IgM or IgG toxoplasma antibodies.
- Toxoplasma antigens in CSF, aqueous humor, or blood.
- Increased TLI may indicate pancreatitis.
- Radiographs often show diffuse opacities in the lungs.

Acetaminophen Toxicity

diagnosis depends on history

Acetaminophen is toxic to cats. Ingestion depletes cellular stores of glutathione, an important agent for detoxification. Because cats are deficient in glucuronyl transferase activity, a moderate ingestion causes liver necrosis, methemoglobinemia, and Heinz-body anemia. Ingestion of 50 mg/kg (1 regular Tylenol tablet) is usually fatal.

Interpretation
The raised liver enzymes indicate liver necrosis. The anemia may be severe. Heinz bodies indicate oxidative degeneration of the hemoglobin. If less than 3 days have elapsed since exposure, there may be no signs of response. When the patient's blood is placed on filter paper, it will have a brown color.

Differential Diagnoses
• Other oxidated agents such as methylene blue, onions

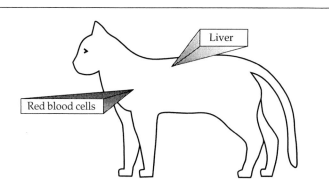

Signs
- Cyanosis
- Brown mucous membranes
- Facial edema

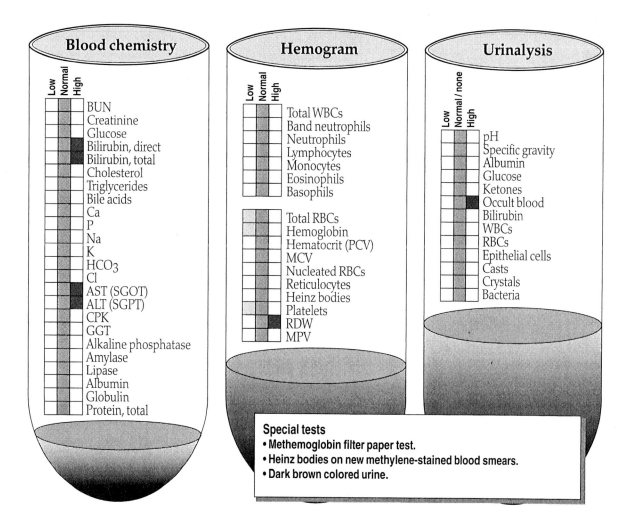

Blood chemistry

	Low	Normal	High	
BUN				
Creatinine				
Glucose				
Bilirubin, direct				
Bilirubin, total				
Cholesterol				
Triglycerides				
Bile acids				
Ca				
P				
Na				
K				
HCO₃				
Cl				
AST (SGOT)				
ALT (SGPT)				
CPK				
GGT				
Alkaline phosphatase				
Amylase				
Lipase				
Albumin				
Globulin				
Protein, total				

Hemogram

	Low	Normal	High	
Total WBCs				
Band neutrophils				
Neutrophils				
Lymphocytes				
Monocytes				
Eosinophils				
Basophils				
Total RBCs				
Hemoglobin				
Hematocrit (PCV)				
MCV				
Nucleated RBCs				
Reticulocytes				
Heinz bodies				
Platelets				
RDW				
MPV				

Urinalysis

	Low	Normal / none	High	
pH				
Specific gravity				
Albumin				
Glucose				
Ketones				
Occult blood				
Bilirubin				
WBCs				
RBCs				
Epithelial cells				
Casts				
Crystals				
Bacteria				

Special tests
- Methemoglobin filter paper test.
- Heinz bodies on new methylene-stained blood smears.
- Dark brown colored urine.

Ethylene Glycol Toxicity

early diagnosis depends on history, fluorescence of the urine, and a positive test for ethylene glycol in the blood

Ethylene glycol is metabolized and causes renal tubular necrosis and later tubular blockage from the formation of calcium oxalate crystals. Successful treatment requires rapid tentative diagnosis from minimal historical and indirect tests with confirmation with a specific ethylene glycol test on whole blood. Usually an animal is seen in renal failure. When this stage is reached, treatment is usually unsuccessful.

Interpretation
Early laboratory tests are normal, so diagnosis is based on history of exposure to antifreeze, fluorescence in the urine, and a positive blood test for propylene glycol. The induction stage of kidney disease may be detected by an increased urine GGT/creatinine ratio and an increased fractional excretion of sodium.

After 72 hours uremia is usually present and a presumptive diagnosis is based on calcium oxalate crystals in the urine and a hyperechoic kidney sonogram.

Differential Diagnoses
- Acute renal failure from other causes: negative tests for propylene glycol, no calcium oxalate crystals
- Diabetes mellitus: hyperglycemia
- CNS disorder: no progression to renal failure

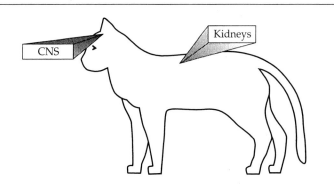

Signs
Early
- History of antifreeze ingestion
- Depression
- Vomiting
- Ataxia
- Nystagmus

Late
- Oliguria or polyuria

Blood chemistry

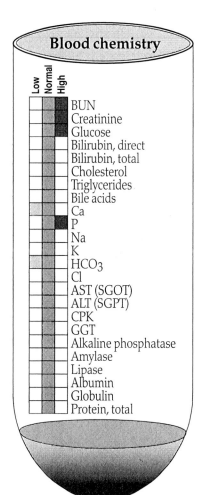

	Low	Normal	High	
			■	BUN
			■	Creatinine
			■	Glucose
				Bilirubin, direct
				Bilirubin, total
				Cholesterol
				Triglycerides
				Bile acids
	▨			Ca
		■		P
				Na
				K
	▨			HCO₃
				Cl
				AST (SGOT)
				ALT (SGPT)
				CPK
				GGT
				Alkaline phosphatase
				Amylase
				Lipase
				Albumin
				Globulin
				Protein, total

Hemogram

	Low	Normal	High	
			■	Total WBCs
			■	Band neutrophils
			■	Neutrophils
	▨			Lymphocytes
				Monocytes
				Eosinophils
				Basophils
				Total RBCs
				Hemoglobin
				Hematocrit (PCV)
				MCV
				Nucleated RBCs
				Reticulocytes
				Heinz bodies
				Platelets
				RDW
				MPV

Urinalysis

	Low	Normal / none	High	
	▨			pH
				Specific gravity
				Albumin
				Glucose
				Ketones
			■	Occult blood
				Bilirubin
				WBCs
			■	RBCs
				Epithelial cells
			■	Casts
			■	Crystals
				Bacteria

Special tests
- Check urine for fluorescence: many antifreeze products contain a fluorescein dye. Urine crystals are calcium oxalate.
- Confirm diagnosis with Ethylene Glycol Test Kit (PRN Pharmco Inc., Pensacola, Fla).
- Ultrasound of kidneys may show hyperechoic renal medulla as a result of calcium oxalate crystals.

Lead Poisoning

lead toxicity
may mimic
myeloproliferative
disease

Although blood abnormalities occur in less than 50% of clinical cases, those showing these changes must be differentiated from other myeloproliferative diseases. Clinical cases often show CNS signs, gastrointestinal signs, and neurologic signs.

Interpretation
When present, immature RBCs in the peripheral blood without a corresponding anemia are key markers. When this is combined with a rise in enzymes, indicating liver necrosis, and urine changes, indicating acute tubular damage, lead exposures should be confirmed with lead blood levels or urine aminolevulinic acid (ALA) levels.

Differential Diagnoses
• Other toxins: normal blood lead levels
• Myeloproliferative disease: anemia, marked left shift in RBC precursors

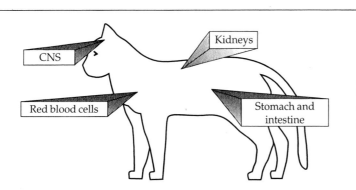

Signs
- Vomiting
- Diarrhea
- Abdominal pain
- Seizures
- Lethargy
- Blindness
- Hysteria

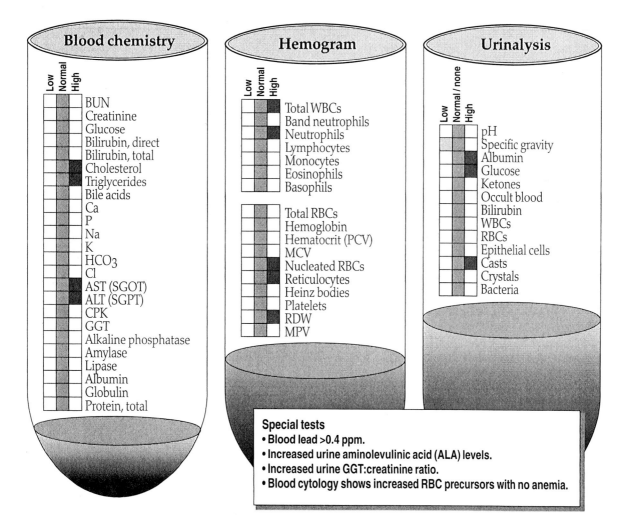

Blood chemistry

	Low	Normal	High	
		▨		BUN
		▨		Creatinine
		▨		Glucose
		▨		Bilirubin, direct
		▨		Bilirubin, total
			▉	Cholesterol
		▨		Triglycerides
		▨		Bile acids
		▨		Ca
		▨		P
		▨		Na
		▨		K
		▨		HCO₃
		▨		Cl
			▉	AST (SGOT)
			▉	ALT (SGPT)
		▨		CPK
		▨		GGT
		▨		Alkaline phosphatase
		▨		Amylase
		▨		Lipase
		▨		Albumin
		▨		Globulin
		▨		Protein, total

Hemogram

	Low	Normal	High	
		▨		Total WBCs
			▉	Band neutrophils
			▉	Neutrophils
		▨		Lymphocytes
		▨		Monocytes
		▨		Eosinophils
		▨		Basophils
		▨		Total RBCs
		▨		Hemoglobin
		▨		Hematocrit (PCV)
		▨		MCV
			▉	Nucleated RBCs
			▨	Reticulocytes
		▨		Heinz bodies
		▨		Platelets
		▉		RDW
		▨		MPV

Urinalysis

	Low	Normal / none	High	
		▨		pH
	▨			Specific gravity
			▉	Albumin
			▉	Glucose
		▨		Ketones
		▨		Occult blood
		▨		Bilirubin
		▨		WBCs
		▨		RBCs
		▨		Epithelial cells
			▉	Casts
		▨		Crystals
		▨		Bacteria

Special tests
- Blood lead >0.4 ppm.
- Increased urine aminolevulinic acid (ALA) levels.
- Increased urine GGT:creatinine ratio.
- Blood cytology shows increased RBC precursors with no anemia.

Vitamin D Toxicosis

excess vitamin D causes hypercalcemia and secondary kidney damage

Vitamin D toxicity is usually caused by ingestion of rodents poisoned with cholecalciferol rodenticides. It is manifest by hypercalcemia and kidney failure. The kidney is particularly vulnerable to the effects of hypercalcemia. Impaired urine-concentrating ability, leading to polyuria and compensatory polydipsia, is an early functional abnormality associated with hypercalcemic nephropathy.

Interpretation
High blood calcium levels in combination with high blood phosphorus levels result in dystrophic calcification. The potential for this is documented by a high Ca $\times$ P product. High GGT:creatinine and high fractional excretions of sodium indicate the induction phase of acute kidney failure. Urinary casts document later stages. High serum cholecalciferol supports a diagnosis.

Differential Diagnoses
• Hyperparathyroidism: high PTH
• Lymphosarcoma: no apparent tumor, lymph node aspiration negative
• Acute renal failure from other causes: no history of vitamin D ingestion

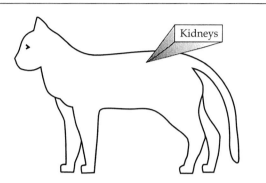

Signs
- Polydipsia
- Polyuria
- ±Bradycardia

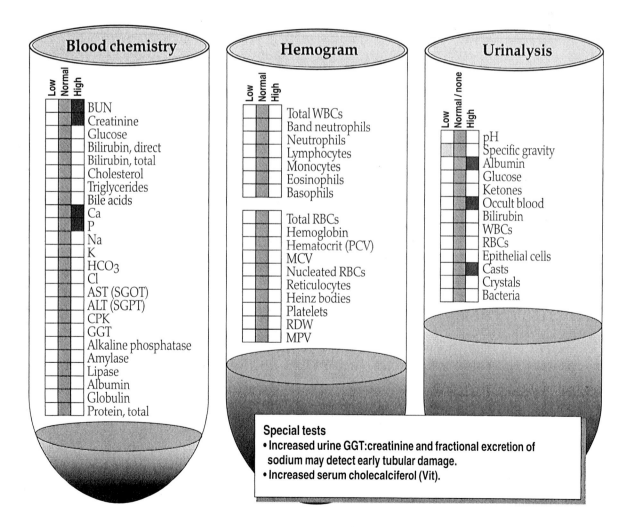

Blood chemistry

	Low	Normal	High	
			■	BUN
		■		Creatinine
		■		Glucose
		■		Bilirubin, direct
		■		Bilirubin, total
		■		Cholesterol
		■		Triglycerides
		■		Bile acids
			■	Ca
			■	P
		■		Na
		■		K
		■		HCO₃
		■		Cl
		■		AST (SGOT)
		■		ALT (SGPT)
		■		CPK
		■		GGT
		■		Alkaline phosphatase
		■		Amylase
		■		Lipase
		■		Albumin
		■		Globulin
		■		Protein, total

Hemogram

	Low	Normal	High	
		■		Total WBCs
		■		Band neutrophils
		■		Neutrophils
		■		Lymphocytes
		■		Monocytes
		■		Eosinophils
		■		Basophils
		■		Total RBCs
		■		Hemoglobin
		■		Hematocrit (PCV)
		■		MCV
		■		Nucleated RBCs
		■		Reticulocytes
		■		Heinz bodies
		■		Platelets
		■		RDW
		■		MPV

Urinalysis

	Low	Normal / none	High	
	■			pH
			■	Specific gravity
		■		Albumin
		■		Glucose
		■		Ketones
			■	Occult blood
		■		Bilirubin
		■		WBCs
		■		RBCs
		■		Epithelial cells
			■	Casts
		■		Crystals
		■		Bacteria

Special tests
- Increased urine GGT:creatinine and fractional excretion of sodium may detect early tubular damage.
- Increased serum cholecalciferol (Vit).

Clinicopathologic Index

Main Index